PROBLEM–BASED PHYSIOLOGY

PROBLEM-BASED PHYSIOLOGY

Robert G. Carroll, PhD

Professor of Physiology
Brody School of Medicine
East Carolina University
Greenville, North Carolina

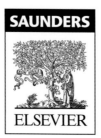

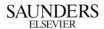

1600 John F. Kennedy Blvd.
Ste 1800
Philadelphia, PA 19103-2899

PROBLEM-BASED PHYSIOLOGY

ISBN 978-1-4160-4217-4

Library of Congress Cataloging in Publication Data
Carroll, Robert G.
Problem-based physiology / Robert G. Carroll. — 1st ed.
p. cm.
Includes bibliographical references and index.
ISBN 978-1-4160-4217-4
1. Physiology, Pathological—Case studies. I. Title.
[DNLM: 1. Pathology—Case Reports. 2. Physiology—Case Reports. QT 104 C319p 2010]
RB113.C25 2010
616.07—dc22
2008040746

Acquisitions Editor: William R. Schmitt
Developmental Editor: Barbara Cicalese
Publishing Services Manager: Hemamalini Rajendrababu
Project Manager: Srikumar Narayanan
Design Direction: Gene Harris

Printed in China

Last digit is the print number: 9 8 7 6 5 4 3 2 1

DEDICATION

To Bettie Ann and to my children Anne Corinne, Elise, and Graham,
for 24 years of love, joy, and friendship

RGC

CONTRIBUTOR

Richard H. Ray PhD
Professor of Physiology
Brody School of Medicine
East Carolina University
Greenville, North Carolina

Preface

A medical student's ability to retain and apply physiological knowledge is improved when information is presented in a contextual format. For medical students, clinical scenarios provide an appropriate springboard for exploring the pathophysiology that leads to the development of specific symptoms, the progression of the disease process, and the appropriate clinical and therapeutic interventions that can be used to treat a patient.

The 88 clinical cases presented in this book are grouped into 10 sections, each loosely tied to an organ system. Each section has an introduction and concept map to help emphasize the interrelatedness of the cases related to that organ system. The integrative nature of physiology and medicine, however, results in complex clinical cases that often extend across multiple organ systems. The advantage of this complexity is that students interpret information across multiple organ systems, as is appropriate for each clinical case.

The individual cases follow a typical clinical scenario. Each case begins with the presenting complaint, followed by a medical history that is limited to events pertinent to the complaint. The physical examination reports vital signs and key physical findings, which is followed by the results from subsequent diagnostic tests. The pathophysiology section expands on the patient presentation and laboratory results, outlining the physiological mechanisms of both the symptom development and the progression of the disease. When appropriate, the pathophysiology section ends with a discussion of the logic that underlies the treatment options and the therapeutic outcomes.

The following aspects of this book make it a unique learning aid:

- Each case study is presented as an unknown to promote active learning. The gradual unfolding of the clinical scenario allows students to test their predictive abilities and to provoke appropriate questions for sequential learning issues and further investigation.

- The integration of basic and clinical sciences is designed to help develop a "big picture" of disease processes.
- Over 135 full-color illustrations reinforce basic physiological mechanisms.
- The 10 section introductions provide a concept map to help organize the physiology underlying multiple clinical presentations.
- Two clinical vignette-based practice questions are derived from each of the 88 cases, illustrating how patient scenarios can be used as a basis for integrative physiology examination questions.

Although medical students are anticipated to be the main benefactors of this book, the format of patient presentation allows the book to be useful to a variety of advanced undergraduate, graduate, and professional students in the health-related professions. The health profession team deals with the same patient, and the clinical scenarios provide useful starting points for discussion by all members of the team.

It is my hope that all students will develop a deeper understanding of concepts of medical physiology but also develop an enthusiasm for the lifelong learning process initiated by complex patient-based problem presentations. Clinical practice is continually improving based on outcomes of medical and physiological research. Health practitioners need to become comfortable with their role as perpetual students.

I invite the readers' suggestions for improvement of this work. The preferred way to submit suggestions or corrections is electronic mail. Enthusiastic readers are advised to include "Problem-Based Physiology" as the subject line and send submissions by email to: carrollr@ecu.edu

Robert G. Carroll, PhD

Acknowledgments

As with most major undertakings, Problem-Based Physiology could not be completed without the help of many individuals. First and foremost, I would like to thank my colleagues within the teaching community of the American Physiological Society, the International Association of Medical Science Educators, and the International Union of Physiological Sciences for educating me about the effectiveness of a "student-centered" teaching style. Teaching and curriculum modifications need to be informed by the results of educational research, and I have benefited from both the knowledge and the enthusiasm of these groups.

For this project, I am particularly indebted to Swapan Nath and Sanjay Revanker for the innovative structure of this series as executed in the "Problem-Based Microbiology" text. I followed their format as closely as possible, but incorporated the unique aspects of physiology.

I am also extremely grateful to my colleagues at the Brody School of Medicine at East Carolina University for the information and expertise they have shared over the years, particularly Dick Ray, Mike Van Scott, Bob Lust, Chris Wingard, Greg Iams, Jitka Virag, Steve Wood, and Ed Seidel. Each of these educators has helped simultaneously reveal the complexity and simplicity of the organ systems and helped me understand the clinical implications of the field of physiology. Dick Ray, in particular, was a huge help in the neurophysiology section, as well as in composing the Practice Questions and Answers tied to each of the clinical cases.

I am particularly grateful to the graduate students in the Physician Assistant Program Pathophysiology courses of 2006 and 2007 for both the clinical scenarios and clinical fact checking for the cases used in this book. Teaching is always a learning experience, and it has been fun learning with this group of talented students.

Many at Elsevier deserve recognition for their role in the production of this book. My heartfelt thanks go to William Schmitt, Acquisitions Editor of Medical Textbooks, for over a decade of support to the teaching section of the American Physiological Society. Barbara Cicalese expertly balanced the demands as Developmental Editor in encouraging timely completion of tasks but also allowed time to develop a quality product.

Finally, I wish to acknowledge the medical and graduate students, past and present, who provided support for the framework of the text in the inception of ideas for this project and provided encouragement and stimulation for completion of Problem-Based Physiology.

Robert G. Carroll, PhD

How to Use This Book

Problem-Based Physiology was written for students with various study goals and learning styles and can be used both in a physiology course and as a review resource for the USMLE Step 1 examination. It might also be used as a reference during the clinical years. There are three parts to each case: patient presentation, physical examination and laboratory results, and pathophysiology. Practice questions at the end of the book allow students to assess their knowledge base. Each of these parts is described next. At the end is a special discussion with suggestions for three ways or tracks that this book might be used, depending on the study goals, preferred learning style, and background of the individual student.

FEATURES

Section Overviews

At the beginning of each section is an overview that includes a concept map of the specific organ system and illustrates where the individual cases fit in the functional aspect of the organ system. This background is built on using the problem-solving exercises in the cases that follow.

Cases

Cases are presented in an "unknown format" intended to immediately engage the reader in thinking about physiology in clinical terms, emphasizing the application facts. Each case includes important pieces of information about the patient's problem that is under discussion.

CASE DESCRIPTION. To obtain the greatest benefit from the problem-based nature of this book, it is advisable that the reader focus separately on each part of the first page of the case, making sure that the information is synthesized and digested before going on to the next. The entirety of the case description has been

kept to the first page of the case as much as possible. In those cases where it has by necessity flowed onto the next page, it is suggested that the reader purposely not read the pathophysiology until a proper synthesis of the case description has been attained.

Clinical Scenario. Each case begins with a presenting symptom in an appropriate clinical setting and includes pertinent history of the patient's problem.

Physical Examination and Laboratory Studies. These features give further information about the specific case and offer a framework for evaluating the situation.

PATHOPHYSIOLOGY OF KEY SYMPTOMS. This section illustrates the mechanisms underlying the presentation of the symptoms and the progression of the disease. Whenever possible, either clinical outcome or treatment options are provided.

FURTHER READING. A short bibliography of current resources is provided to allow the student to more fully explore the case.

Practice Questions and Answers

NBME-style practice questions can be used for preparing for course examinations and for readiness assurance for the USMLE. Each clinical case is used as the basis for two questions, one usually emphasizing mechanisms for symptom development and the other emphasizing the pathophysiology of the disease. These questions are grouped in the same sequence as the presented cases and, consequently, all are clustered around individual organ systems. This grouping may be particularly useful for student self-assessment of learning in problem-based learning (PBL) pathways and integrated curricula. When laboratory values are given, normal values are provided in parentheses.

TRACKS OF STUDY

Before plunging into the first case, readers are encouraged to evaluate their fund of knowledge and think about how they should best approach this book. Three "Tracks" of study are described here, designed to give readers an appropriate experience, based on the level of understanding.

Self-motivated learners with a strong basic science background who enjoy the freedom of a non-traditional curriculum and who learn best through self-directed reading and problem solving may wish to approach the book using the **Track 1** philosophy. These individuals might read the Section Overviews for each organ system and then delve into the investigative study of a patient problem. The goal would be to focus on the clinical scenario and related information available on the first page of the case, using them to define the diagnosis before reading on to verify the diagnosis. Once the mechanism of the disease has been determined, students can turn to the pathophysiology section, which expands on the underlying physiology and mechanisms of the therapeutic options available for treating this particular patient's problem.

Track 2 can be used by small groups of students in a PBL setting, where student-centered, self-directed learning is emphasized. Here, a faculty facilitator might present the first page of a case over the course of three discussion sessions. For instance, the presenting symptoms and medical/social history could be presented and progressively disclosed in Session 1 and physical examination and laboratory results in Session 2. This would leave the follow-up materials for student self-study and group discussion in Session 3. During the first session, students might also discuss open-ended learning issues that are outside the scope of this book. Students might further refine their learning in the context of the problem and the open-ended issues by focusing on biology, diagnostics, pathophysiology, and management in the second, and possibly a third, session. This PBL track is appropriate for students who are flexible in their learning goals and who want a strong clinical context for their learning.

Track 3 is appropriate for students who learn well from a more traditional combination of presentations (e.g., lectures) and readings and are more comfortable in a teacher-directed environment. Students using Track 3 may save the first-page patient scenario and other information for the end of their study to be used for assessment of recall and application of processed information.

In all cases, using any of the Tracks, self-evaluation using the practice questions will help the reader recall important information and identify areas for further study.

Contents

SECTION I

Nerves and Muscles

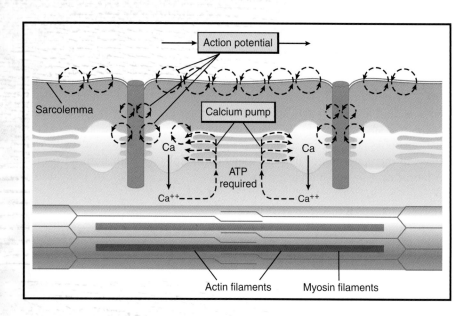

Voluntary movement requires a successful interplay of central nervous system components, peripheral nervous system components, muscles, and joints of the skeleton. Abnormalities in movement include disorders of coordination as well as of muscle weakness. Movement disorders provide a complex diagnostic challenge because defects in the chain of events can occur in any one region or multiple locations. Consequently, this introduction is organized around the physiology of normal voluntary muscle movement involved in picking up a pencil from a desk.

Voluntary movement originates in the planning regions of the accessory motor cortex. The first region of the brain to become activated is the sensory cortex, specifically the area receiving proprioception input from the periphery. Before movement can be initiated, it is first necessary to know where in three-dimensional space both the hand and the object are located. Proprioception plays a continuing and important role throughout voluntary muscle movement.

Voluntary muscle activity also integrates activity from the cerebellum and the basal ganglia. Coordination of central nervous system activities and symptoms arising from specific defects are addressed in neuroscience textbooks. Here, clinical problems arising from defects in the upper motor neuron, spinal cord, alpha (α)-motor neuron, and muscle are addressed.

Cell electrical activity underlies neuromuscular function. Both nerves and muscle cells have negative resting membrane potentials, resulting from both the differential distribution of ions across the cell membrane and the relative conductance for these ions based on ion channels. At rest, the cell is most permeable to K$^+$ and, consequently, resting membrane potential is close to the K$^+$ Nernst (equilibrium) value of –90 mV. Any changes in plasma K$^+$ values can impact both nerve and muscle function.

Depolarization of the cell can result in a local potential or an action potential. Local potentials are more common and are found in the neuron dendrites, cell body, and regions of the axon covered by the myelin sheath. Action potentials are a marked depolarization of the axon regions not covered by myelin (or the entire axon in unmyelinated axons), due to the opening of voltage-gated Na$^+$ channels. Local potentials decrease over time and distance, but action potentials regenerate without any decrease in amplitude. Consequently, action potentials allow neuronal electrical activity to be conducted over long distances. Myelinated nerves have the fastest conduction velocity (see Case 3).

The axons of upper motor neurons extend from the motor cortex to the spinal cord, where they synapse with both an α-motor neuron and spinal cord interneurons (see Case 1). The axon of the upper motor

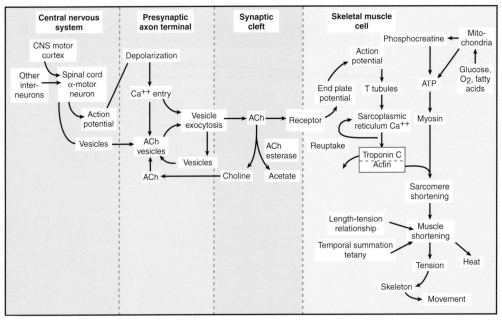

FIGURE I–1 Skeletal muscle physiologic processes can be grouped according to the region in which they occur. The neural signal for voluntary movement originates in the central nervous system (CNS) and passes along the motor neurons to the neuromuscular junction. Acetylcholine, released from the presynaptic neuron, depolarizes the muscle cell and initiates muscle contraction.

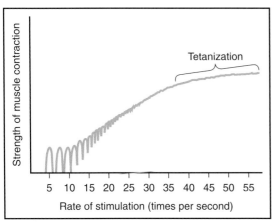

FIGURE I–2 Frequency summation and tetanization.

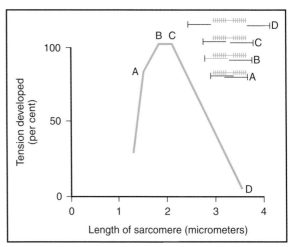

FIGURE I–3 Length-tension diagram for a single fully contracted sarcomere, showing maximum strength of contraction when the sarcomere is 2.0 to 2.2 μm in length. At the upper right are the relative positions of the actin and myosin filaments at different sarcomere lengths from point A to point D. *(Modified from Gordon AM, Huxley AF, Julian FJ: The length-tension diagram of single vertebrate striated muscle fibers. J Physiol 171:28P, 1964.)*

neuron is myelinated, and the action potential is transmitted by saltatory conduction.

The α-motor neuron, sometimes called the lower motor neuron, receives descending input from the upper motor neurons of the corticospinal tract, as well as multiple inputs from spinal cord interneurons. Spinal cord interneurons coordinate and integrate a variety of muscle activities, from the simple monosynaptic patellar tendon stretch reflex to the more complex polysynaptic flexor withdrawal reflex.

The axon of the α-motor neuron extends from the spinal cord to the muscle fibers (see Case 2). The α-motor neuron is myelinated, and action potentials are transmitted by saltatory conduction.

The axon and all of the muscle fibers that it innervates represent the "motor unit." Some axons, such as the motor units of the hand that are used in writing, innervate only a few muscle fibers and provide fine control. Other axons innervate a large number of muscle fibers, such as the motor units of the leg that are used for lifting.

The α-motor neuron synapses with a skeletal muscle cell at the neuromuscular junction. The neuromuscular junction consists of the presynaptic axon terminal, the synaptic cleft, and the postsynaptic "end plate" region of the skeletal muscle cell.

Neuromuscular transmission begins with the action potential arriving at the axon terminal of the α-motor neuron (Fig. I-1). Depolarization of the axon terminal opens voltage-sensitive calcium channels, leading to the influx of calcium into the axon terminal. Calcium entry causes the docking and fusion of

acetylcholine-containing vesicles, resulting in the exocytosis of acetylcholine (see Case 4). Acetylcholine diffuses across the synaptic cleft, where it binds with a nicotinic receptor on the skeletal muscle cell (see Case 5). Receptor binding opens a nonspecific cation channel, leading to a depolarization of the end plate region and the development of an action potential within the skeletal muscle cell.

The action potential in a skeletal muscle cell is transmitted to the interior of the muscle cell along the T tubules. Depolarization of the T tubules stimulates the release of calcium from the sarcoplasmic reticulum. Calcium binds with troponin C, exposing the active sites on the actin protein. The myosin binds to actin and, in the presence of adenosine triphosphate (ATP), contracts according to the sliding filament theory, causing the muscle to develop tension and to shorten (see Case 6).

Skeletal muscle contraction occurs by a tetany or sustained contraction (Fig. I-2). For an individual fiber, the strength of contraction is determined in part by the length-tension relationship (Fig. I-3). Increases in contractile force for an entire muscle can also be achieved by activating a larger number of motor units and, consequently, contracting a larger number of fibers within the muscle.

CASE 1

A 42-year-old man comes to his primary care physician complaining of awkwardness when running or walking.

The patient indicates that he noticed trouble with cramping and weakness in his right leg 4 months ago but attributed that to a change in his exercise habits. The weakness is progressing despite continued exercise, and now the left leg is beginning to show signs of weakness. He was last seen for a routine physical examination 3 years ago, and no abnormalities were noted at that time.

PHYSICAL EXAMINATION

VS: T 37°C, P 68/min, R 14/min, BP 110/60 mm Hg, BMI 25

PE: Neuromuscular examination reveals a positive Babinski sign on the right foot but not the left foot. Patient has some slurring of speech (dysarthria) and awkwardness when asked to run down a hallway. Patellar tendon reflex on the right leg is exaggerated (hyperreflexia). There were no other significant findings. Patient is referred for muscle biopsy and neuromuscular study.

LABORATORY STUDIES

Muscle biopsy: Normal

Electromyography: As disease progresses, muscle fibrillation, increased amplitude and duration of action potentials may be found.

Nerve conduction studies: Normal early, then defective as disease progresses to a lower motor neuron disease

DIAGNOSIS

Amyotrophic lateral sclerosis (ALS)

PATHOPHYSIOLOGY OF KEY SYMPTOMS

The diagnosis of ALS is achieved by eliminating the variety of other causes of muscle weakness. This diagnosis is complicated by the fact that the appearance of clinical symptoms and the time course for the progression of the disease are quite variable. One diagnostic approach involves beginning with skeletal muscle function and assessing function from the periphery back to the central nervous system.

Skeletal muscles elsewhere in the body are functioning normally. This indicates that the muscles are capable of maintaining a normal resting membrane potential and that cellular and extracellular electrolyte concentrations are within the normal range. The muscle biopsy rules out any protein-related defects in the muscle contractile and structural proteins. Electromyography confirms that the muscle is still able to contract when directly electrically stimulated. The defect in nerve traffic, however, eventually leads to atrophy of the skeletal muscle and exacerbates the weakness associated with the progression of the disease.

An appropriate patellar tendon reflex requires afferent input from the muscle spindles, transmission of the afferent action potential to the spinal cord, a monosynaptic reflex within the spinal cord, efferent action potential transmission by the alpha (α)-motor neuron, transmission across the neuromuscular synapse, activation of the skeletal muscle, and, finally, contraction (Fig. 1-1). This patient shows a hyperreflexive response in the right leg. Normally, the α-motor neurons receive descending inhibitory input from upper motor neurons and both inhibitory and stimulatory input from interneurons (Figs. 1-2 and 1-3). Hyperreflexia can be an indication that the normal descending input is diminished, which is characteristic of an upper motor neuron disease.

The finding of a positive Babinski sign is also characteristic of a defect in the upper motor neurons.

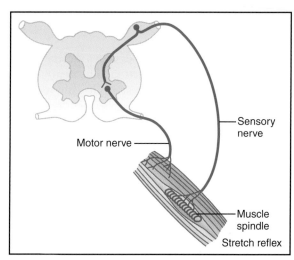

FIGURE 1-1 Neuronal circuit of the stretch reflex.

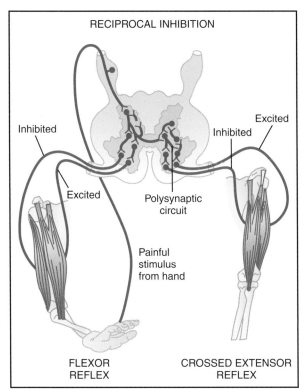

FIGURE 1–2 Flexor reflex, crossed extensor reflex, and reciprocal inhibition.

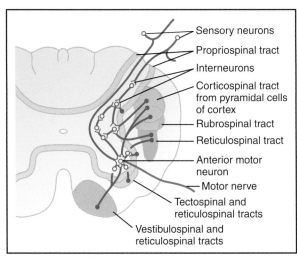

FIGURE 1–3 Convergence of different motor control pathways on the anterior motor neurons.

The Babinski sign is elicited by stroking the sole of the foot. When only lower motor neurons are functional, the big toe extends as part of a spinal cord reflex. The upper motor neurons usually inhibit the flaring response. When the upper motor neurons are functional, stroking the sole of the foot causes the big toe to contract. The Babinski sign is present in infants until about 2 years of age, when the upper motor neuron development becomes complete. Prior to the complete development of the upper motor neurons, stroking the sole of the foot causes the big toe to contract.

Nerve conduction velocity assessment is normal, indicating that the transmission of the action potential along the α-motor neuron by saltatory conduction is normal.

ALS is a motor neuron disease and does not involve other types of neurons. Consequently, ALS is characterized by progressive muscle weakness but no defects in intelligence, memory, or sensory discrimination. ALS begins as an upper motor neuron disease and then progresses to a complete loss of upper motor neuron input, resulting in a spastic or rigid paralysis. As the disease progresses, lower motor neurons may become involved, leading first to muscle weakness, then to fasciculations, and ultimately to a complete loss of muscle control and spinal cord reflexes.

The progressive loss of motor neurons ultimately involves the phrenic nerve, which innervates the diaphragm. Consequently, death results from respiratory muscle paralysis unless the patient is placed on an artificial ventilator.

Three to 10 percent of ALS cases are due to a dominant genetic defect, some of which involve a mutation of the superoxide dismutase 1 gene. The etiology of the remaining 90% to 97% of the cases is unknown.

Patients with ALS sometimes show elevated levels of glutamate in blood and spinal fluid. Excessive activation of the excitatory glutaminergic nerves is associated with neuronal damage, and, consequently, glutamate is suspected to be a contributing or causative agent.

OUTCOME

Riluzole (Rilutek), a glutamate antagonist, slows the progression of ALS. Although the exact mechanism of benefit is unknown, riluzole inhibits glutamine release and also blocks the activity of excitatory amino acids. Riluzole also inactivates voltage-gated sodium channels and interferes with intracellular events that follow transmitter binding and excitatory amino acid receptors.

Riluzole is the only approved treatment for ALS. Patient management is directed at relieving the symptoms and maintaining the quality of life. Physical therapy can help maintain some muscle and joint motility. Ultimately, death results from the loss of phrenic nerve function and respiratory paralysis.

FURTHER READING

Web Sources

http://www.ninds.nih.gov/disorders/amyotrophiclateralsclerosis/detail_amyotrophiclateralsclerosis.htm

Rilutek information. Available at http://products.sanofi-aventis.us/rilutek/rilutek.html

MDConsult: ALS: Possible role of environmental influences. Neurol Clin 23:2, 2005.

MDConsult: Protein interaction may be key to apoptosis in ALS. Lancet Neurol 3:9, 2004.

Text Sources

Carroll RG: Elsevier's Integrated Physiology. Philadelphia, Elsevier, 2007.

Copstead L, Banasik J: Pathophysiology, 3rd ed. Philadelphia, Saunders, 2005.

Dudek RW, Louis TM: High-Yield Gross Anatomy, 3rd ed. Philadelphia, Lippincott Williams & Wilkins, 2008, p 21.

Guyton AC, Hall JE: Textbook of Medical Physiology, 11th ed. Philadelphia, Saunders, 2006.

McPhee SJ, Papadakis MA, Tierney LM Jr: Current Medical Diagnosis and Treatment, 46th ed. New York, McGraw-Hill, 2007.

A 54-year-old woman returns to her oncologist for continuing treatment of recurrent ovarian cancer. It is 2 days since treatment, and she is now complaining of paresthesia of the hands and feet and difficulty in fastening buttons due to muscle weakness in the hands.

The patient began treatment for recurrent ovarian cancer 2 months ago. The treatment regimen includes paclitaxel, 150 mg/m^2; gemcitabine, 800 mg/m^2; and cisplatin, 75 mg/m^2, three times a week for 6 cycles. She was diagnosed with diabetes mellitus type 2 at age 35 and has been successfully managed with Ultralente insulin. The patient has lost body hair due to the chemotherapy. Her appetite remains good, and nausea is managed.

PHYSICAL EXAMINATION

VS: T 37°C, P 75/min, R 18/min, BP 128/84 mm Hg, BMI 34

PE: Sensory neuropathy (tingling) present in the hands. Deep tendon reflexes were diminished bilaterally.

LABORATORY STUDIES

None ordered

DIAGNOSIS

Taxol-induced peripheral neuropathy

COURSE

The sensory and motor neuropathies resolved over the next 5 days.

PATHOPHYSIOLOGY OF KEY SYMPTOMS

Normal neuromuscular transmission requires the release of acetylcholine from the synaptic vesicles in the alpha (α)-motor neuron presynaptic nerve terminal (Fig. 2-1), diffusion across the synaptic cleft, and binding to the receptors at the motor end plate region of the skeletal muscle cell. The acetylcholine is degraded by the enzyme acetylcholinesterase into acetate and choline. The choline is transported back into the presynaptic terminal and returned to the recycled portion of the vesicle. Acetylcholine is resynthesized, and the vesicle is ready for reuse.

The vesicles and associated vesicle proteins are synthesized in the cell body of the α-motor neuron.

The vesicles are transported to the axon terminal by microtubules. Once reaching the axon terminal, the vesicles are acidified and loaded with acetylcholine for synaptic release.

Cisplatin and paclitaxel both disrupt microtubule function by polymerizing the tubules and, therefore, block cellular mitosis. Consequently, rapidly dividing cells are targeted and killed. Neuromuscular symptoms develop because of the depletion of the vesicles that release acetylcholine. Disruption of the microtubules reduces the rate of vesicle arrival at the presynaptic axon and can lead to a reduction in the number of vesicles released during depolarization of the axon terminal.

Muscle electrical activity consists of miniature end plate potentials and end plate potentials. The miniature end plate potentials result from the release of a single vesicle of acetylcholine, usually causing a 0.4-mV depolarization in the muscle cell. The magnitude of the miniature end plate potentials will not be altered, because each vesicle contains a normal amount of acetylcholine, but their frequency may be diminished.

A normal α-motor neuron action potential normally causes the release of about 125 vesicles. That quantity of acetylcholine released into the synaptic cleft causes a 40-mV depolarization at the muscle end plate, which is sufficient to elicit an action potential and a contraction of the muscle. In this patient, the end plate potentials will be diminished because the total number of vesicles released during any one action potential will be diminished. Consequently, every α-motor neuron action potential does not result in a muscle cell contraction. This results in the weakness in the muscles.

Paclitaxel can also damage Schwann cells, leading to diminished nerve conduction velocity of both motor and sensory nerves, particularly the large myelinated nerves.

Sensory nerve conduction is more acutely altered, because the cell body of the sensory nerves is not behind the blood-brain barrier and, consequently, is more completely exposed to the paclitaxel.

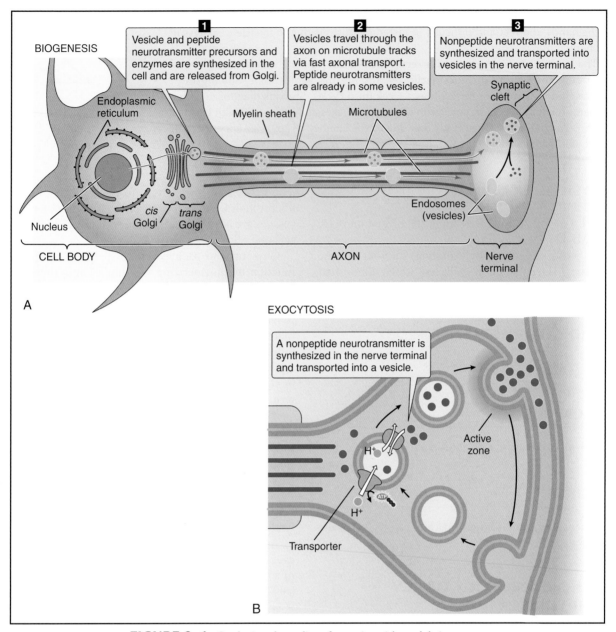

FIGURE 2–1 Synthesis and recycling of synaptic vesicles and their content.

Symptoms develop gradually, as the majority of the neurotransmitter vesicles in the axon are recycled and recovered after exocytosis. Only a small portion of the vesicles are lost and have to be replaced by vesicles synthesized in the cell body. Consequently, the onset of muscle weakness occurs 1 to 3 or more days after paclitaxel treatment.

The muscle groups involved also illustrate the pathophysiology. Axons innervating distal muscles have the longest distance for vesicle transport and, consequently, are more sensitive to microtubule disruption.

OUTCOME

Paclitaxel neuropathies normally (but not always) resolve over 1 week. Excessive alcohol use and diabetes are risk factors for the development of permanent neuropathies.

FURTHER READING

Web Sources

Argyriou A, Polychronopoulos P, Koutras A, et al: Clinical and electrophysiological features of peripheral neuropathy induced by administration of cisplatin plus paclitaxel-based chemotherapy. Eur J Cancer Care 16:231-237, 2007. Available at http://gateway.tx.ovid.com.jproxy.lib.ecu.edu/gw1/ovidweb.cgi

Postma TJ, Vermorken JB, Liefting AJ, et al: Paclitaxel-induced neuropathy. Ann Oncol 6:489-494, 1995. Available at http://gateway.tx.ovid.com.jproxy.lib.ecu.edu/gw1/ovidweb.cgi

Text Sources

Brunton L, Lazo J, Parker K: Goodman & Gilman's The Pharmacological Basis of Therapeutics, 11th ed. New York, McGraw-Hill Professional, 2005.

Carroll RG: Elsevier's Integrated Physiology. Philadelphia, Elsevier, 2007.

Copstead L, Banasik J: Pathophysiology, 3rd ed. Philadelphia, Saunders, 2005.

Guyton AC, Hall JE: Textbook of Medical Physiology, 11th ed. Philadelphia, Saunders, 2006.

McPhee SJ, Papadakis MA, Tierney LM Jr: Current Medical Diagnosis and Treatment, 46th ed. New York, McGraw-Hill, 2007.

A 35-year-old woman comes to her primary care physician complaining of difficulty in walking.

On questioning, the patient indicates she had trouble walking for 5 days last month and also that she has experienced pain and prickly sensations that come and go, as well as occasional muscle weakness.

PHYSICAL EXAMINATION

VS: T 36.5°C, P 70/min, R 15/min, BP 124/80 mm Hg, BMI 27

PE: Muscle strength testing: Normal. Deep tendon reflexes: Normal. When asked to walk, the patient had difficulty in balancing and maintaining a normal gait. Patellar tendon reflexes were normal. The muscles, however, were weak.

LABORATORY STUDIES

MRI: Gadolinium-enhancing brain lesions, as well as one lesion in the brain infratentorium and three periventricular lesions

Cerebrospinal fluid analysis: Oligoclonal IgG band

Edrophonium (Tensilon) test: Normal

Nerve conduction velocity test: Normal

Electromyography: Normal

DIAGNOSIS

Multiple sclerosis

PATHOPHYSIOLOGY OF KEY SYMPTOMS

Outflow from the upper motor neurons of the cerebral motor cortex travels by the corticospinal tracts to synapse with an alpha (α)-motor neuron. Each muscle fiber is innervated by a single α-motor neuron; however, a single α-motor neuron can innervate one or many muscle fibers. The motor unit consists of the α-motor neuron and all of the muscle fibers that it innervates. The strength of muscle contraction depends in part on the number of motor units activated. Smaller motor units are activated first, followed by larger ones.

Complex activities such as walking require the coordinated, sequential activation of multiple motor units. The sequence of activation is determined by neurons in the cerebellum, basal ganglia, and premotor cortex that synapse with the upper motor neurons. This results in the appropriate sequential activation of the muscles involved in walking and in balance, producing a smooth gait.

Action potential transmission depends on the diameter of the axon and on the presence of myelination. Myelination restricts the regions of the axon capable of producing an action potential to the nodes of Ranvier, where the myelin sheath is absent (Fig. 3-1). The wave of depolarization that initiates in the axon hillock travels by local conduction in the region of the axon beneath the myelin and is regenerated as an action potential at the nodes. This form of transmission is called "saltatory" conduction, because the action potential appears to jump from node to node along the length of the axon. Myelinated axons have much faster conduction velocities than do axons that lack myelin.

Multiple sclerosis is thought to be an autoimmune disease that leads to loss of myelin from central nervous system axons. The lost myelin is replaced by scar tissue called sclerosis. The central nervous system damage results in multiple lesions that are visible on magnetic resonance imaging.

Demyelinating diseases diminish the speed of axonal transmission. Consequently, this negatively impacts the coordinated and sequential activation of motor neurons necessary for walking. The difficulty

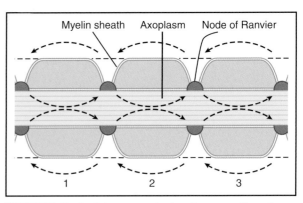

FIGURE 3–1 Saltatory conduction along a myelinated axon. Flow of electrical current from node to node is illustrated by the *arrows*.

in walking is likely due to damage to the myelinated axons of the basal ganglia or the cerebellum.

Deep tendon reflexes are normal because the neuromuscular transmission is working normally in the early stage of the disease. Similarly, muscle weakness may not be apparent. However, over time, the degeneration of the nerves will lead to muscle atrophy and weakness.

OUTCOME

Currently there is no cure for multiple sclerosis. The frequency and intensity of symptoms, however, can be diminished with interferon drugs that diminish the activity of the immune system. In addition, relapses may be shortened by treatment with corticosteroids. Symptoms can be helped by physical therapy.

FURTHER READING

Web Sources

Campellone J: U.S. National Library of Medicine. Nerve conductivity test. Accessed April 30, 2007. Available at http://www.nlm.nih.gov/medlineplus/ency/article/003927.htm

Goetz C: Textbook of Clinical Neurology, 3rd ed., Philadelphia, Saunders, 2007. Available at http://www.mdconsult.com/das/book/body/79885428-3/0/1488/402.html?#4-u1.0-B978-1-4160-3618-0.10048-7–s0030_3250

Multiple Sclerosis Foundation. Accessed October 16, 2007. Available at http://www.msfocus.org/info_diagnosed.php

Wrongdiagnosis.com. Deep tendon reflexes. Accessed October 2007. Available at http://www.wrongdiagnosis.com/t/tendinitis/book-diseases-14b.htm

Text Sources

Carroll RG: Elsevier's Integrated Physiology. Philadelphia, Elsevier, 2007.

Copstead L, Banasik J: Pathophysiology, 3rd ed. Philadelphia, Saunders, 2005.

Guyton AC, Hall JE: Textbook of Medical Physiology, 11th ed. Philadelphia, Saunders, 2006.

McPhee SJ, Papadakis MA, Tierney LM Jr: Current Medical Diagnosis and Treatment, 46th ed. New York, McGraw-Hill, 2007.

C A S E 4

A 48-year-old man comes to the emergency department complaining of trouble seeing and has difficulty swallowing.

The patient is not from the area but is visiting friends who live on a commune. On questioning, the patient indicates that approximately 24 hours earlier he ate some green beans that were canned at the commune. Symptoms began 3 hours ago, and the decision to come to the emergency department was made because of his difficulty in swallowing. The patient is now anxious and easily excited.

PHYSICAL EXAMINATION

VS: T 37°C, P 90/min, R 19/min, BP 145/100 mm Hg
PE: Physical examination reveals double vision and drooping of the eyelids. The patient is slurring his speech and has difficulty swallowing. He shows signs of muscle weakness. Deep tendon reflexes are diminished in the legs and arms.

LABORATORY STUDIES

CBC, electrolytes: Normal
Brain CT and MRI: Normal (rule out cerebrovascular accident)
Cerebrospinal fluid examination: Normal
Electromyography: Nerve conduction velocity and amplitude normal; neuromuscular junction impaired
Edrophonium (Tensilon) test: Normal (rule out myasthenia gravis, myasthenic syndrome)

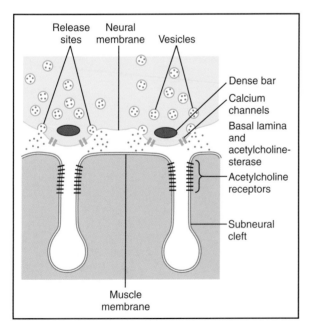

FIGURE 4–1 Release of acetylcholine from synaptic vesicles at the neural membrane of the neuromuscular junction. Note the proximity of the release sites in the neural membrane to the acetylcholine receptors in the muscle membrane, at the mouths of the subneural clefts.

Stool sample: Positive for *Clostridium botulinum*

DIAGNOSIS

Botulism toxicity

COURSE

Botulism is a paralytic illness caused by a neurotoxin released from *Clostridium botulinum*. There are seven types of *C. botulinum* bacteria, identified by the letters A through G. The bacteria grow best in low oxygen conditions, and food-borne botulism is usually caused by eating contaminated foods canned at home.

PATHOPHYSIOLOGY OF KEY SYMPTOMS

Acetylcholine is stored in vesicles in the presynaptic terminal of alpha (α)-motor neurons. After an action potential arrives, calcium enters the presynaptic

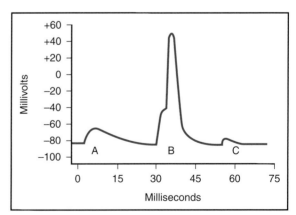

FIGURE 4–2 End plate potentials (in millivolts). A, Weakened end plate potential recorded in a curarized muscle, too weak to elicit an action potential. B, Normal end plate potential eliciting a muscle action potential. C, Weakened end plate potential caused by botulinum toxin that decreases end plate release of acetylcholine, again too weak to elicit a muscle action potential.

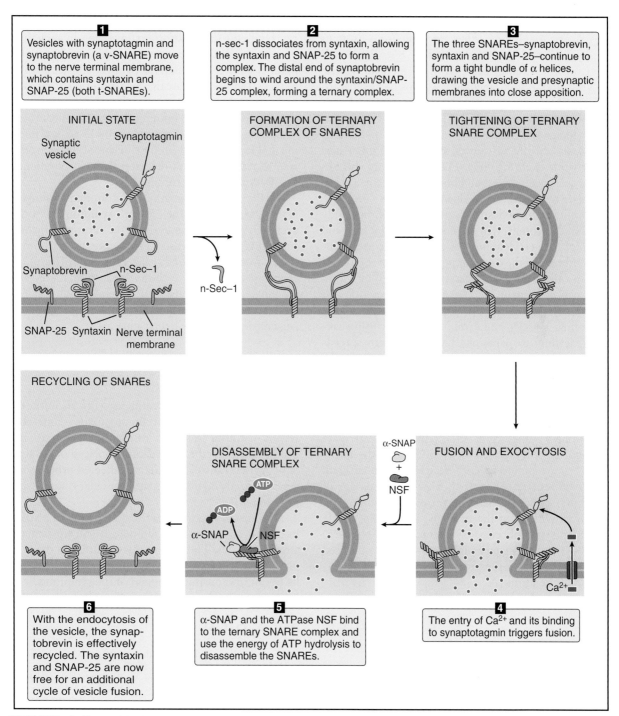

FIGURE 4–3 Model of synaptic-vesicle fusion and exocytosis. ADP, adenosine diphosphate; ATP, adenosine triphosphate; NSF, N-ethyl maleimide-sensitive factor; SNAP-25, synaptosome-associated protein-25kDa; α-SNAP, soluble NSF-attachment protein; SNARE, SNAP receptor.

terminal, causing the vesicles to migrate toward the presynaptic membrane. There are numerous proteins involved in vesicle exocytosis. The SNAP-SNARE mechanism includes proteins that mediate vesicle docking and fusion, including synapsin 1, synapto-brevin, SNAP-25, syntaxin, synaptotagmin, and syn-aptophysin. The series of SNAP and SNARE proteins allow docking of the vesicles with the cell membrane, fusion, and, finally, exocytosis of the acetylcholine into the synaptic cleft (Fig. 4-1). The acetylcholine diffuses across the synaptic cleft and binds to receptors on the end plate region of the skeletal muscle cell.

Botulinum toxin destroys one or more of the family of "SNAP" proteins that are essential for docking and fusion of the acetylcholine vesicles with the presynap-tic membrane of the α-motor neuron. In the absence of these proteins, acetylcholine is not released by action potentials arriving at the neuromuscular junction and flaccid paralysis occurs. The paralysis is first evident in the cranial muscles and exhibits a symmetrical weak-ening, leading to paralysis. The impairment spreads to other proximal muscles and finally will include the distal muscles.

Impaired acetylcholine release by botulinum toxin depresses the end plate potential amplitude, an event tied to the exocytotic release of acetylcholine-containing vesicles (Fig. 4-2). Miniature end plate potential amplitude, which is a function of the quan-tity of acetylcholine in each vesicle, is not affected. The toxin is extremely potent, with a lethal dosage of 2 to 3 mg. There are many forms of botulinum toxin, but all cleave one of the proteins involved in vesicle priming (synaptobrevin, syntaxin, and SNAP-25) (Fig. 4-3) and subsequent inhibition of Ca^{++}-induced vesicle release from presynaptic terminals and degen-eration of the terminals.

Very dilute preparations of botulinum toxin (Botox) can be used to treat disorders involving hyperactivity of neuromuscular junctions. In addition, botulinum toxin is used cosmetically to paralyze muscles, which reduces the wrinkles in the face resulting from con-traction of the underlying muscles. Recovery of func-tion after exposure to botulinum toxin requires weeks to months and depends on the synthesis of new dock-ing and fusion proteins in the nucleus of the neuron as well as transport along the axon for incorporation at the presynaptic nerve terminal.

The loss of function at the neuromuscular junction is the basis for all of the patient's symptoms. Droopy eyelids result from paralysis of the levator palpebrae superioris (eyelid) muscle. Difficulty in swallowing results from paralysis of the skeletal muscle of the upper esophagus. Impaired α-motor neuron function also accounts for the diminished deep tendon reflexes. The double vision and the blurred vision are the result of partial paralysis of the ocular muscles.

OUTCOME

Early diagnosis allows treatment with an antitoxin directed against the botulinum toxin. Untreated severe botulism leads to respiratory paralysis and death. However, the patient can be placed on a venti-lator for several weeks while the affected proteins are resynthesized and normal neuromuscular transmission is reestablished.

Administration of the antitoxin resulted in a stabi-lization of the patient but did not reverse any damage already present. The patient was admitted to the hos-pital for observation for 4 days and was released when he began to show improvement of the symptoms.

FURTHER READING

Web Source
http://www.bt.cdc.gov/agent/botulism/

Text Sources
Carroll RG: Elsevier's Integrated Physiology. Philadelphia, Elsevier, 2007.
Copstead L, Banasik J: Pathophysiology, 3rd ed. Philadelphia, Saunders, 2005.

Goldman L, Ausiello D: Clostridial infections. Cecil Medicine, 23rd ed. Philadelphia, Saunders, 2007.
Guyton AC, Hall JE: Textbook of Medical Physiology, 11th ed. Philadelphia, Saunders, 2006.
Horowitz B: Botulinum toxin. Crit Care Clin 21:825–839, 2005.
McPhee SJ, Papadakis MA, Tierney LM Jr: Current Medical Diag-nosis and Treatment, 46th ed. New York, McGraw-Hill, 2007.
Salzman M, Madsen JM, Greenberg MI: Toxins: Bacterial and marine toxins. Clin Lab Med 26:397–419, 2006.

A 65-year-old man comes to his primary care physician complaining of a decreasing ability to read that is more pronounced in the evening. The difficulty is due to a combination of diplopia and blurred vision.

The patient has a 15-year history of hypertension that is being managed with diuretics and a low salt diet. He began using bifocals for reading about 10 years ago, and his current eyeglass prescription allows him to see comfortably.

PHYSICAL EXAMINATION

VS: T 37°C, P 75/min, R 15/min, BP 130/90 mm Hg, BMI 28

PE: Neurologic examination indicated normal sensory responses. Deep tendon reflexes were normal, although a small amount of muscle weakness was present.

LABORATORY STUDIES

Edrophonium (Tensilon) test: Positive

Repetitive nerve stimulation test on the biceps: Response to the fifth stimulus in the train of stimuli was decreased by 20%.

Plasma testing: Presence of antibodies directed against the acetylcholine receptor (normal < 0.03 mmol/L)

DIAGNOSIS

Myasthenia gravis

COURSE

Myasthenia gravis is an autoimmune disease in which antibodies attack the acetylcholine receptors on the motor end plate region of the muscle cell. The symptoms are due to both the inactivation of the acetylcholine receptors and to the disruption of the histology of the motor end plate region.

PATHOPHYSIOLOGY OF KEY SYMPTOMS

Neuromuscular transmission requires the release of an appropriate amount of acetylcholine into the synaptic cleft, the diffusion of the acetylcholine across the cleft, and the binding of the acetylcholine to the receptors on the motor end plate region of the skeletal muscle cell. Binding of acetylcholine to the receptors opens a cation channel that is equally selective for Na^+ and K^+, and there is a subsequent depolarization of the end plate region to –15 mV. The depolarization generates an action potential that spreads along the skeletal muscle cell, causing Ca^{++} release from the sarcoplasmic reticulum and inducing a contraction.

Myasthenia gravis is a chronic autoimmune disease leading to destruction of the acetylcholine receptors on the motor end plate region of muscle cells. Acetylcholine release from the α-motor neuron synapse, however, remains normal.

Normally, the amount of acetylcholine released by an α-motor neuron action potential is in excess of the amount needed to generate a skeletal muscle action potential. The threshold for an action potential in skeletal muscle is about –40 mV, so there is a large safety factor in neuromuscular transmission. Consequently, a noticeable impairment of neuromuscular transmission does not occur until approximately 70% of the acetylcholine receptors have been damaged.

Although acetylcholine release is normal, the absence of functional receptors on the motor end plate region of the muscle cell means that the biologic response is diminished. Normally, acetylcholine is degraded in the synaptic cleft by the activity of the enzyme acetylcholinesterase. Drugs such as edrophonium inhibit acetylcholinesterase. Therefore, an improvement in function after edrophonium confirms a defect in acetylcholine/receptor interaction.

Sequential nerve stimulation results in a reduced amount of acetylcholine released from the nerve terminal. This is not normally evident because of the large safety factor for neuromuscular transmission. However, when the number of receptors on the muscle cell is diminished there is a reduction in the strength of contraction that is detected by the repetitive nerve stimulation test.

The diagnosis of myasthenia gravis is based on the presence of antibodies against the acetylcholine receptor. The disruption of the motor end plate region of the skeletal muscle cell can also be detected histologically from a biopsy.

Myasthenia gravis is often associated with a tumor of the thymus gland. For these patients, thymectomy can provide significant relief or complete remission of symptoms.

OUTCOME

Acutely, symptoms can be diminished by increasing the amount of acetylcholine in the synaptic cleft. This is done by administering pyridostigmine, an acetylcholinesterase inhibitor. Blocking the degradation of acetylcholine acts to increase the effective concentration of acetylcholine in the synapse and therefore activates a greater percentage of the remaining functional acetylcholine receptors.

Plasma exchange has caused an acute diminishment of symptoms as the acetylcholine receptor antibodies are removed from the circulation.

Chronically, treatments that diminish the activity of the immune system will diminish the destruction of the acetylcholine receptors, allowing the muscle cell to replace the receptors by synthesis of new receptor proteins. These treatments include corticosteroids, immunosuppressive drugs, or thymectomy.

FURTHER READING

Web Sources

http://www.emedicine.com
http://www.medscape.com
Ocular aspects of myasthenia gravis. Available at http://www.medscape.com/viewarticle/410859
Thymectomy and myasthenia gravis. Available at http://www.medscape.com/viewarticle/524436
Thymus and lesions. Available at http://www.emedicine.com/radio/topic693.HTM

Text Sources

Carroll RG: Elsevier's Integrated Physiology. Philadelphia, Elsevier, 2007.
Copstead L, Banasik J: Pathophysiology, 3rd ed. Philadelphia, Saunders, 2005.
Guyton AC, Hall JE: Textbook of Medical Physiology, 11th ed. Philadelphia, Saunders, 2006.
LeBlond R, DeGowin R, Brown D: DeGowin's Diagnostic Examination, 8th ed. New York, McGraw-Hill, 2004.
McPhee SJ, Papadakis MA, Tierney LM Jr: Current Medical Diagnosis and Treatment, 46th ed. New York, McGraw-Hill, 2007.
Pagana K, Pagana T: Mosby's Diagnostic and Laboratory Test Reference, 8th ed. St. Louis, Mosby, 2007.

A 3-year-old boy is brought to the clinic for physical examination. His mother reports that the child has difficulty in walking and he appears clumsy compared with other boys his age.

The patient learned to stand and walk about 8 months after the three boys in his play group who are the same age. Both parents appear normal, and the father has no known family history of musculoskeletal problems. The mother was adopted and does not know the medical history of her family of origin.

PHYSICAL EXAMINATION

VS: T 37°C, P 80/min, R 15/min, BP 90/70 mm Hg, BMI 22, height and weight 40th percentile, normal growth curve

PE: Muscle coordination is low for age. Muscles are weak, and grip strength is weak. Muscles of the calf appear hypertrophied.

LABORATORY STUDIES

Plasma analysis: Elevated creatine kinase level
Muscle biopsy: Confirmed the diagnosis of Duchenne muscular dystrophy

DIAGNOSIS

Duchenne muscular dystrophy

PATHOPHYSIOLOGY OF KEY SYMPTOMS

Muscle tension development depends on the contraction of the muscle filaments as described by the sliding filament model. Depolarization of the muscle cell causes Ca^{++} to be released from the sarcoplasmic reticulum (Fig. 6-1). The Ca^{++} binds to troponin C, pulling the tropomyosin away from the G-actin site. Myosin binds to the exposed actin site, and the myosin head pivots using adenosine triphosphate (ATP) as an energy source. The pivoting of the myosin head causes the actin filaments to slide past the myosin filaments, shortening the muscle (Fig. 6-2). This shortening is transmitted to the muscle cell cytoskeleton by a number of proteins, including the elastic protein titin.

Dystrophin is a protein that anchors the cytoskeleton of the muscle cell to the extracellular matrix. An abnormal dystrophin molecule alters the transmission of tension from the contracting muscle

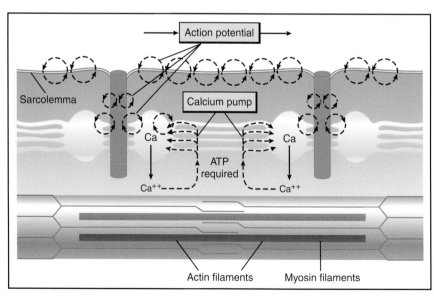

FIGURE 6–1 Excitation-contraction coupling in the muscle, showing (1) an action potential that causes release of calcium ions from the sarcoplasmic reticulum and then (2) reuptake of the calcium ions by a calcium pump.

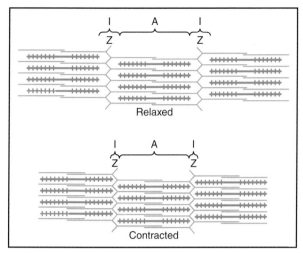

FIGURE 6–2 Relaxed and contracted states of a myofibril showing *(top)* sliding of the actin filaments *(pink)* into the spaces between the myosin filaments *(red)*, and *(bottom)* pulling of the Z membranes toward each other.

filaments through the cell membrane to the extracellular matrix. The contractile actin and myosin proteins still function and shorten normally. The abnormal dystrophin results in both muscle weakness and damage to the cell membrane. Creatine kinase leaks from the damaged muscle cells and consequently is found in abnormally high levels in the plasma. Diagnosis is confirmed by detecting the abnormal dystrophin protein from a muscle biopsy.

The pseudohypertrophy of the calf muscles is due to an inflammatory response generated by the damaged muscle cells and the replacement of damaged muscle cells with scar tissue. Consequently, although the muscles appear hypertrophied, there is actually a deficit in functioning contractile filaments in the muscle and the muscles are weak.

Duchenne muscular dystrophy is transmitted from mother to son as an X-linked recessive trait. As a recessive trait, women with one copy of the defective gene are carriers who exhibit no signs of the disease. There is a 50% chance of the transmission of the disease to sons and a 50% chance that daughters will be asymptomatic carriers.

OUTCOME

There is currently no cure for any form of muscular dystrophy. Current treatment is designed to relieve the symptoms, including diminishing deformities in the joints and spine. Severe cardiac and respiratory problems develop during the late teen years and early 20s.

FURTHER READING

Text Sources
Behrman RE, Kliegman RM, Jenson HB: Nelson Textbook of Pediatrics, 16th ed. Philadelphia, Saunders, 2000.
Brambrink AM, Kirsch JR: Perioperative care of patients with neuromuscular disease and dysfunction. Anesthesiol Clin 25:483-509, 2007.
Carroll RG: Elsevier's Integrated Physiology. Philadelphia, Elsevier, 2007.

Copstead L, Banasik J: Pathophysiology, 3rd ed. Philadelphia, Saunders, 2005.
Deconinck N, Dan B: Pathophysiology of Duchenne muscular dystrophy: current hypotheses. Pediatr Neurol 36:1-7, 2007.
Guyton AC, Hall JE: Textbook of Medical Physiology, 11th ed. Philadelphia, Saunders, 2006.
McPhee SJ, Papadakis MA, Tierney LM Jr: Current Medical Diagnosis and Treatment, 46th ed. New York, McGraw-Hill, 2007.

Section II

Cardiology

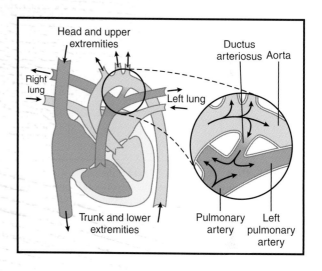

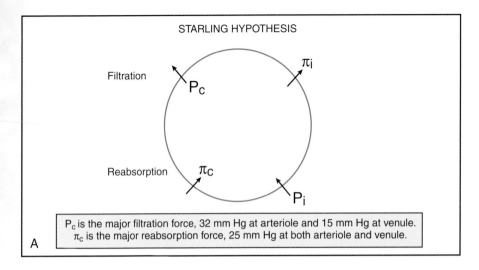

STARLING HYPOTHESIS

P_c is the major filtration force, 32 mm Hg at arteriole and 15 mm Hg at venule.
π_c is the major reabsorption force, 25 mm Hg at both arteriole and venule.

A

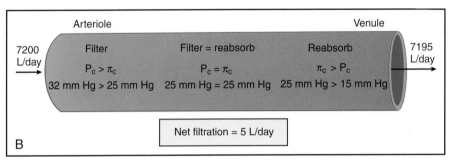

Arteriole   Venule

7200
L/day

Filter   Filter = reabsorb   Reabsorb

$P_c > \pi_c$ $P_c = \pi_c$ $\pi_c > P_c$

32 mm Hg > 25 mm Hg   25 mm Hg = 25 mm Hg   25 mm Hg > 15 mm Hg

7195
L/day

Net filtration = 5 L/day

B

FIGURE II–1   **A,** Filtration of fluid at the capillary is increased by increases in capillary hydrostatic pressure or interstitial fluid oncotic pressure. Reabsorption is increased by increases in capillary oncotic pressure or by increases in interstitial fluid pressure. **B,** The balance between hydrostatic and colloid osmotic pressures favors filtration at the arteriolar end of the capillaries. The drop in pressure along the length of the capillary reverses this balance, and absorption occurs at the venous end of the capillaries. Any change in hydrostatic pressure or colloid osmotic pressure can change the fluid balance between the capillaries in the tissues.

The functional role of the cardiovascular system is to provide an adequate tissue blood flow to support cellular metabolism. The cardiovascular system transports nutrients to the tissues of the body and removes metabolic waste products. Compounds are exchanged between the blood and the cells mostly at the capillary level by the processes of diffusion and filtration. Diffusional movement of a compound, described by Fick's law of diffusion,

$$J = -DA(\Delta\text{Concentration}/\Delta\text{Distance})$$

is increased by increasing the concentration gradient, by increasing the surface area participating in exchange, and by decreasing the distance. Filtration is a net movement of water based on the balance of hydrostatic and oncotic pressures, as described by the Starling hypothesis (Fig. II-1).

Tissue blood flow depends on the pressure gradient and the vascular resistance, as described by the equation

$$\text{Flow} = \text{pressure gradient/resistance}$$
$$Q = \Delta P/R.$$

Resistance to blood flow is locally determined in the microcirculation by the contraction or relaxation of vascular smooth muscle, which controls arteriolar diameter (see Case 11). Depletion of nutrients, or accumulation of metabolic wastes, leads to a dilation of the vascular smooth muscle and an increase in tissue blood flow.

Adequate blood flow depends on a relatively constant arterial pressure to provide the pressure gradient. Arterial pressure is a regulated variable in the cardiovascular system (see Case 7). The arterial

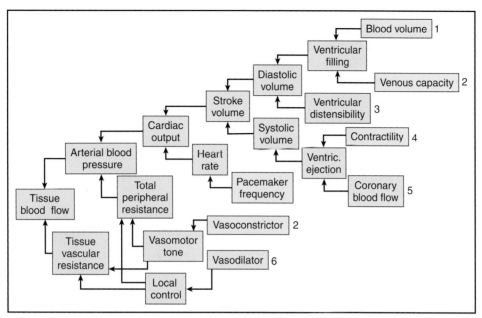

FIGURE II–2 Map of the cardiovascular system. This diagram illustrates the causal relationships of various cardiovascular parameters. *Blue-shaded boxes* indicate targets of the sympathetic nervous system. *Numbers* indicate initial disturbances that can lead to shock. 1, Blood or plasma loss; 2, vasodilation (neurogenic); 3, pericardial tamponade; 4, heart failure; 5, myocardial infarction; 6, peritonitis, anaphylaxis.

baroreceptor reflex provides acute (within seconds) control of blood pressure by appropriately adjusting the balance of sympathetic and parasympathetic nervous system output (see Case 13). Endocrine control systems, particularly angiotensin II, provide blood pressure control in the intermediate time frame, and the renal regulation of circulating blood volume provides chronic regulation of blood pressure.

Arterial blood pressure is determined by the volume of blood entering the arteries (cardiac output), the volume of blood exiting the arteries (determined by total peripheral resistance), and arterial compliance (decreases with age and atherosclerosis). Contraction of cardiac muscle generates the pressure in the arterial system, and, consequently, impaired pumping ability in the heart causes a drop in arterial blood pressure (see Cases 10 and 12). The major determinants of cardiac output are preload in the ventricle (see Case 9), afterload created by arterial blood pressure (see Case 14), and contractility (Case 8) (Fig. II-2).

Ischemia occurs when tissue blood flow is insufficient to match tissue metabolic needs (see Case 16). Ischemia results in impaired organ function and possibly cellular death. The coronary and the cerebral circulations are particularly susceptible to interruptions in blood flow (see Case 15).

A 31-year-old man arrived by ambulance at the emergency department after suffering a laceration to the left thigh in an industrial accident that cut the femoral artery.

The patient was working in a metal fabrication plant. A falling piece of steel lacerated the artery in his left thigh, causing the loss of 1.5 L of blood, an estimated 30% of blood volume. Bleeding was controlled by direct pressure, and the patient received 2 L of 0.9% saline during transport.

PHYSICAL EXAMINATION

VS: T 35.5°C, P 120/min and weak, R 22/min and shallow, BP 80/60 mm Hg
PE: Height 68 in, weight 155 lb (70 kg), BMI 25

The patient was pale, diaphoretic, and anxious. He was transferred to the trauma room, where arterial, Swan-Ganz, and bladder catheters were inserted and a pulse oximeter was placed on the fourth finger of the left hand.

LABORATORY STUDIES

Pulse oxymetry: 92% saturated
Arterial blood gases: P_{O_2} 90 mm Hg, P_{CO_2} 32 mm Hg, pH 7.45
Venous blood gases: P_{O_2} 25 mm Hg, P_{CO_2} 47 mm Hg, pH 7.32
Cardiac output: 3 L/min
Hematocrit: 35%
Plasma protein concentration: 5 mg/dL
Urine production: Minimal

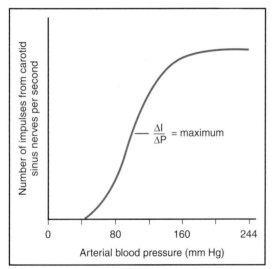

FIGURE 7–1 Activation of the baroreceptors at different levels of arterial pressure. ΔI, change in carotid sinus nerve impulses per second; ΔP, change in arterial blood pressure in millimeters of mercury.

DIAGNOSIS

Hemorrhagic shock

COURSE

The patient was infused with 2 L of typed and cross-matched blood. This restored the blood pressure toward normal, and pulse and respiratory rates declined. Mixed venous blood gas values returned toward normal. The patient was transferred to surgery for repair of the damaged artery.

PATHOPHYSIOLOGY OF KEY SYMPTOMS

Arterial blood pressure is the regulated variable in the cardiovascular system. Arterial pressure results from the accumulation of blood in the aorta and large arteries. Consequently, arterial blood pressure represents a balance between the volume entering the aorta (cardiac output of the left ventricle) and the volume leaving the artery and flowing into the capillaries (determined by total peripheral resistance).

Cardiac output is determined by the pumping ability of the heart and is limited by the venous return. Pumping ability of the heart is a function of heart rate and stroke volume, and stroke volume is a function of the ventricular preload and the cardiac contractility. Venous return ultimately limits cardiac output because as cardiac output exceeds venous return the preload on the ventricle falls, resulting in a reduced cardiac output. The heart cannot pump more blood than the volume that flows into it from the vena cava.

Arterial blood pressure is sensed by the stretch receptors of the aortic arch and the carotid sinus, collectively called arterial baroreceptors. A drop in arterial blood pressure unloads the baroreceptors and causes a sympathetic activation and a parasympathetic inhibition (Fig. 7-1). Sympathetic activation causes increases in heart rate, ventricular contractility, and total peripheral resistance and a decrease in venous capacitance (Table 7-1).

TABLE 7–1	**Autonomic Effects on Various Organs of the Body**	
Organ	**Effect of Sympathetic Stimulation**	**Effect of Parasympathetic Stimulation**
Eye		
Pupil	Dilated	Constricted
Ciliary muscle	Slight relaxation (far vision)	Constricted (near vision)
Glands	Vasoconstriction and slight secretion	Stimulation of copious secretion
Nasal		(containing many enzymes for
Lacrimal		enzyme-secreting glands)
Parotid		
Submandibular		
Gastric		
Pancreatic		
Sweat glands	Copious sweating (cholinergic)	Sweating on palms of hands
Apocrine glands	Thick, odoriferous secretion	None
Blood vessels	Most often constricted	Most often little or no effect
Heart		
Muscle	Increased rate	Slowed rate
	Increased force of contraction	Decreased force of contraction (especially of atria)
Coronaries	Dilated (β_2); constricted (α)	Dilated
Lungs		
Bronchi	Dilated	Constricted
Blood vessels	Mildly constricted	? Dilated
Gut		
Lumen	Decreased peristalsis and tone	Increased peristalsis and tone
Sphincter	Increased tone (most times)	Relaxed (most times)
Liver	Glucose released	Slight glycogen synthesis
Gallbladder and bile ducts	Relaxed	Contracted
Kidney	Decreased output and renin secretion	None
Bladder		
Detrusor	Relaxed (slight)	Contracted
Trigone	Contracted	Relaxed
Penis	Ejaculation	Erection
Systemic arterioles		
Abdominal viscera	Constricted	None
Muscle	Constricted (adrenergic α)	None
	Dilated (adrenergic β_2)	
	Dilated (cholinergic)	
Skin	Constricted	None
Blood		
Coagulation	Increased	None
Glucose	Increased	None
Lipids	Increased	None
Basal metabolism	Increased up to 100%	None
Adrenal medullary secretion	Increased	None
Mental activity	Increased	None
Piloerector muscles	Contracted	None
Skeletal muscle	Increased glycogenolysis	None
	Increased strength	
Fat cells	Lipolysis	None

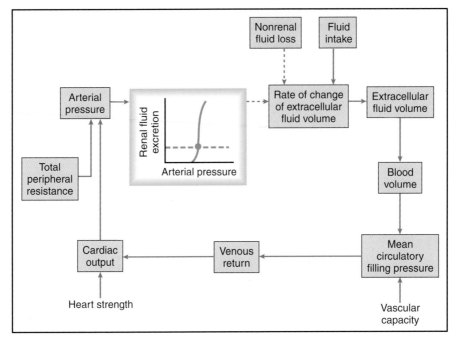

FIGURE 7–2 Basic renal body fluid feedback mechanism for control of blood volume, extracellular fluid volume, and arterial pressure. *Solid lines* indicate positive effects, and *dashed lines* indicate negative effects.

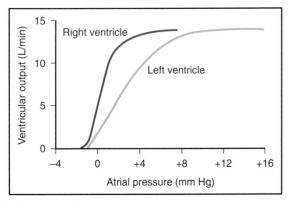

FIGURE 7–3 Approximate normal right and left ventricular volume output curves for the normal resting human heart as extrapolated from data obtained from dogs and humans.

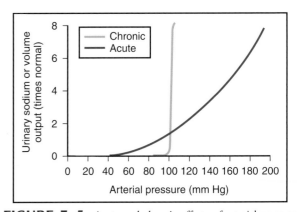

FIGURE 7–5 Acute and chronic effects of arterial pressure on sodium output by the kidneys (pressure natriuresis). Note that chronic increases in arterial pressure cause a much greater increase in sodium output than those measured during acute increases in arterial pressure.

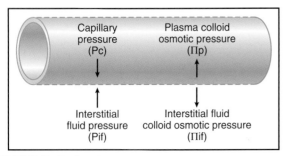

FIGURE 7–4 Fluid pressure and colloid osmotic pressure forces operate at the capillary membrane, tending to move fluid either outward or inward through the membrane pores.

These changes cause an increase in cardiac output and a reduction in the volume of blood exiting the arteries. Consequently, arterial pressure recovers toward normal.

The initial event in this patient was the loss of circulating blood volume. Estimated blood volume for this individual is 5 L, which accounts for 8% of body weight. Blood loss caused a drop in venous volume and venous pressure and, consequently, a fall in cardiac preload (see Fig. II-2, p. 21). The fall in preload causes a drop in cardiac output and, therefore, a drop in arterial blood pressure (Fig. 7-2).

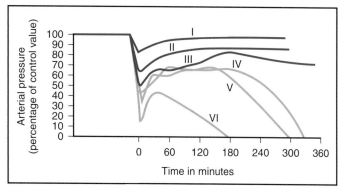

FIGURE 7–6 Time course of arterial pressure in dogs after different degrees of acute hemorrhage. Each curve represents average results from six dogs.

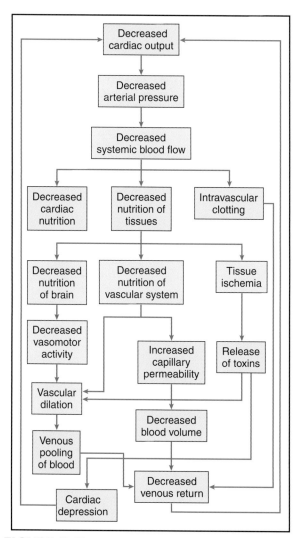

FIGURE 7–7 Different types of "positive feedback" that can lead to progression of shock.

Sympathetic nerve activation causes the observed increases in heart rate, respiratory rate, and anxiety. In addition, sympathetic nerves to the skin cause vasoconstriction of the blood vessels, accounting for the loss of skin color. Sympathetic cholinergic nerves activate sweat glands, causing diaphoresis. The common description of a patient in shock is "pale and sweaty." Arterioles of the cerebral and coronary circulations respond more strongly to local control than to sympathetic activity. Consequently, blood flow to the brain and heart are not diminished by increases in sympathetic nerve activity.

Arteriolar constriction also causes a decrease in capillary blood pressure. Capillary blood pressure is one of the Starling forces that determine the balance of fluid exchange between the blood and the interstitial space of the microcirculation. A drop in capillary pressure causes the reabsorption of fluid from the interstitial space back into the circulation, helping to restore blood volume back toward normal (Fig. 7-3).

The drops in hematocrit and in plasma protein concentration are due to two separate events. First, sympathetic arteriolar constriction causes a drop in capillary blood pressure, enhancing reabsorption in interstitial fluid at the capillary level. The reabsorbed interstitial fluid lacks the red blood cells and large molecular weight proteins that are found in blood. Consequently, blood cell and protein concentrations are diluted. In addition, infusion of the 0.9% saline during transport also dilutes the blood cell and plasma protein components.

Arterial oxygen levels and pulse oxymetry values were normal, reflecting adequate gas exchange at the lungs. The anxiety actually causes a slight hyperventilation and a consequent fall in arterial P_{CO_2} and results in respiratory alkalosis. Mixed venous blood gases show a hypoxia and hypercapnia, both characteristic of the tissue ischemia that occurs during periods of low cardiac output.

Hemorrhage stimulates the release of adrenal catecholamines, antidiuretic hormone from the pituitary, and renin from the kidney, leading to angiotensin II synthesis. These hormones both acutely constrict vascular smooth muscle and, in the longer term, stimulate the renal retention of water and sodium.

Urine production also depends on an adequate arterial pressure. Severe hypotension acutely causes a marked drop in urine production. Restoration of arterial pressure after control of the hemorrhage and replacement of circulating blood volume allows normal urine production to resume (Fig. 7-4).

OUTCOME

Restoration of circulating blood volume and sealing of the damaged vessel resulted in a complete recovery. An even greater loss of blood (40% of estimated circulating volume) can be fatal (Figs. 7-5 to 7-7).

FURTHER READING

Web Sources

eMedicine. Hypovolemic shock. Accessed Oct. 16, 2007. Available at http://www.emedicine.com/EMERG/topic531.htm
Perez E: U.S. National Library of Medicine. Hypovolemic shock. Accessed July 2006. Available at http://www.nlm.nih.gov/medlineplus/ency/article/000167.htm

Text Sources

Carroll RG: Elsevier's Integrated Physiology. Philadelphia, Elsevier, 2007.

Copstead L, Banasik J: Pathophysiology, 3rd ed. Philadelphia, Saunders, 2005.
Guyton AC, Hall JE: Textbook of Medical Physiology, 11th ed. Philadelphia, Saunders, 2006.
Marx J, Hockberger R, Walls R: Rosen's Emergency Medicine: Concepts and Clinical Practice, 6th ed. St. Louis, Mosby, 2006.
McPhee SJ, Papadakis MA, Tierney LM Jr: Current Medical Diagnosis and Treatment, 46th ed. New York, McGraw-Hill, 2007.

A 68-year-old man comes to his primary care physician complaining of tiredness and difficulty sleeping.

Six months earlier, the patient experienced myocardial infarction of the anterior wall of the left ventricle. A stent was placed in the occluded coronary artery, reestablishing perfusion. The patient now complains of difficulty sleeping at night, awakening with shortness of breath. He reports that he is able to sleep better using pillows to elevate his chest and head. The moderate exercise regimen that he followed after the myocardial infarction is now causing him to become progressively more short of breath.

PHYSICAL EXAMINATION

VS: T 37°C, P 80/min, R 18/min and shallow, BP 100/70 mm Hg, BMI 29
PE: A third heart sound is evident. Auscultation reveals crackles at the base of the lung, and there is dullness to percussion at the base of the lung.

LABORATORY STUDIES

Chest radiography: Enlarged left atrium and ventricle, interstitial pulmonary edema, and consolidation of the lower lung fields
Echocardiography: Ejection fraction of 40%
Arterial blood gases: Po_2 85 mm Hg, Pco_2 40 mm Hg, pH 7.38

DIAGNOSIS

Congestive heart failure (after a myocardial infarction)

PATHOPHYSIOLOGY OF KEY SYMPTOMS

Blood entering the right atrium flows progressively through the right ventricle, pulmonary circulation, left atrium, and left ventricle before exiting the heart into the aorta. The ventricles are the power pumps in the heart. Ventricular output is determined by the preload on the ventricle and ventricular contractility.

The volume that flows through each of the cardiac chambers has to be equal or a fluid imbalance develops. This balance is achieved by the effect of preload on ventricular pumping. If the left ventricle pumps less blood than the right ventricle, the left ventricular end-diastolic volume will gradually increase. Left ventricular end-diastolic volume is "preload," and an increase in preload will increase the pumping capability of the left ventricle. Left ventricular output increases, and the imbalance is corrected.

Echocardiography permits calculation of chamber size, chamber shape, wall thickness, and valvular function. This information can be used to calculate ejection fraction, which is the ratio of the stroke volume to the ventricular end-diastolic volume. The calculated left ventricular ejection fraction of 40% in this patient indicates that there is a systolic dysfunction of the left ventricle. Systolic dysfunction accounts for 60% to 70% of heart failure cases.

The presenting complaints of fatigue and nocturnal dyspnea are caused by impaired oxygen exchange at the alveolar capillaries. The impaired gas exchange is secondary to pulmonary edema, resulting from an impaired pumping ability of the left ventricle.

Myocardial infarction causes damage to the ventricular tissue and impairs the pumping ability. Because the infarct was in the left ventricle in this patient, left ventricular pumping is impaired. This results in a decreased arterial blood pressure and an elevated

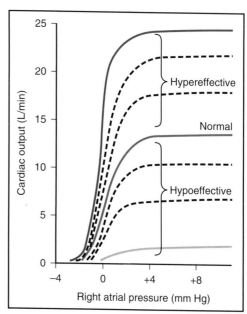

FIGURE 8–1 Cardiac output curves for the normal heart and for hypoeffective and hypereffective hearts. (*Redrawn from Guyton AC, Jones CD, Coleman TB: Circulatory Physiology: Cardiac Output and Its Regulation, 2nd ed. Philadelphia, WB Saunders, 1973.*)

pressure in the left atrium and pulmonary circulation. The elevated volume in the left atria causes the appearance of a third heart sound owing to the turbulent flow of blood during atrial filling (Fig. 8-1).

The decreased arterial blood pressure causes a renal retention of volume and a consequent expansion of the body fluid volume. This volume expansion (preload) increases the pumping ability of the right ventricle. The preload, however, is not capable of restoring the

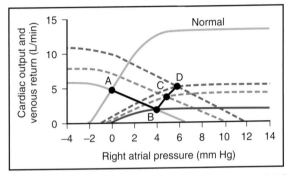

FIGURE 8–2 Progressive changes in cardiac output and right atrial pressure during different stages of cardiac failure.

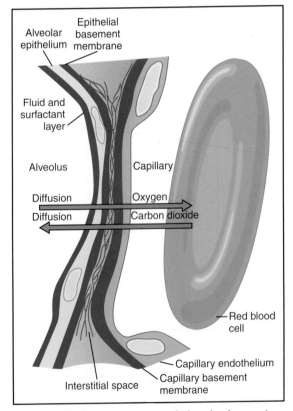

FIGURE 8–3 Ultrastructure of the alveolar respiratory membrane, shown in cross section.

pumping ability of the left ventricle, and the kidneys continue to retain fluid because of the arterial hypotension (Fig. 8-2). Blood accumulates within the pulmonary vasculature, and the increase in pulmonary capillary pressure causes excessive filtration into the pulmonary interstitial space. This leads to the accumulation of fluid both in the space between the alveoli and the pulmonary capillaries and in some of the alveoli (Fig. 8-3). This free fluid is evident as interstitial edema on chest radiography, causing crackles and dullness to percussion at the base of a lung.

Pulmonary edema increases the distance over which gas must exchange in the lung. Because oxygen is less soluble in water than is carbon dioxide, a deficit in oxygen exchange occurs earlier than a carbon dioxide exchange deficit. This is evidenced by the low oxygen partial pressure and normal CO_2 partial pressure in the arterial blood gas sample (Fig. 8-4).

When the patient lies down at night, the excess fluid redistributes from the base of the lung throughout the dependent portions of a lung. Consequently, there is a greater deficit in gas exchange and nocturnal dyspnea develops. The hypoxemia awakens the patient, preventing a restful sleep. Sleeping in a partially upright position is achieved with the use of pillows and helps to ameliorate these symptoms.

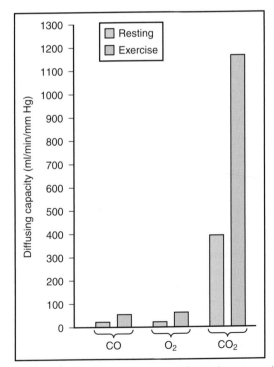

FIGURE 8–4 Diffusing capacities for carbon monoxide, oxygen, and carbon dioxide in the normal lungs under resting conditions and during exercise.

OUTCOME

The patient is started on a beta-adrenergic blocker with an initial low dose. If symptoms of heart failure persist, a diuretic and a cardiac glycoside can be added to the treatment.

The patient is encouraged to continue to exercise as is possible and to maintain a low-salt diet.

FURTHER READING

Web Source
http://www.emedicinehealth.com/congestive_heart_failure/article_em.htm

Text Sources
Carroll RG: Elsevier's Integrated Physiology. Philadelphia, Elsevier, 2007.

Copstead L, Banasik J: Pathophysiology, 3rd ed. Philadelphia, Saunders, 2005.

Davidoff AW, Boyden PA, Schwartz K, et al: Congestive heart failure after myocardial infarction in the rat: cardiac force and spontaneous sarcomere activity. Ann NY Acad Sci 1015:84–95, 2004.

Guyton AC, Hall JE: Textbook of Medical Physiology, 11th ed. Philadelphia, Saunders, 2006.

McPhee SJ, Papadakis MA, Tierney LM Jr: Current Medical Diagnosis and Treatment, 46th ed. New York, McGraw-Hill, 2007.

Zipes DP, Libby P, Bonow R, et al: Braunwald's Heart Disease, a Textbook of Cardiovascular Medicine. Philadelphia, Saunders, 2005.

A 45-year-old man comes to the emergency department complaining of sharp, stabbing chest pain beneath the sternum.

The patient is anxious, and his cognitive abilities are slightly impaired. The pain is relieved by sitting upright. He has a dry cough and is recovering from an upper respiratory tract infection.

PHYSICAL EXAMINATION

VS: T 38.5°C, P 85/min, R 22/min and shallow, BP 105/55 mm Hg during expiration and 90/40 mm Hg during inspiration (pulsus paradoxus). Jugular veins are distended and enlarge during inspiration (Kussmaul sign).

PE: All heart sounds are muffled. A pericardial rub can be heard on the lower left sternal border.

LABORATORY STUDIES

Echocardiogram: Enlargement of the heart
ECG: Normal sinus rhythm with no abnormalities
CK-MB: Normal troponin I and myoglobin levels
CBC: Elevated white blood cell count

DIAGNOSIS

Pericardial tamponade

COURSE

Pericardiocentesis was performed under echocardiographic guidance. Symptoms were relieved with removal of 300 mL of fluid. The patient was admitted to the hospital for treatment and observation.

PATHOPHYSIOLOGY OF KEY SYMPTOMS

Preload is one of the main determinants of cardiac output. It is the volume of blood in the ventricle before ventricular contraction. Left ventricular end-diastolic volume, left ventricular end-diastolic pressure, and the "upstream" pressures in the left atrium, pulmonary vein, or pulmonary capillary all provide useful indices of left ventricular preload.

Ventricular filling occurs at low pressures (5 to 10 mm Hg), in contrast to the high pressures (120 mm Hg) generated by the left ventricle during systole. The low filling pressures mean that ventricular filling can be impaired by a relatively low pressure external compression (Fig. 9-1).

The heart sits within a fibrous pericardium, with between 20 and 50 mL of fluid in the pericardial space. Pericardial fluid lubricates the heart and diminishes frictional damage to the epicardial surface of the heart as it moves during cardiac contraction. Although the pericardium can in theory limit the expansion of the heart during diastolic filling, the fibrous connective tissue in the myocardium is the more important source that limits cardiac filling at high atrial pressures.

The underlying cause for the symptoms in this patient is the accumulation of fluid in the pericardial space. Tamponade results from an increase in intrapericardial pressure greater than 15 mm Hg. This fluid prevents the expansion of the ventricles during ventricular diastole and consequently diminishes ventricular preload. The lack of preload leads to a deficit in cardiac output, causing a pronounced hypotension.

Pulsus paradoxus is defined as greater than a 10-mm Hg variation in arterial blood pressure during respiration. Inspiration normally causes a small drop in blood pressure because the retention of blood in the pulmonary vasculature during pulmonary inflation leads to a small drop in left ventricular filling. Pericardial tamponade accentuates this drop, and, consequently, arterial pressure measured during inspiration is much lower than that measured during expiration.

Arterial blood pressure is sensed by stretch receptors in the aortic arch and carotid sinus. A decrease in stretch diminishes the nerve traffic in the baroreceptor afferent nerves to the cardiovascular centers of the medulla and results in an increase in sympathetic nerve activity and a decrease in parasympathetic nerve activity. Increased sympathetic nerve activity and decreased parasympathetic nerve activity increases the firing rate of the sinoatrial pacemaker cells, causing an increased heart rate. Hypotension also causes anxiety and, if severe, some impairment of cognitive function.

refilling   contract

*Where is
Hr sounds
where Do things
open close?
relaxation?
contraction?*

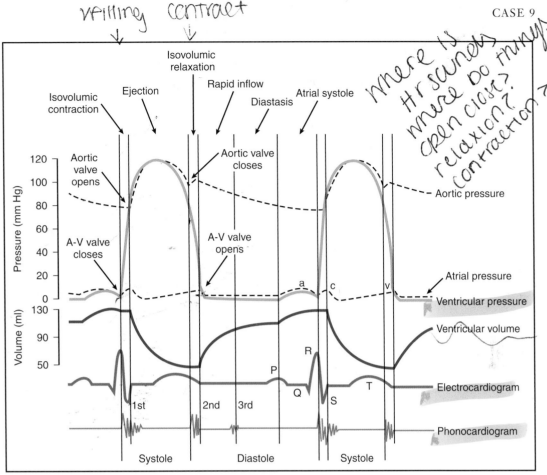

FIGURE 9-1 Events of the cardiac cycle for left ventricular function, showing changes in left atrial pressure, left ventricular pressure, aortic pressure, ventricular volume, the electrocardiogram, and the phonocardiogram.

The muffled heart sounds heard during auscultation are due to the accumulation of fluid within the pericardial sac. This fluid acts as an acoustic insulator and diminishes the heart sounds in all locations. Movement of the heart within the pericardium normally does not produce a sound. When excess fluid is present, however, movement of the heart against the pericardium does generate a high-pitched sound called a pericardial rub.

The diminished flow of blood into the ventricle during diastole leads to an accumulation of volume in the systemic and pulmonary veins. Elevation of pulmonary venous pressure can lead to signs and symptoms of congestive heart failure. Elevated central venous pressure will lead to distention of the jugular veins and, possibly, hepatomegaly and ascites.

Combination of chest pain, hypotension, and elevated jugular venous pressure is also characteristic of myocardial infarction of the right ventricle. The electrocardiogram and cardiac enzymes help rule out that possibility.

The low-grade fever and the elevated white blood cell count are characteristic of persistent infection that has spread to the pericardial space.

OUTCOME

Pericardiocentesis relieves the acute symptoms, and the patient should be monitored to make sure that additional fluid does not accumulate in the pericardial space.

FURTHER READING

Web Sources

Lee JA: Cardiac tamponade. Last update 7/14/2006. Medline Plus
http://www.nlm.nih.gov/medlineplus/ency/article/000194.htm
Pericarditis and pericardial tamponade. Last Updated 6/15/2006.
eMedicine http://www.emedicine.com/emerg/topic412.htm

Text Sources

Carroll RG: Elsevier's Integrated Physiology. Philadelphia,
Elsevier, 2007.

Copstead L, Banasik J: Pathophysiology, 3rd ed. Philadelphia,
Saunders, 2005.
Guyton AC, Hall JE: Textbook of Medical Physiology, 11th ed.
Philadelphia, Saunders, 2006.
McPhee SJ, Papadakis MA, Tierney LM Jr: Current Medical Diag-
nosis and Treatment, 46th ed. New York, McGraw-Hill, 2007.

A 58-year-old woman comes to her primary care physician complaining of shortness of breath and difficulty sleeping at night, especially while lying down. She complains of coughing at night that awakens her.

FLUID

The patient first reports having symptoms 3 days ago. The symptoms do not appear to be worsening. She has a history of mitral valve prolapse in the past, but this has not been symptomatic.

PHYSICAL EXAMINATION

VS: T 37°C, P 80/min, R 15/min, BP 100/70 mm Hg, BMI 24
PE: The patient has a systolic murmur that is heard best at the apex of the heart. The intensity of the murmur is constant throughout systole. The patient has rales during inspiration bilaterally in the base of the lung. There is no sign of peripheral edema.

LABORATORY STUDIES

ECG: Normal, including no displacement of the ST segment
Plasma analysis: CK-MB normal.
Echocardiogram: Left atrial enlargement.

DIAGNOSIS

Mitral valve regurgitation

PATHOPHYSIOLOGY OF KEY SYMPTOMS

The mitral valve usually closes and isolates the left atrium from the left ventricle during ventricular systole. In patients with mitral valve regurgitation the high pressures generated during left ventricular systole lead to the ejection of blood into the aorta (normal) as well as the backward flow of blood from the left ventricle into the left atrium (abnormal). Retrograde blood flow through the mitral valve is turbulent and can be heard as a systolic murmur (see Fig. 9-1, p.30 in Case 9).

The intensity of the murmur is fairly constant (holosystolic), reflecting the significant pressure gradient across mitral valve during ventricular systole. In addition, the timing of the murmur extends throughout the interval between the first and second heart sounds (pansystolic), because the pressure gradient exists during this entire interval. These characteristics distinguish the murmur of the mitral valve regurgitation from that of the other systolic murmur, aortic stenosis.

Mitral valve regurgitation can occur after rupture of the chordae tendineae or papillary muscles. The initiating event can be a myocardial infarction, infective endocarditis, trauma, or, in this case, degeneration of the valvular tissue in patients with mitral valve prolapse.

Normal functioning of the cardiac valves is essential to the pumping ability of the heart. Normally, the left ventricular and diastolic volume is about 150 mL and 60% of this volume is ejected into the aorta during ventricular systole (60% ejection fraction) and 40% remains in the left ventricle as the end-systolic left ventricular volume. In this patient, blood in the left ventricle at the end of diastole can (1) be pumped into the aorta, (2) be pumped retrograde back into the left atrium, or (3) remain in the left ventricle. The ejection fraction is reduced because of the retrograde flow of blood through the mitral valve. In addition, the left atrium now has two sources of filling: the normal filling of blood flowing from the pulmonary vein and the retrograde filling of blood flowing from the left ventricle during ventricular systole. Consequently, the left atrium is enlarged and left atrial pressures are elevated (Fig. 10-1).

The elevation of left atrial pressure causes an increase in pressure in the pulmonary veins and pulmonary capillaries. An increase in pulmonary capillary pressure causes an increase in filtration at the pulmonary capillaries, leading to pulmonary edema, often called pulmonary congestion. Pulmonary edema impairs gas exchange across the pulmonary capillary/alveolar interface. This defect in gas exchange impacts oxygen exchange more than carbon dioxide exchange because of the relatively low solubility of oxygen in water. Pulmonary J receptor activation by the edema contributes to the cough reflex and also to the dyspnea.

The impaired oxygen exchange accounts for the patient's presenting symptoms: shortness of breath and nocturnal dyspnea. The shortness of breath is due to hypoxia and is exacerbated whenever there is an increased oxygen utilization, such as during exercise. The nocturnal dyspnea occurs because of the

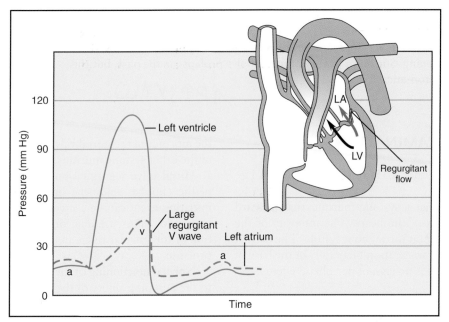

FIGURE 10–1   Mitral regurgitation causes characteristic giant v waves on the left atrial (LA) pressure monitor. LV, Left ventricle.

gravity-induced distribution of pulmonary blood flow. In an upright individual, pulmonary capillary pressure and blood flow are highest at the base of the lung and lowest at the apex. When an individual lies down, the pulmonary capillary pressures are high throughout the lung and the consequent edema impairs gas exchange. Patients find that they are able to sleep more comfortably in a semi-upright state, either in a chair or by using pillows to prop themselves up.

Acute mitral valve regurgitation causes an acute onset of congestive heart failure. Consequently, the presenting symptoms are those of congestive heart failure. The negative findings on the electrocardiogram in cardiac enzymes rule out acute myocardial infarction as the initiating event for the regurgitation. If the mitral regurgitation would become more severe, the fluid back up may extend through the right side of the heart, ultimately causing peripheral edema.

OUTCOME

The patient was admitted to the cardiac care unit of the hospital. Doppler echocardiogram revealed a significant (20%) retrograde flow across the mitral valve during systole. The patient underwent annuloplasty (surgical repair of the mitral valve) and was discharged 2 weeks later.

FURTHER READING

Web Source
Mitral valve regurgitation. Available at http://www.mayoclinic.com/health/mitral-valve-regurgitation/DS00421/DSECTION=8

Text Sources
Carroll RG: Elsevier's Integrated Physiology. Philadelphia, Elsevier, 2007.

Copstead L, Banasik J: Pathophysiology, 3rd ed. Philadelphia, Saunders, 2005.
Guyton AC, Hall JE: Textbook of Medical Physiology, 11th ed. Philadelphia, Saunders, 2006.
McCance K, Huether S: Pathophysiology: The Biological Basis for Disease in Adults and Children, 5th ed. St. Louis, Mosby, 2006.
McPhee SJ, Papadakis MA, Tierney LM Jr: Current Medical Diagnosis and Treatment, 46th ed. New York, McGraw-Hill, 2007.

A 4-day-old female infant is seen by the cardiologist, having been referred because of suspicion of a patent ductus arteriosus.

The infant was delivered by cesarean section at 32 weeks' gestational age because of preeclampsia in the mother. The APGAR score was 7 at 1 minute and improved to 9 at 5 minutes. The pediatrician noted a machine-like murmur extending through both the systole and diastole.

PHYSICAL EXAMINATION

VS: T 36°C, P 115/min, R 35/min, BP 65/35 mm Hg
PF: The infant still exhibits the systolic and diastolic murmur but otherwise appears healthy. Cyanosis is not present.

LABORATORY STUDIES

Doppler echocardiography: Continuous flow of blood from the aorta into the pulmonary artery through the ductus arteriosus.

DIAGNOSIS

Patent ductus arteriosus

COURSE

Blockade of prostaglandin production removes the vasodilatory prostaglandins, allowing the smooth muscle of the ductus to contract and close the vessel.

PATHOPHYSIOLOGY OF KEY SYMPTOMS

In utero, the ductus arteriosus allows the flow of blood from the pulmonary artery into the aorta, so that 90% of the right ventricular output bypasses the lungs. Blood flowing through the ductus arteriosus joins with the blood pumped by the left ventricle into the aorta to provide blood flow to most of the body. Vessels that originate from the aorta before the juncture with the ductus arteriosus carry relatively well oxygenated blood to the brain and heart (Fig. 11-1).

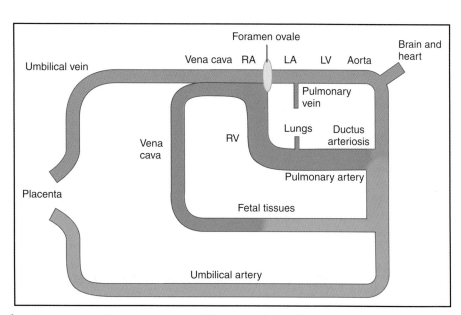

FIGURE 11-1 Fetal circulation directs the oxygenated blood from the umbilical vein to the blood vessels supplying the heart and brain. The O$_2$-rich blood from the umbilical vein is directed through the foramen ovale into the left atrium (LA), left ventricle (LV), and out the aorta. The O$_2$-depleted blood from the superior and inferior vena cava flows through the right atrium (RA), right ventricle (RV), and out the pulmonary artery before passing through the ductus arteriosus and joining the fetal systemic circulation.

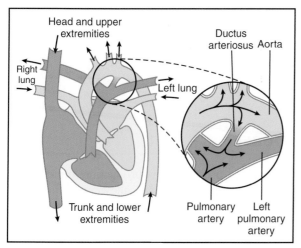

FIGURE 11–2 Patent ductus arteriosus. The intensity of the pink color shows that dark venous blood changes into oxygenated blood at different points in the circulation. The right-hand diagram shows backflow of blood from the aorta into the pulmonary artery and then through the lungs for a second time.

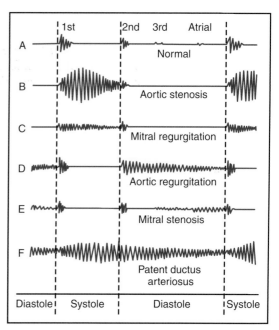

FIGURE 11–3 Phonocardiograms from normal and abnormal hearts.

At birth, the inflation of the lungs reduces pulmonary vascular resistance and the constriction of the umbilical artery increases systemic vascular resistance. Consequently, aortic pressure becomes higher than pulmonary artery pressure and oxygenated blood flows from the aorta into the pulmonary artery. The presence of oxygenated blood in the ductus arteriosus normally inhibits the production of the vasodilator prostaglandins, and the ductus arteriosus closes. Closure of the ductus arteriosus, along with closure of the foramen ovale, effectively isolates the pulmonary circulation from the systemic circulation. Remnants of the ductus arteriosus persist throughout life and are identified as the ligamentum arteriosus connecting the pulmonary artery and the aorta.

When the ductus arteriosus remains patent, or "open," blood flow from the aorta into the pulmonary artery persists after birth. There may not be any apparent symptoms, because this congenital defect does not impair oxygenation of blood pumped by the left ventricle. Instead, blood flowing through the ductus arteriosus actually passes through the lungs for a second time before being pumped into the systemic circulation (Fig. 11-2).

APGAR is an assessment of a neonate at 1 minute and 5 minutes after birth. The acronym stands for Activity, Pulse, Grimace, Appearance, and Respiration. The maximum score is 10, and a score of 7 to 10 is considered normal. Because oxygenation is not impaired by a patent ductus arteriosus, the APGAR score can be normal.

Vital signs are normal for a 4-day-old infant. There is a gradual drop in pulse and respiratory rate, and an increase in blood pressure, during the first years of life.

Cardiac murmurs are caused by the turbulent flow of blood through a narrow opening. Murmurs associated with a cardiac valve defect are usually limited to either the systolic or the diastolic portion of the cardiac cycle. The pressure gradient between the aorta and the pulmonary artery persists throughout systole and diastole. Consequently, the murmur associated with a patent ductus arteriosus is continuous but is more prominent during the systolic portion of the cardiac cycle. This type of murmur is often called "machine-like" because of the regular cyclic changes in intensity (Fig. 11-3).

The underlying problem is either (1) the continued production of vasodilator prostaglandins or (2) the persistence of the ductus even in the absence of the prostaglandins. Premature infants often exhibit continuing vasodilator prostaglandin production, and full-term infants often have the structural abnormality. Consequently, drugs that block prostaglandin production are used for treatment in premature infants. Infants born at full term with a patent ductus arteriosus usually require transcatheter device closure or, after 6 months of age, surgical correction.

Patent ductus arteriosus occurs in about 1 of every 2000 births. It is more common in preterm infants. Often the ductus will spontaneously close during the first 1 to 2 years of life.

OUTCOME

Indomethacin treatment (10 mg/kg bolus, 5 mg/kg for next 2 days) was initiated.

The ductus arteriosus gradually closed over the next 2 days, and the infant was discharged from the hospital.

FURTHER READING

Web Source

www.mayoclinic.com/health/patent-ductus-arteriosus/DS00631

Text Sources

Behrman RE, Kliegman RM, Jenson HB: Nelson Textbook of Pediatrics, 16th ed. Philadelphia, Saunders, 2000.

Carroll RG: Elsevier's Integrated Physiology, Philadelphia, Elsevier, 2007.

Clyman RI, Chorne N: Patent ductus arteriosus: evidence for and against treatment, J Pediatr 150:216–219, 2007.

Copstead L, Banasik J: Pathophysiology, 3rd ed. Philadelphia, Saunders, 2005.

Guyton AC, Hall JE: Textbook of Medical Physiology, 11th ed. Philadelphia, Saunders, 2006.

McPhee SJ, Papadakis MA, Tierney LM Jr: Current Medical Diagnosis and Treatment, 46th ed. New York, McGraw-Hill, 2007.

Perloff JK: The Clinical Recognition of Congenital Heart Disease, Philadelphia, Saunders, 1994.

A 73-year-old man comes to the emergency department complaining of chest pain, shortness of breath on exertion, and syncope.
The patient has poorly managed hypercholesterolemia and a 10-year history of hypertension.

[handwritten: Syncope, angina, dysphea — A valve stenosis.]

PHYSICAL EXAMINATION

VS: T 37°C, P 85/min, R 18/min, BP 100/75 mm Hg

PE: A systolic murmur is present, loudest over the aorta and peaking at mid systole. Palpitation of the carotid upstroke reveals a pulse that is both decreased and late relative to the apical impulse. Palpation of the chest reveals an apical impulse that is laterally displaced. Lungs are clear, and there are no rales.

LABORATORY STUDIES

ECG: Left axis deviation but no abnormalities in the ST segment.

Chest radiography: Enlarged left ventricle and calcification of the aortic valve

Doppler ultrasonography: A greatly increased velocity of flow during the systolic portion of the cardiac cycle. The left atrium and left ventricle chambers are enlarged, and left ventricular hypertrophy is present.

Cardiac enzymes: CK-MB, troponin I, and myoglobin levels are normal.

DIAGNOSIS

Aortic valve stenosis

PATHOPHYSIOLOGY OF KEY SYMPTOMS

The normal function of the aortic valve is to isolate the aortic and left ventricular chambers during ventricular diastole and to open so as not to impede ventricular ejection during ventricular systole. Aortic valve stenosis is a narrowing of the aortic valve so that ventricular ejection is impeded. Aortic stenosis often occurs as a result of calcium deposits on the leaflets of the aortic valve (see Fig. 9-1, p.31).

The symptoms are due to an impaired ability to eject blood from the left ventricle into the aorta. Impaired ventricular ejection, combined with the normal inflow of blood from the left atrium, results in an increased volume in the left ventricle during diastolic filling. The increase in preload causes an increase in left ventricular pressure generation during systole. The increased left ventricular systolic pressure can overcome the resistance caused by the stenotic aortic valve, which allows a partial recovery of left ventricle cardiac output. In patients with this disease, left ventricular systolic pressures are much higher than aortic systolic pressures and there is a pressure gradient across the aortic valve throughout systole (Fig. 12-1).

Impaired cardiac pumping by the left ventricle also causes an increase in volume and pressure upstream of the left ventricle, in the left atrium and in the pulmonary circulation. Although not yet evident in this patient (no rales), congestive heart failure can develop if pressures in the pulmonary capillaries rise.

The cardiac murmur occurs during the period of time when the aortic valve is open and is classified as a systolic murmur. The murmur does not begin immediately after the first heart sound, and it increases in intensity during the midpoint of the systolic interval. These characteristics, along with a location along the aortic outflow tract (right of the sternum), distinguish this murmur from the systolic murmur caused by mitral regurgitation.

The obstruction to ventricular outflow leads to the carotid pulse being diminished and delayed. Normally, the increase in arterial pressure during the early stages of ventricular ejection is quite rapid. This is because of the rapid ejection of blood from the left ventricle. The resistance to blood flow caused by the stenotic aortic valve delays and slows that ejection and, as a consequence, the normal rise in arterial pressure during systole is delayed and is slower than normal.

The chest pain noted by the patient is a result of the increased metabolic demands of the ventricle. Even though aortic pressure remains low, the pressure generated by the ventricle is abnormally high, and it is generation of ventricular pressure that is the primary determinant of cardiac work. The elevated ventricular work leads to hypertrophy of the left ventricle, as evidenced by (1) the left axis deviation on

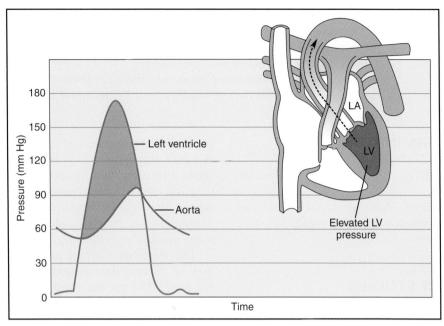

FIGURE 12–1   Aortic stenosis is characterized by an abnormal left ventricular (LV)-to-aortic pressure gradient *(shaded area)*. LA, left atrium.

the electrocardiogram, (2) the lateral displacement of the cardiac impulse, and (3) the enlarged ventricular chamber in cardiac imaging. The chest pain is not due to myocardial ischemia, as is indicated by the normal cardiac enzymes and the absence of ST segment shifts.

The shortness of breath on exertion and syncope are characteristics of impaired cardiac pumping ability. It is cardiac output that normally limits exercise performance. For this patient, the impaired ventricular pumping limits cardiac output more severely than normal. Syncope can result from a drop in aortic pressure, particularly when peripheral metabolic demands cause a vasodilation that is not matched by an increase in cardiac output.

Hypertension, diabetes, hyperlipidemia, and age are all risk factors for the development of aortic stenosis, as is a prior history of rheumatic fever.

OUTCOME

The patient was admitted to the cardiac care unit. Cardiac surgery was performed to replace the aortic valve, and the patient was discharged.

FURTHER READING

Web Source
Shipton B, Wahba H: Valvular heart disease: review and update, American Academy of Family Physicians. Available at http://www.aafp.org/afp/20010601/2201.html

Text Sources
Alpert JS, Figer MA: Aortic stenosis and regurgitation. In: Cardiology for the Primary Care Physician, 4th ed. New York, Springer, 2005.

Carroll RG: Elsevier's Integrated Physiology. Philadelphia, Elsevier, 2007.

Copstead L, Banasik J: Pathophysiology, 3rd ed. Philadelphia, Saunders, 2005.

Goldman L, Ausiello D: Cecil Medicine, 23rd ed. Philadelphia, Saunders, 2007.

Guyton AC, Hall JE: Textbook of Medical Physiology, 11th ed. Philadelphia, Saunders, 2006.

McPhee SJ, Papadakis MA, Tierney LM Jr: Current Medical Diagnosis and Treatment, 46th ed. New York, McGraw-Hill, 2007.

CASE

13

A 22-year-old female college student comes to the university clinic complaining of palpitations.

The patient has had occasional incidences of rapid heart rates but never lasting for more than 2 minutes. In this instance, the heart rate has been elevated for 15 minutes. The patient has only been sleeping 4 hours a night while studying for examinations and is consuming "more than the usual amount" of coffee to help her remain alert. Her father died of a heart attack 3 years ago at the age of 55.

PHYSICAL EXAMINATION

VS: T 37°C, P 180/min, R 22/min and shallow, BP 95/80 mm Hg

PE: Patient is anxious. Pulse is extremely rapid and regular. No murmurs are present, and the lungs are clear.

LABORATORY STUDIES

ECG: Ventricular tachycardia, characterized by narrow QRS complexes at a rate of 180/min. Atrial P waves are also present at a rate of 180/min, but the QRS complexes precede the P wave.

DIAGNOSIS

Paroxysmal supraventricular tachycardia

PATHOPHYSIOLOGY OF KEY SYMPTOMS

Cardiac depolarization normally begins in the sino-atrial (SA) node, passes through the atria to the atrio-ventricular (AV) node, and, after a delay, enters the ventricle through the common bundle of His and proceeds through the bundle branches and Purkinje fibers, ultimately reaching the ventricular muscle cells. The AV node is characterized by a slow conduction rate. A slow conduction through the AV node normally allows the atria to finish their contraction before the ventricles begin their period of contraction.

The electrocardiogram provides a record of the flow of current that accompanies depolarization of the heart. The normal electrocardiogram consists of a P wave, representing atrial depolarization, a QRS complex representing ventricular depolarization, and a T wave representing ventricular repolarization. This sequence is termed "normal sinus rhythm." Spread of the depolarization through the AV node is contained within the PR interval (Fig. 13-1).

Paroxysmal super ventricular tachycardia occurs when the origin of the tachycardia is in the atria or the AV node ("above" the ventricles, or "supraventricular"). One possibility is the occurrence of a reentry loop of depolarization within the AV node (AV nodal reentrant tachycardia). In this instance, a wave of depolarization originating in the atria is split within the node and a portion flows retrogradely in the node until it encounters tissue outside its refractory period. The circuit then becomes self-propagating (Fig. 13-2).

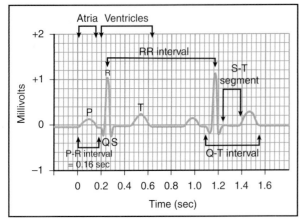

FIGURE 13–1 Normal electrocardiogram.

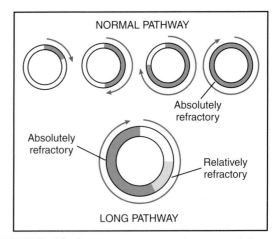

FIGURE 13–2 Circus movement, showing annihilation of the impulse in the short pathway and continued propagation of the impulse in the long pathway.

Because the electrical impulse arises within the AV node it spreads through the ventricles following the normal conducting pathway. Consequently, the QRS complexes appear normal. In contrast, the tachycardia of ventricular origin would be due to an ectopic pacemaker developing within the ventricles and likely be characterized by an abnormally wide QRS complex. The origin of the electrical impulse within the AV node, rather than the SA node, alters the relationship between the P wave and the QRS complex. For this patient, the ventricles have completely depolarized before the wave of depolarization retrogradely excites the atria. Consequently, the QRS complex precedes the P wave in the electrocardiogram.

The severe tachycardia can diminish the duration of the cardiac diastole. The short diastolic interval may not allow for sufficient ventricular filling (for heart rates > 200 beats/min), and, consequently, cardiac output decreases in spite of the rapid heart rate. The low cardiac output contributes to the drop in aortic pressure, while the diminished stroke volume and elevated heart rate both cause the arterial pulse pressure to be narrowed. For this patient, a heart rate of 180 beats/min is not sufficient to cause hypotension and syncope.

Thus, the only presenting complaint is "palpitations" and anxiety from being aware of the rapid heart rate.

Abnormal cardiac electrical activity is increased by smoking, caffeine ingestion, sleep deprivation, and anxiety.

Therapeutic intervention is centered on disrupting the self-propagating electrical circuit. Agents that decrease conduction velocity through the AV node, such as beta-adrenergic blocking drugs or calcium channel blockers, can slow the spread of depolarization and disrupt the circuit. Alternatively, vagal stimulation caused by pressure on the eyeball or massage of the carotid sinus baroreceptors can also be used to slow the spread of depolarization.

OUTCOME

The area of carotid arteries near the bifurcation is massaged, stimulating the stretch receptors in the carotid sinus. The increase in vagal activity slows the conduction in the atrioventricular node, breaking the abnormal conduction circuit. Heart rate reverts to a normal sinus rhythm of 72 beats/min.

FURTHER READING

Web Sources
Haro LH, Hess EP, Whatt WW: Arrhythmias in the office. Med Clin North Am 90(3), 2006. Available at http://www.mdconsult.com .jproxy.lib.ecu.edu/das/article/body/80268304-3/jorg=clinics& source=MI&sp=16010415&sid=635600823/N/521377/1.html

Kadish A, Passman R: Mechanisms and management of paroxysmal supraventricular tachycardia. Cardiol Rev 7:254-264, 1999. Available at http://gateway.tx.ovid.com.jproxy.lib.ecu.edu/gw1/ovidweb.cgi

Text Sources
Braunwald E, Zipes DP, Libby P: Heart Disease, A Textbook of Cardiovascular Medicine, 6th ed. Philadelphia, Saunders, 2001.

Carroll RG: Elsevier's Integrated Physiology. Philadelphia, Elsevier, 2007.

Copstead L, Banasik J: Pathophysiology, 3rd ed. Philadelphia, Saunders, 2005.

Guyton AC, Hall JE: Textbook of Medical Physiology, 11th ed. Philadelphia, Saunders, 2006.

McPhee SJ, Papadakis MA, Tierney LM Jr: Current Medical Diagnosis and Treatment, 46th ed. New York, McGraw-Hill, 2007.

A 45-year-old man presents at the clinic after having a reading of elevated blood pressure at a health department screening. His blood pressure is 160/110 and is equal in both arms and legs. He has no other health concerns.

He is alert and cooperative but appears to be anxious. The patient reports being a social drinker and smokes 1½ packs of cigarettes a day. He indicates that he is too busy to exercise. There is a family history of heart disease but no family history of diabetes.

PHYSICAL EXAMINATION

VS: T 37°C, P 80/min, R 15/min, BP 165/110 mm Hg
PE: BMI 32

LABORATORY STUDIES

SMA-12: All within normal ranges
ECG: Left axis deviation

DIAGNOSIS

Essential hypertension

PATHOPHYSIOLOGY OF KEY SYMPTOMS

Arterial blood pressure is determined by the volume of blood in the arterial system and the arterial compliance. Volume of blood in the arteries reflects the inflow from the cardiac output and the outflow, determined by total peripheral resistance (see Fig. II-2)

Hypertension has few, if any, symptoms. It is only when systolic blood pressure is in the range of 200 mm Hg that symptoms of headache, nausea, and dizziness become apparent. Most instances of hypertension are discovered at screenings or when the patient is at the health care provider for unrelated problems.

There are numerous endocrine problems that are characterized by intermittent or persistent hypertension. These include pheochromocytoma, excessive aldosterone production, and excessive angiotensin II production. These hormone levels can be measured to rule out secondary causes of the hypertension.

Acute alterations in arterial blood pressure are buffered by the arterial baroreceptor reflex. When blood pressure in the carotid sinus or aortic arch falls there is a reflex activation of the sympathetic nervous system and inhibition of the parasympathetic nervous system. The resultant increases in heart rate, ventricular contractility, arteriolar constriction, and venous constriction all act to restore blood pressure back toward normal (Fig. 14-1).

Persistent hypertension, however, is tied more closely to renal regulation of circulating blood volume. The arterial baroreceptors adapt over time, resetting to the new blood pressure level. Blood volume regulation by the kidneys does not show that adaptation and, consequently, is the dominant long-term regulator of arterial blood pressure.

The patient shows signs of anxiety, which causes an increase in sympathetic activity. A diagnosis of hypertension is confirmed after separate determinations of an elevated blood pressure. Anxiety can be a confounding factor, as the increase in sympathetic nervous system activity can cause an acute increase in blood pressure. Consequently, a determination of hypertension is made only after three separate readings of an elevated blood pressure. The need for an accurate diagnosis must be balanced against the potential risk to the patient. If left untreated for 3 months, there is a twofold increase in cardiovascular morbidity and mortality in high-risk hypertensive patients.

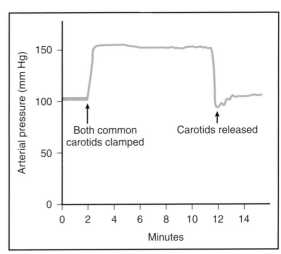

FIGURE 14–1 Typical carotid sinus reflex effect on aortic arterial pressure caused by clamping both common carotids (after the two vagus nerves have been cut).

Essential hypertension is a diagnosis of exclusion. Physical examination and diagnostic testing rule out secondary causes of hypertension, because the treatment options need to be directed against the underlying cause for the elevated blood pressure.

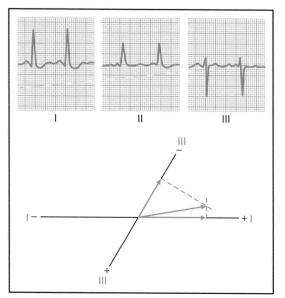

FIGURE 14–2 Left axis deviation in a hypertensive heart (hypertrophic left ventricle). Note the slightly prolonged QRS complex as well.

Chronic hypertension results in a hypertrophy of the left ventricle. This hypertrophy can be evident on cardiac imaging or can be manifested by a left axis deviation of the electrocardiogram. The ventricular hypertrophy results from the increased work load imposed on the left ventricle due to the elevated afterload (arterial pressure). This ventricular remodeling occurs only after many months of persistent hypertension (Fig. 14-2).

Blood volume regulation is tied to the renal processes of pressure natriuresis and pressure diuresis. Any time arterial blood pressure changes from the renal set point, the renal excretion of water and sodium is adjusted to help bring blood pressure back to normal. The treatment of hypertension with diuretics helps to artificially lower circulating blood volume and therefore lower blood pressure (Fig. 14-3).

Angiotensin II and dietary sodium intake also play an important role in the renal regulation of blood pressure. Angiotensin II, by direct vascular actions and through renal actions, increases blood pressure. Inhibition of angiotensin I converting enzyme leads to a decrease in angiotensin II levels and a decrease in blood pressure. Diminishing sodium intake has a somewhat smaller blood pressure–lowering effect but can augment the effectiveness of the angiotensin-converting enzyme inhibition and the diuretic (Fig. 14-4).

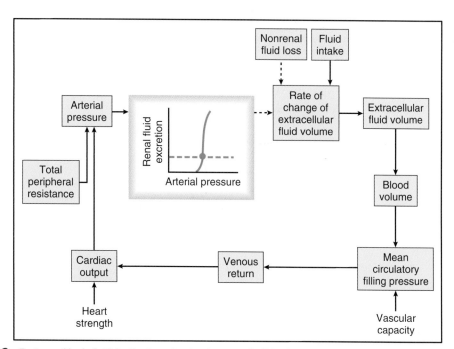

FIGURE 14–3 Basic renal body fluid feedback mechanism for control of blood volume, extracellular fluid volume, and arterial pressure. *Solid lines* indicate positive effects, and *dashed lines* indicate negative effects.

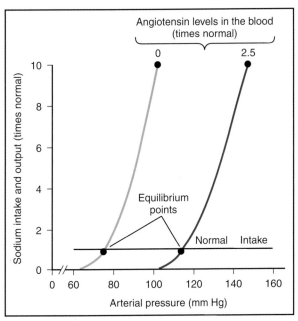

FIGURE 14–4 Effect of two angiotensin II levels in the blood on the renal output curve, showing regulation of the arterial pressure at an equilibrium points of 75 mm Hg when the angiotensin II level is low and at 115 mm Hg when the angiotensin level is high.

Hypertension is managed by the medication, not cured. If the patient stops taking the medication, the blood pressure will likely revert back to the hypertensive levels.

The patient has some risk factors for the development of hypertension. These include obesity, lack of exercise, a diet high in sodium, stress, smoking and alcohol consumption.

OUTCOME

The patient begins treatment with an angiotensin I converting enzyme (ACE) inhibitor and a thiazide diuretic and begins a low-salt diet. The patient should be encouraged to stop smoking and to incorporate exercise into his daily routine. When he returns to the clinic 1 month later for follow-up, he has lost 5 lb and has a blood pressure of 130/85 mm Hg. Both thiazide treatment and sodium restriction are continued.

FURTHER READING

Web Sources

Essential hypertension. Medline Plus Medical Encyclopedia. National Library of Medicine, 6/4/2007. Available at http://www.nlm.nih.gov/medlineplus/ency/article/000153.htm

Primary prevention of essential hypertension. Med Clin North Am 88(1), 2004. Available at http://www.mdconsult.com.jproxy.lib.ecu.edu/das/article/body/80142229-3/jorg=clinics&;source=MI&sp=14306113&sid=634838464/N/399282/1.html

Text Sources

Carroll RG: Elsevier's Integrated Physiology. Philadelphia, Elsevier, 2007.

Copstead L, Banasik J: Pathophysiology, 3rd ed. Philadelphia, Saunders, 2005.

Guyton AC, Hall JE: Textbook of Medical Physiology, 11th ed. Philadelphia, Saunders, 2006.

LeBlond RF, DeGowin RL, Brown DD: DeGowin's Diagnostic Examination, 8th ed. New York, McGraw-Hill, 2004.

McPhee SJ, Papadakis MA, Tierney LM Jr: Current Medical Diagnosis and Treatment, 46th ed. New York, McGraw-Hill, 2007.

A 66-year-old woman presents to the emergency department complaining of shortness of breath and chest pain that extends to her neck.

The patient has had difficulty sleeping for the past few nights and reports being more tired than usual. She is a retired office worker who smokes (1 pack/day) and drinks socially. Her body mass index (BMI) is 33, and she had been taking captopril, an angiotensin I converting enzyme (ACE) inhibitor to control her blood pressure. She ran out of captopril 2 weeks ago and has not refilled the prescription.

PHYSICAL EXAMINATION

VS: T 37°C, P 88/min, R 23/min, BP 150/105 mm Hg
PE: The patient is pale and diaphoretic. Neurologic examination is normal, but the patient is anxious.

LABORATORY STUDIES

ECG: Wide Q wave in leads I and aVL; ST segment elevation in leads I, aVL, and V_{2-5}
Blood tests (CBC, chem panel, cardiac markers): Elevated troponin and CK-MB
Lipid panel: Cholesterol high, HDL low, LDL high

DIAGNOSIS

Coronary artery disease

COURSE

Electrocardiographic findings and patient symptoms are consistent with a recent anteroapical infarction. Cardiac catheterization showed atherosclerosis in all major vessels with a 99% occlusion of the left anterior descending coronary artery. A stent was successfully inserted, and the patient was transferred to the coronary care unit.

PATHOPHYSIOLOGY OF KEY SYMPTOMS

Myocardial infarction results from interruption of blood flow through the coronary blood vessels. About 95% of the oxygen contained in the arterial blood is extracted as blood flows through the coronary circulation. Therefore, any increase in myocardial metabolism must be balanced by an equivalent increase in coronary blood flow and oxygen delivery.

Ischemia results when oxygen delivery is no longer adequate to meet myocardial oxygen demand, and an infarction occurs when blood flow is reduced so that myocardial function is impaired. One common cause of myocardial infarction is the development of a clot or thrombus at the site of an atherosclerotic plaque. The atherosclerotic plaque extends into the lumen of the coronary arteries, causing a partial occlusion. A thrombus formed at the side of the plaque can abruptly occlude the blood vessel, creating an area of infarcted tissue downstream from the occlusion.

Myocardial infarction causes a referred pain that often presents as a crushing pain in the chest that radiates to the left arm. However, many patients, particularly women, experience a less prominent set of symptoms. Symptoms in women may include a burning sensation in the upper abdomen, lightheadedness, and upset stomach or a sudden weakness or unexplained tiredness. This patient also shows many risk factors for coronary artery disease, including smoking, elevated cholesterol, high BMI, and hypertension.

The pain and other symptoms cause a pronounced activation of the sympathetic nervous system. The presenting appearance of elevated blood pressure, elevated heart rate, elevated respiratory rate, and diaphoresis all reflect the actions of the sympathetic nerves.

The initial treatment of a suspected myocardial infarction is to help restore adequate oxygen delivery to the damaged area of the heart. This requires

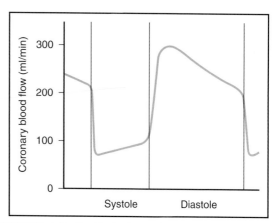

FIGURE 15–1 Phasic flow of blood through the coronary capillaries of the human left ventricle during cardiac systole and diastole (as extrapolated from measured flows in dogs).

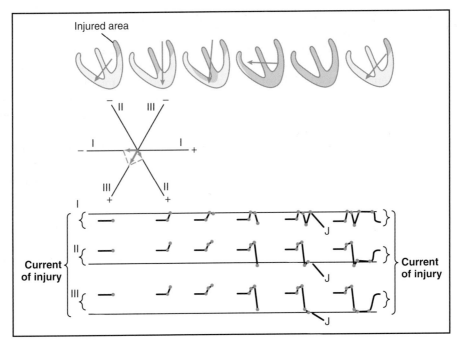

FIGURE 15–2 Effect of a current of injury on the electrocardiogram.

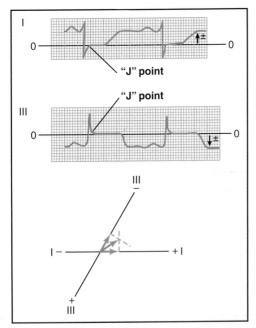

FIGURE 15–3 J point as the zero reference potential of the electrocardiograms for leads I and II. Also, the method for plotting the axis of the injury potential is shown by the lowermost panel.

adequate oxygenation, adequate blood flow, and diminished metabolic need.

Supplemental oxygen ensures that the arterial blood is well oxygenated. Nitroglycerin acts to increase nitric oxide formation, and nitric oxide is a potent vasodilator in the circulation. Aspirin or some other cyclooxygenase inhibitor is used to diminish the formation of platelet plugs, which can occlude vascular segments. If a thrombus is suspected, a clot-dissolving compound such as tissue plasminogen activator (tPA) can also be administered. Early (within 1 hour) restoration of coronary blood flow greatly limits the damage and increases the chance of recovery.

Morphine is useful for pain relief and is particularly important because pain increases sympathetic nervous system (SNS) activity, exacerbating the progression of myocardial damage through multiple pathways. SNS activation increases arterial blood pressure and thus increases the workload on the left ventricle. The majority of blood flow to the left ventricle occurs during diastole, and the SNS-mediated increase in heart rate diminishes diastolic duration and impairs blood flow particularly to the left ventricle. SNS activation also increases ventricular contractility and, therefore, ventricular work load (Fig. 15-1).

Damage to the myocardium results in the plasma appearance of enzymes that are normally contained within the myocardial cells. Troponin appears in the plasma soon after damage and is an early indicator of an infarction. Creatinine kinase is an enzyme normally in all muscle cells, and the isoenzyme form characteristic of myocardium is termed CK-MB, the creatinine kinase-myocardial band. CK-MB normally first appears in the plasma about 4 hours after injury and increases progressively, reaching a peak at 24 hours after injury.

The presence of an infarction is confirmed by the ECG and the elevated troponin and CK-MB. Ischemic and infracted areas of the heart do not repolarize, and, consequently, a current of injury is apparent as a "shift" in the ST segment (Figs. 15-2 and 15-3). The appearance of the ST segment shift in leads I, aVL, and V_{2-5} places the damaged area in the anteroapical portion of the left ventricle.

OUTCOME

Atherosclerotic plaques are difficult to treat. The most common process is to isolate them from the blood, either by placing a stent inside of the vessel or by removing the vessel and replacing it with another (often a vein) through coronary artery bypass graft surgery.

Pharmacologic management is centered on (1) anticoagulant therapy to reduce the chance of additional platelet plug or clot formation and (2) reduction of myocardial work load by reduction in arterial pressure.

The patient is immediately treated with morphine, nitroglycerin, and aspirin and placed on supplemental oxygen. Pulse oximetry shows O_2 saturation of 95%.

FURTHER READING

Web Source
http://www.med.umich.edu/1libr/wha/wha_myoinf_car.htm

Text Sources
Carroll RG: Elsevier's Integrated Physiology. Philadelphia, Elsevier, 2007.

Copstead L, Banasik J: Pathophysiology, 3rd ed. Philadelphia, Saunders, 2005.
Guyton AC, Hall JE: Textbook of Medical Physiology, 11th ed. Philadelphia, Saunders, 2006.
McPhee SJ, Papadakis MA, Tierney LM Jr: Current Medical Diagnosis and Treatment, 46th ed. New York, McGraw-Hill, 2007.

A 67-year-old man presents to his physician complaining of sharp cramps and pains in his legs while exercising. He states that the pain is relieved by rest but begins again when he continues exercising.

The patient was diagnosed with hypertension 25 years ago and smoked cigarettes (two packs/day) up until 10 years ago. He was also diagnosed with type 2 diabetes 10 years ago. At the request of his physician and wife, he has been trying to incorporate more exercise into his daily regimen. The cramping is occurring in the calf area and occurs at any exercise intensity greater than walking at a moderate pace. There is a history of cardiovascular disease in both parents.

PHYSICAL EXAMINATION

VS: T 37°C, P 80/min, R 15/min, BP 165/100 mm Hg
PE: BMI 35; there is a slight ulceration of the skin on the lower left leg, and the toes on both feet show signs of cyanosis. The lower legs appear shiny and feel cool to the touch. Elevation of the calf causes the skin color to become pale.

LABORATORY STUDIES

Segmental blood pressure readings show a marked decrease in blood pressure when measured at the calf. Pulse volume readings are also reduced at the calf. The ankle-brachial index is 0.8 (normal: 0.95 to 1.20). Duplex ultrasound imaging shows an increased lumen blood flow velocity in both calves, indicating areas of stenosis. Contrast angiography reveals widespread arterial calcifications in the arteries below the knee.

DIAGNOSIS

Intermittent claudication

COURSE

Angioplasty of the lesions was performed, resulting in improved leg blood flow and restoring the ability to exercise.

PATHOPHYSIOLOGY OF KEY SYMPTOMS

Tissue blood flow is determined by the pressure gradient and the vascular resistance. The pressure gradient remains fairly constant, unless there is an abrupt decrease in arterial pressure. Vascular resistance,

however, is regulated by local metabolic control, sympathetic nerves, and circulating vasoactive hormones.

During exercise there has to be an increase in muscle blood flow to provide sufficient oxygen and other nutrients and to remove metabolic wastes. Exercise results in an increase in adenosine triphosphate (ATP) consumption, and replenishing the ATP stores requires increased oxygen delivery to the muscle (Fig. 16-1). Hypoxia is a powerful local vasodilator, and a decrease in vascular resistance results in an increase in blood flow to the exercising muscle. Metabolic wastes also serve as vasodilators, and metabolic control results in the autoregulation of tissue blood flow (Fig. 16-2).

At rest, only 25% of the capillaries in the skeletal muscle are perfused. During exercise, skeletal muscle blood flow can increase tenfold, both from perfusion of all of the capillaries in skeletal muscle bed as well as vasodilation of the arterioles in the precapillary sphincters.

The growth of atherosclerotic plaques results in a narrowing of the lumen of the arteries or a stenosis. The reduction in arterial diameter increases resistance

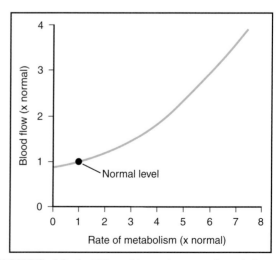

FIGURE 16–1 Effect of increasing rate of metabolism on tissue blood flow.

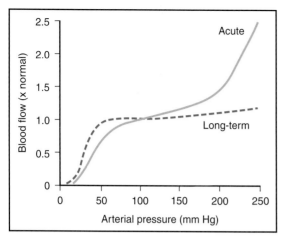

FIGURE 16–2 Effect of different levels of arterial pressure on blood flow through a muscle. The *solid red curve* shows the effect if the arterial pressure is raised over a period of a few minutes. The *dashed green curve* shows the effect if the arterial pressure is raised extremely slowly over a period of many weeks.

to blood flow. During this time, metabolic control dilates the vasculature downstream from the stenosis, and, consequently, blood flow is maintained. As an individual begins to exercise, however, the vasodilation from local metabolic control is already at a maximum and cannot contribute to any further vasodilation. In this case, blood flow cannot increase to match the increased metabolic demands caused by exercise. The resulting hypoxia and buildup of metabolites causes the muscle to cramp and to be painful.

The stenosis is impeding blood flow even at rest. The patient's symptoms of pale skin in the legs, cyanosis of the toes, and the ulceration are all evidence of insufficient vascular perfusion. Diagnostic testing reveals reduced blood pressure and pulse volume readings in the calves, which indicate a vascular blockage. The ankle-brachial index, calculated as the ankle blood pressure divided by the higher of the blood pressures in the two arms, confirms a significant vascular resistance in the larger arteries of the legs. Doppler ultrasonography reveals an increase in the velocity of blood flow in the region of the stenosis, and arteriography shows multiple sites where the atherosclerotic plaque is narrowing the lumen of the arteries and impeding blood flow.

This patient has numerous risk factors for the development of atherosclerotic plaques. This includes hypertension, type 2 diabetes, a past history of smoking, and his age.

OUTCOME

Angioplasty uses a catheter threaded through the lumen of the artery to dilate the artery and to remove the stenosis. Once the stenosis is removed, normal tissue perfusion is reestablished, as is the ability to appropriately increase blood flow during exercise.

FURTHER READING

Web Source
www.mayoclinic.com/health/peripheral-arterial-disease/DS00537

Text Sources
Carroll RG: Elsevier's Integrated Physiology. Philadelphia, Elsevier, 2007.

Copstead L, Banasik J: Pathophysiology, 3rd ed. Philadelphia, Saunders, 2005.

Guyton AC, Hall JE: Textbook of Medical Physiology, 11th ed. Philadelphia, Saunders, 2006.

Izquierdo-Porrera AM, Gardner AW, Powell CC, et al: Effects of exercise rehabilitation on cardiovascular risk factors in older patients with peripheral arterial occlusive disease. J Vasc Surg 31:670-677, 2000.

McDaniel MD, Cronenwett JL. Basic data related to the natural history of intermittent claudication. Ann Vasc Surg 3:273-327, 1989.

McPhee SJ, Papadakis MA, Tierney LM Jr: Current Medical Diagnosis and Treatment, 46th ed. New York, McGraw-Hill, 2007.

SECTION III

Nephrology and Electrolyte Balance

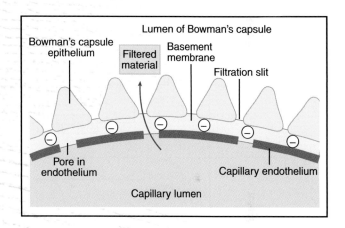

Bowman's capsule epithelium

Filtered material

Lumen of Bowman's capsule

Basement membrane

Filtration slit

Pore in endothelium

Capillary endothelium

Capillary lumen

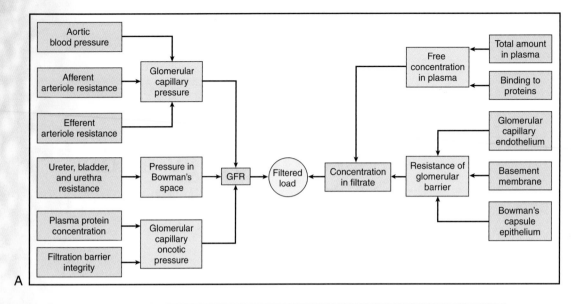

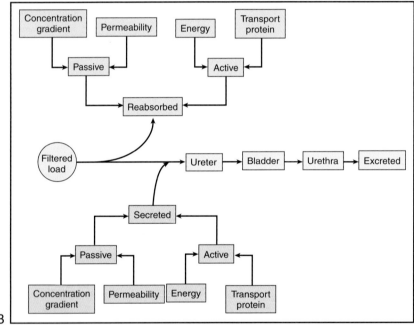

FIGURE III–1 The renal physiology map illustrates major renal processes. Conceptually, renal processes can be split into those creating the filtered load at the renal glomerulus and those modifying the filtered load as it passes through the renal tubule system.

The major function of the kidney is the production of the physiologically appropriate volume and composition of urine. The initial step in urine formation is the formation of an ultrafiltrate of plasma in the renal glomerular capillaries. The ultrafiltrate passes through a series of histologically and functionally distinct renal tubules. The renal tubules are lined by epithelial cells, and the glomerular ultrafiltrate is modified by transport across the epithelium. Filtrate then exits the renal collecting duct as the final urine, because the epithelial lining of the ureter, bladder, and urethra does not have transport capabilities (Fig. III-1).

Fluid and electrolyte balance in the body is achieved by regulating gain (ingestion and production) against loss (excretion or consumption) (see Case 24). Complex regulatory systems allow the independent control of urinary output of water, sodium, potassium, and calcium. For example, ingestion of 1 L of water leads

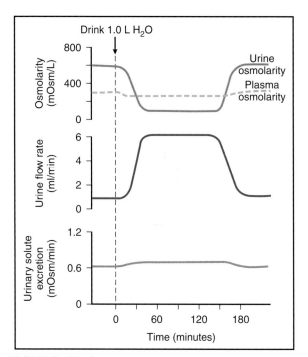

FIGURE III–2 Water diuresis in a human after ingestion of 1 liter of water. Note that after water ingestion, urine volume increases and urine osmolarity decreases, causing the excretion of a large volume of dilute urine; however, the total amount of solute excreted by the kidneys remains relatively constant. These responses of the kidneys prevent plasma osmolarity from decreasing markedly during excess water ingestion.

to a large increase in urine production and a large drop in urine osmolarity with minimal changes in urinary solute excretion (Fig. III-2).

Renal pathophysiologies can loosely be grouped as extrarenal, glomerular, tubular, or urinary. Extrarenal events that alter renal function include severe hypotension or alterations in the production of the regulatory hormones antidiuretic hormone (ADH), aldosterone, and parathyroid hormone. Glomerular disturbances include those that alter the glomerular capillary pressure (see Cases 17 and 18), glomerular capillary protein content, or the integrity of the filtration barrier that separates the glomerular capillaries from Bowman's space (see Case 20). Tubular disturbances include disorders of specific transport proteins, disorders of the hormones regulating transport (see Case 21), or damage to the integrity of the tubule cells (see Case 22). Urinary disorders include the obstruction of the ureters or urethra (see Case 19), as well as impairment of the micturition reflex or bladder function (see Case 23).

The kidneys also serve other important functions, such as the production of the hormone erythropoietin and the conversion of amino acids into glucose through gluconeogenesis. The kidneys synthesize renin, an enzyme that catalyzes the initial step leading to the formation of angiotensin II.

A 60-year-old woman being treated for hypertension returns to her physician's office for treatment.

The patient is a smoker (45 packs/year) and social drinker and walks for exercise three times per week. She reports that her calves begin to ache 15 minutes after exercise but the pain quickly resolves when exercise stops. Past radiologic studies identified cholelithiasis, which was treated by laparoscopic surgery. Radiologic findings included an abnormal finding of an asymmetric right kidney.

PHYSICAL EXAMINATION

VS: T 37.2°C, P 70/min, R 20/min, BP 180/120 mm Hg, weight 135 lb, BMI 22

PE: Patient does not exhibit distress. She has a raspy voice due to smoking. During physical examination, the aorta is palpated superior to the navel. The patient has abnormalities of the optic fundi showing hypertensive retinopathy. She has been treated in the past for hypertension and is currently experiencing intolerance to her angiotensin I converting enzyme (ACE) inhibitor.

LABORATORY STUDIES

Abdominal ultrasound: No abdominal aortic aneurysm

Renal artery ultrasonography: Decreased size of the left kidney, increase in blood flow velocity at the left proximal renal artery, and decreased blood flow through the left renal artery

Renal arteriography: Stenosis of the left renal artery

DIAGNOSIS

Renal artery stenosis

PATHOPHYSIOLOGY OF KEY SYMPTOMS

The kidneys are a major determinant of arterial blood pressure through the regulation of body fluid volume. This regulation is evidenced by both pressure diuresis and pressure natriuresis, where a decrease in renal perfusion pressure results in the retention of both sodium and water (Fig. 17-1).

Glomerular capillary blood pressure is determined in part by the aortic pressure and by the preglomerular vascular resistance. The preglomerular vascular resistance is predominantly at the afferent arteriole; however, a constriction in any vessel between the heart and the glomerular capillaries is also characterized as a preglomerular vascular resistance.

A stenosis in the renal artery introduces a preglomerular vascular resistance and decreases glomerular capillary pressure. The decrease in glomerular capillary pressure results in the fall in glomerular filtration rate and the shift toward retention of sodium and water. Retention of water and sodium causes an increase in systemic arterial blood pressure; and as soon as the blood pressure is sufficiently high, glomerular capillary pressure returns to normal. In this instance, sodium and water are in balance but only because the patient is hypertensive. For example, aortic stenosis above the origin of the renal arteries will result in hypertension but aortic stenosis below the origin of the renal arteries will not cause hypertension (Fig. 17-2).

Renal ultrasound confirmed the left artery stenosis. The narrowed renal artery lumen at the site of the stenosis causes a large increase in velocity of blood flow in that region and pressure waveforms in the renal artery, both evident on the Doppler ultrasound. This increase in velocity leads to turbulent flow, and a bruit can often be heard over the affected kidney with a stethoscope.

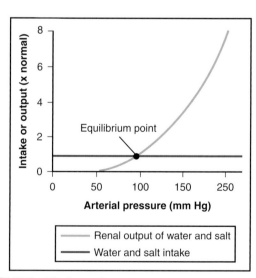

FIGURE 17–1 Analysis of arterial pressure regulation by equating the "renal output curve" with the "salt and water intake curve." The equilibrium point describes the level to which the arterial pressure will be regulated.

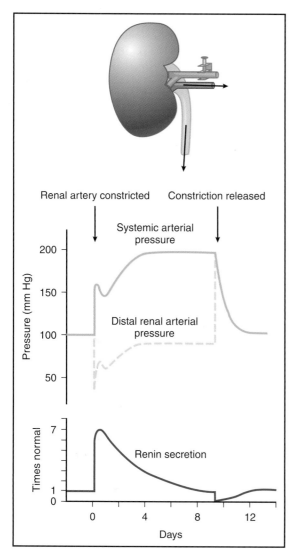

FIGURE 17–2 Effect of placing a constricting clamp on the renal artery of one kidney after the other kidney has been removed. Note the changes in systemic arterial pressure, renal artery pressure distal to the clamp, and rate of renin secretion. The resulting hypertension is called "one-kidney" Goldblatt hypertension.

The left kidney is more commonly affected than is the right kidney. The reason for the more common left kidney involvement may be due to both structural and functional differences between the two kidneys. There is a large reserve in renal function, and total body renal function may be normal. Therefore, it is important to study the function of each kidney separately when underlying renal disease is suspected.

Renal artery constriction also limits blood flow to the kidney and can result in a failure of the kidney to grow and develop normally in children. Adults with significant renal artery stenosis often exhibit an asymmetric or smaller than normal kidney.

Hypertension caused by renal artery stenosis is often refractory to treatment. This is because the underlying defect persists and any successful treatment of systemic hypertension results in a lower renal perfusion (glomerular capillary) pressure and shifts the renal fluid balance into retention of sodium and water.

OUTCOME

Renal artery stenosis occurs in 1% to 2% of hypertensive patients. If sufficiently severe, renal artery stenosis can be surgically corrected or angiography and stent placement can be used to remove the constriction. Successful surgical correction of the renal artery stenosis should also correct the hypertension. If untreated, a progressive stenosis can result in unilateral renal failure. The loss of one kidney, however, is not life threatening, because the remaining kidney undergoes a compensatory hypertrophy to restore renal function back toward "normal."

Balloon angioplasty was used to reestablish normal vessel diameter. There was a 48-hour period of diuresis and natriuresis, with a return of arterial blood pressure back to the normal range.

FURTHER READING

Web Sources
Tentori F: Focus on hypertension. J Nephrol 20:135-140, 2007. Available at http://www.mdconsult.com/das/citation/body/81726043-8/jorg=journal&source=MI&sp=19679170&sid=643753876/N/19679170/1.html
VanOnna M, Houbens J, Kroon A, et al: Asymmetry of renal blood flow in patients with moderate to severe hypertension. Am Heart Assoc J 41:108, 2003. Available at http://hyper.ahajournals.org/cgi/content/full/41/1/108

Text Sources
Carroll RG: Elsevier's Integrated Physiology. Philadelphia, Elsevier, 2007.
Copstead L, Banasik J: Pathophysiology, 3rd ed. Philadelphia, Saunders, 2005.
Guyton AC, Hall JE: Textbook of Medical Physiology, 11th ed. Philadelphia, Saunders, 2006.
Kasper DL: Harrison's Principles of Internal Medicine, 16th ed. New York, McGraw-Hill, 2005, vol II.
McPhee SJ, Papadakis MA, Tierney LM Jr: Current Medical Diagnosis and Treatment, 46th ed. New York, McGraw-Hill, 2007.

C A S E
18

A 40-year-old male comes to his primary care physician complaining of blurred vision and a headache.

The patient has a 6-year history of hypertension and hyperlipidemia. The hypertension has been poorly controlled because of noncompliance. The patient works in a manufacturing plant and has smoked 1 pack of cigarettes per day for the past 20 years.

PHYSICAL EXAMINATION

VS: T 37°C, P 68/min, R 22/min, BP 210/150 mm Hg and the same in all four extremities, BMI 28

PE: The patient is anxious and complains of an inability to concentrate because of the headaches. He does not remember urinating during the past day and is unable to provide a urine sample for analysis. A presystolic murmur (fourth heart sound) is evident. Funduscopic examination shows swelling of the optic nerve in both eyes (papilledema).

LABORATORY STUDIES

SMA-12: BUN 160 mg/dL (normal: 7-20 mg/dL); Creatinine: 8.2 mg/dL (normal: 0.8 to 1.4 mg/dL)

Blood gas analysis: Po_2 90 mm Hg, Pco_2 33 mm Hg, HCO_3^- 12 mEq, pH 7.30

Plasma renin activity: 25 ng/mL/hr (normal: 1.9 to 3.7 ng/mL/hr)

ECG: Normal sinus rhythm, left axis deviation, no shift in ST segment

Cardiac enzymes (myosin, CK-MB): Normal

DIAGNOSIS

Malignant hypertension

PATHOPHYSIOLOGY OF KEY SYMPTOMS

The kidneys provide chronic regulation of blood pressure through the processes of pressure diuresis and pressure natriuresis. Normally, hypertension produces few if any symptoms. Malignant hypertension is an example of a hypertensive emergency in which the elevated blood pressure is life threatening.

The presenting symptoms of blurred vision and headache are caused by cerebral edema. The abnormally large arterial pressure exceeds the autoregulatory range of the cerebral circulation and results in an increase in cerebral capillary pressure. Increasing capillary pressure causes a net filtration of plasma into the central nervous system (CNS), resulting in cerebral edema. Increased pressure within the cranial vault causes neurologic impairment and papilledema, a bulging of the optic nerve that is visible through a funduscope.

Malignant hypertension causes target organ damage, particularly to the kidney. The patient is likely in renal failure, indicated by the elevation in blood urea nitrogen and creatinine, the lack of urine production, and the metabolic acidosis. Metabolic acidosis is characterized by an acidic pH, a decrease in plasma HCO_3^- levels, and a compensatory decrease in Pco_2. The kidneys normally excrete slightly acidic urine, and, consequently, impaired renal function usually leads to a metabolic acidosis (Fig. 18-1).

In this patient there is not yet any damage to the myocardium, as indicated by the normal cardiac enzymes and the lack of an ST segment shift. The left axis deviation in the electrocardiogram is consistent with the poorly controlled hypertension, because the left ventricle will hypertrophy to produce a sufficient cardiac output.

Plasma renin activity is increased in this patient, indicating increased angiotensin II production. In malignant hypertension, angiotensin II is not the cause of the hypertension but rather results from the decrease in glomerular filtration rate (GFR). Attempted treatment of malignant hypertension with angiotensin I converting enzyme (ACE) inhibitors can cause complete renal failure because of the loss of efferent arteriole constriction (Fig. 18-2).

Therapy is directed at a gradual lowering of blood pressure, usually using a vasodilator such as nitroprusside. The hypertension is supported by significant increase in total peripheral resistance. If blood pressure is lowered too quickly, tissue blood flow may be compromised, leading to central nervous system, coronary, or renal ischemia.

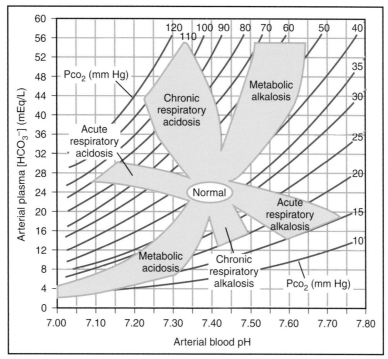

FIGURE 18–1 Acid-base nomogram showing arterial blood pH, arterial plasma HCO₃⁻, and Pco₂ values. The *central open circle* shows the approximate limits for acid-base status in normal people. The *shaded areas* show the approximate limits for the normal compensations caused by simple metabolic and respiratory disorders. For values lying outside the shaded areas, one should suspect a mixed acid-base disorder. (*Adapted from Cogan MG, Rector FC Jr: Acid-Base Disorders in the Kidney, 3rd ed. Philadelphia, WB Saunders, 1986.*)

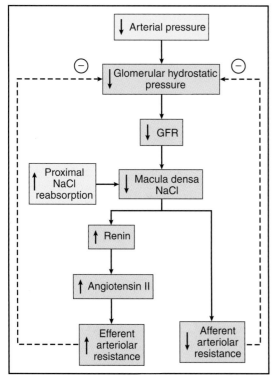

FIGURE 18–2 Macula densa feedback mechanism for autoregulation of glomerular hydrostatic pressure and glomerular filtration rate (GFR) during decreased renal arterial pressure.

OUTCOME

Arterial and venous catheters are inserted on the right arm, and 0.9% saline is administered. The patient is admitted to the intensive care unit for continuous cardiac monitoring and frequent assessment of neurologic status and urine output. Sodium nitroprusside is used to gradually reduce blood pressure over the first 48 hours. The patient was discharged 2 weeks later.

FURTHER READING

Web Sources

Bosignano JD, Orsini AN: Malignant hypertension. Accessed October 2006. Available at http://www.emedicine.com/med/topic1107.htm

Kaplan NM, Rose BD: Hypertensive emergencies. Accessed April 2007. Available at http://63.240.11.74/topic.asp?file=hyperten/15683

Text Sources

Carroll RG: Elsevier's Integrated Physiology. Philadelphia, Elsevier, 2007.

Copstead L, Banasik J: Pathophysiology, 3rd ed. Philadelphia, Saunders, 2005.

Gavras H, Brunner HR, Laragh JH, et al: Malignant hypertension resulting from deoxycorticosterone acetate and salt excess: role of renin and sodium vascular change. Circ Res 36:300-309, 1975.

Guyton AC, Hall JE: Textbook of Medical Physiology, 11th ed. Philadelphia, Saunders, 2006.

Kitiyakara C, Guzman NJ: Malignant hypertension and hypertensive emergencies. J Am Soc Nephrol 9:133-142, 1998.

McCance K, Huether S: Pathophysiology: The Biological Basis for Disease in Adults & Children, 3rd ed. St. Louis, Mosby, 1998.

McPhee SJ, Papadakis MA, Tierney LM Jr: Current Medical Diagnosis and Treatment, 46th ed. New York, McGraw-Hill, 2007.

A 45-year-old man comes to the emergency department complaining of severe pain on his right flank.

There is no evidence of injury. The patient has been working in the yard all day and appears dehydrated. He is capable of providing a small volume of urine for analysis.

PHYSICAL EXAMINATION

VS: T 38°C, P 100/min, R 22/min, BP 130/100 mm Hg
PE: The patient describes the colicky pain that has a sudden onset. On examination, the pain is localized to the flank area, particularly with pressure. During the examination, the patient appears extremely restless and unable to find a comfortable position.

LABORATORY STUDIES

Urinalysis: Urine pH is 4.3 and osmolality is 1200 mOsm/L. Abnormal findings include microscopic hematuria (red blood cells) and small calcium oxalate crystals (kidney stones).
Noncontrast spiral CT scan: Stone in the right kidney

DIAGNOSIS

Kidney stones

COURSE

The patient received 1 L of 0.45% saline and additional water to drink. He was given ketorolac for pain management. He was sent home with instructions to drink lots of fluids until the kidney stone passes and to take Vicodin as needed for pain. He is to pass urine through a strainer and bring in any excreted stones to be sent to the pathology laboratory.

PATHOPHYSIOLOGY OF KEY SYMPTOMS

Fluid balance within the body requires adjusting accumulation, through ingestion and metabolism, against elimination in the urine, feces, breath, skin, and sweat. Excessive sweating in the absence of additional water ingestion results in dehydration, characterized by a decrease in both the extracellular and cell water stores (Fig. 19-1).

Although sweat does contain NaCl, sweat is hypotonic compared with plasma. Consequently, excessive sweating results in an increase in osmolality in the body fluid compartments. The increase in osmolality stimulates the release of antidiuretic hormone (ADH, vasopressin) from the posterior pituitary. ADH increases the permeability of the distal tubule and collecting duct to water and urea and results in the production of a very small volume of highly concentrated urine. In this patient, the urine osmolality of 1200 mOsm/L is close to the maximum urine concentrating ability (Fig. 19-2).

One unintended consequence of the production of highly concentrated urine is the precipitation of salt

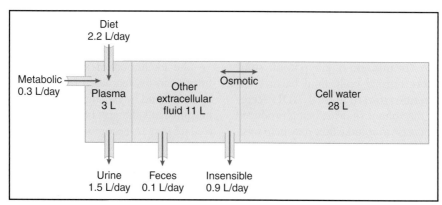

FIGURE 19–1 Body water balance requires the regulation of intake (thirst) and renal excretion to compensate for the unregulated loss of water through respiration and sweating.

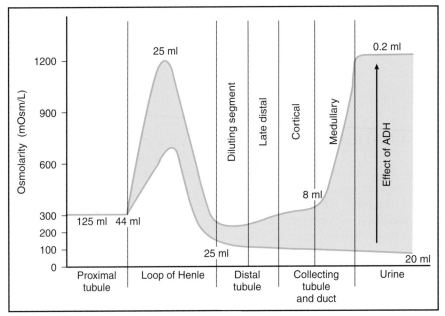

FIGURE 19–2 Changes in osmolarity of the tubular fluid as it passes through the different tubular segments in the presence of high levels of antidiuretic hormone (ADH) and in the absence of ADH. (Numerical values indicate the approximate volumes in milliliters per minute of fluid flowing along the different tubular segments.)

crystals in renal calyces. Uric acid crystals form the pH more acidic than 5.5, and these crystals then layer to form calcium oxalate stones. The pH more alkaline than 7.2 suggests a struvite stone.

Urine in the renal calyx passes successively through the ureter, bladder, and urethra before exiting the body. Urine movement through the ureter is accomplished by peristalsis of the smooth muscle of the ureter. Kidney stones can become lodged in the ureter, especially at the ureteropelvic junction, where the ureters cross the pelvic inlet, and at the ureterovesical junction. Lodging of kidney stones causes significant pain and possibly causes damage to the ureter. Damage to the endothelium of the urinary tract results in the appearance of a small number of red blood cells in the urine called microscopic hematuria. The associated pain likely underlies the elevation in blood pressure and heart rate shown by the patient.

Ingestion of water or infusion of a hypotonic solution can help restore normal body fluid balance. As plasma osmolality returns toward normal, ADH secretion is reduced and the volume of urine being produced will increase. The increase in volume flow may help wash the stone through the urinary tract and out of the body.

The severe pain characteristic of kidney stone presence is caused by distention, often of the ureter. While the stones are within the kidney they are usually, but not always, painless. Kidney stone formation in susceptible individuals is increased by dehydration.

OUTCOME

Initial treatment of kidney stones consists of fluid hydration, bed rest, and pain management. This will usually allow urinary excretion of small (<4 mm) stones and often excretion of stones from 4 to 7 mm diameter. Stones larger than 7 mm usually cannot pass through the urinary system. The average time for passage of a kidney stone is 7 to 21 days.

If this does not result in excretion of the kidney stones, options include (1) extracorporeal shockwave lithotripsy, in which the patient is immersed in water and exposed to shock waves, (2) retrieval of the stone using a ureteroscope advanced through the urethra and bladder, or (3) surgical removal via percutaneous nephrolithotomy or flank incision.

If the endothelium of the ureter is damaged, a stent may be inserted to protect the epithelium during repair.

The likelihood of kidney stone formation in the future can be decreased by having the patient remain hydrated and by having a diet containing citrate, magnesium, and dietary fiber. In addition, foods low in oxalate may be recommended.

The majority of cases of kidney stones spontaneously resolve with excretion of the stone.

FURTHER READING

Web Sources

Mushnick R. U.S. National Library of Medicine. Kidney stones. Accessed August 2007. Available at http://www.nlm.nih.gov/medlineplus/ency/article/000458.htm#Signs%20and%20tests

National Kidney and Urologic Diseases Information Clearing House. Accessed October 2007. Available at http://kidney.niddk.nih.gov/kudiseases/pubs/stonesadults/index.htm

Wein A, ed. Campbell-Walsh Urology, 9th ed. Philadelphia, Saunders, 2007. Available at http://www.mdconsult.com/about/book/79902754-9/instruct.html?DOCID=1445

Text Sources

Carroll RG: Elsevier's Integrated Physiology. Philadelphia, Elsevier, 2007.

Copstead L, Banasik J: Pathophysiology, 3rd ed. Philadelphia, Saunders, 2005.

Guyton AC, Hall JE: Textbook of Medical Physiology, 11th ed. Philadelphia, Saunders, 2006.

McPhee SJ, Papadakis MA, Tierney LM Jr: Current Medical Diagnosis and Treatment, 46th ed. New York, McGraw-Hill, 2007.

A 5-year-old boy presents to the urgent care clinic because his mother noticed that the child is not going to the bathroom and his feet are swollen.

Two weeks earlier the child was treated for strep throat with penicillin. The mother admits to ceasing administering the medication to the child after a couple of days because she thought the child was better.

PHYSICAL EXAMINATION

VS: T 37°C, P 78/min, R 15/min, BP 120/90 mm Hg
PE: The patient is oliguric and has a slight fluid accumulation in the lower extremities and periorbital region. There is palpable peripheral edema in both feet.

LABORATORY STUDIES

Urinalysis: Very dark urine, presence of red blood cells, red blood cell casts, and protein (>3 g/day)
Serum complement C3, C4, CH50 levels: Low
ASO titer: 250 Todd units/mL (normal: <160 units/mL)
Anti DNase-B level: >60 units
BUN: 32 mg/dL (normal: 7-18 mg/dL)
Creatinine: 2.0 mg/dL (normal: 0.6-1.2 mg/dL)

DIAGNOSIS

Poststreptococcal glomerulonephritis

PATHOPHYSIOLOGY OF KEY SYMPTOMS

The first step in urine formation is the ultrafiltration of plasma in the glomerular capillaries. Filtration across the glomerular capillaries depends on the balance of hydrostatic pressure (blood pressure) and colloid osmotic pressure (oncotic) pressure. Blood pressure within the glomerular capillaries is around 55 mm Hg, much higher than any other capillary bed in the body. This hydrostatic pressure is the major force driving filtration in the renal glomerulus. Albumin and other plasma proteins normally do not cross the glomerular barrier. Consequently, they provide an osmotic (oncotic) pressure in the capillary, a reabsorptive pressure that diminishes glomerular filtration. The net filtration pressure is about 10 mm Hg favoring filtration, accounting for glomerular capillary blood pressure, Bowman's capsule hydrostatic pressure, and the capillary oncotic pressure (Fig. 20-1).

The glomerular filtration barrier consists of the capillary endothelium and basal lamina (basement membrane) and the epithelium of Bowman's capsule. Plasma proteins have a net negative charge, and the negative charge on the proteins of the basement membrane is a significant impediment to the movement of proteins into Bowman's capsule. Plasma proteins exert an oncotic pressure because they cannot cross the glomerular barrier. Proteins are not a normal component of the urine, and their presence in the urine indicates damage to either the glomerular barrier or the endothelial cells lining the urinary tract (Fig. 20-2).

The streptococcus rods can become trapped in the glomerular basement membrane pores. Antibodies synthesized to combat the infection attach to the streptococci and initiate an immune response that damages the basement membrane. Consequently, proteins and red blood cells can now pass into Bowman's capsule and become lodged in the lumen of the tubules and occlude the lumen. Children have small glomerular basement membrane pores, and the streptococci can become more easily trapped in the basement membrane

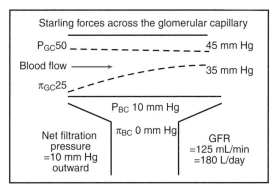

FIGURE 20–1 Hydrostatic and oncotic pressures determine filtration across the glomerular capillary (GC). Glomerular capillary filtration depends on the balance of the hydrostatic and the oncotic pressures. Hydrostatic pressure at the afferent end of the glomerular capillaries is high and decreases slightly along the length of the glomerular capillary. Plasma oncotic pressure in the glomerular capillary increases along the length of the glomerular capillary as plasma is filtered, but the large proteins remain within the capillary. The net balance of pressures ensures that only filtration occurs in the glomerular capillaries.

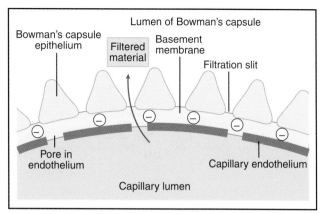

FIGURE 20–2   The glomerular filtration barrier impedes filtration of large proteins. Plasma in the glomerular capillaries must pass through the capillary endothelium, a basement membrane, and Bowman's capsule epithelium before it becomes glomerular filtrate. The negatively charged basement membrane impedes the movement of proteins into the glomerular filtrate.

of children. Poststreptococcal glomerulonephritis occurs more frequently in children, with a peak incidence between the ages of 5 and 15 years.

The patient's symptoms are characteristic of a nephritis. Damage to the tubule segments causes a reduction in glomerular filtration rate (GFR), indicated by the increase in blood urea nitrogen (BUN) and creatinine. Creatinine and the GFR are inversely related, so a twofold increase in creatinine is a reflection of a 50% drop in GFR. Creatinine provides a quick index of renal function, but when serum creatinine levels are rapidly changing, urinary creatinine clearance is an unreliable marker of GFR. As renal function returns during the recovery phase, plasma creatinine levels will fall back toward normal.

Nephritis is also characterized by an increase in blood pressure and an increase in circulating body fluid volume. The normal 5-year-old's blood pressure is 95/53 mm Hg, so 120/90 mm Hg represents hypertension for this patient. Both the loss of plasma protein in the urine and the retention of fluid contribute to the development of peripheral edema. Plasma proteins normally provide an oncotic pressure in all capillary beds of the body. As plasma protein levels fall, the fluid balance in the microcirculation is altered so that more fluid is filtered and is reabsorbed, leading to a generalized edema. Water retention because of the oliguria also contributes to the edema.

The red blood cell "casts" are structures formed by the accumulation of red blood cells within the tubule lumen. The casts are cylindrical structures that are formed from the mucoproteins in the urine to which red blood cells adhere. These casts, or models of the tubule lumen of the distal tubule and collecting duct, are flushed through the remainder of the tubule segment by the flow of filtrate.

Reabsorbing antigen activates the alternative complement cascade, and the low complement levels indicate an antigen/antibody reaction. The ASO titers and anti-DNase-B confirm the prior streptococcal infection.

OUTCOME

The infective process has ended and recovery has begun before a patient presents with poststreptococcal glomerulonephritis. If unsure, antibiotic treatment should be initiated to kill any remaining active streptococci. Treatment is centered on reducing any severe symptoms (exceptional hypertension, anuria, painful edema), reducing salt intake, limiting water ingestion, and allowing the recovery process to proceed.

FURTHER READING

Web Source

Hahn RG, Knox LM, Forman TA: Evaluation of poststreptococcal illness. Am Fam Physician 71:1949-1954, 2005. Available at http://www.aafp.org

Text Sources

Carroll RG: Elsevier's Integrated Physiology, Philadelphia, Elsevier, 2007.

Copstead L, Banasik J: Pathophysiology, 3rd ed. Philadelphia, Saunders, 2005.

Eaton DC, Pooler JP: Renal Access, Blood Flow, and Glomerular Filtration. In: Lange Medical Books, 6th ed. New York, McGraw-Hill, 2004.

Guyton AC, Hall JE: Textbook of Medical Physiology, 11th ed. Philadelphia, Saunders, 2006.

McPhee SJ, Papadakis MA, Tierney LM Jr: Current Medical Diagnosis and Treatment, 46th ed. New York, McGraw-Hill, 2007.

Schrier RW: Diseases of the Kidney and Urinary Tract, 8th ed. Philadelphia, Lippincott Williams & Wilkins, 2001, vol. II.

A 42-year-old woman experiencing peripheral edema is referred to the nephrologist for evaluation of renal function.

The patient was diagnosed with type 1 diabetes mellitus at the age of 12 and has been managing her blood glucose with three daily injections of insulin. Over the past 5 years, the blood glucose has not been as well managed, and 2 years ago urinalysis showed microalbuminuria.

PHYSICAL EXAMINATION

VS: T 37°C, P 72/min, R 15/min, BP 140/95 mm Hg
PE: Peripheral edema, particularly around eyes and feet. Fundoscopy reveals diabetic retinopathy.

LABORATORY STUDIES

Plasma analysis:

- Fasting glucose: 300 mg/dL (normal: 60-110 mg/dL)
- BUN: 32 mg/dL (normal: 7-18 mg/dL)
- Creatinine: 2.0 mg/dL (normal: 0.6-1.2 mg/dL)
- Plasma albumin: 1.5 g/dL (normal: 3.5-5 g/dL)
- Glycosylated hemoglobin: A1c (HbA1c) levels 7.8 (normal: <6)

Urinalysis:

- Glucose: +3 (normal: 0)
- Albuminuria: 200 mg/24 hr (normal: 0)

DIAGNOSIS

Diabetic nephropathy

PATHOPHYSIOLOGY OF KEY SYMPTOMS

The hormone insulin stimulates glucose uptake by a number of tissues, especially skeletal muscle and adipose. Diabetes mellitus is a chronic disease characterized by impaired uptake of glucose by the tissues. The disease can be caused either by a deficiency in insulin production or by the loss of tissue responsiveness to insulin. In either case the underlying cause of diabetic neuropathy is the elevated blood glucose levels characteristic of diabetes.

Glucose is a relatively small molecule that is freely filtered at the renal glomerulus. The filtered glucose load, or tubular glucose load, is the product of the glomerular filtration rate (GFR) × plasma glucose concentration. Once filtered, glucose is reabsorbed by the sodium-coupled transport mechanism (secondary active transport) in the proximal tubule.

The renal glucose transport capacity is determined by the number of transport protein molecules. The maximum glucose transport capacity is about twice as high as the normal filtered load of glucose. Consequently, glucose is not normally excreted in the urine. When the filtered load exceeds the glucose reabsorption, some glucose remains in the tubular filtrate and ultimately is excreted in the urine. For most individuals, the glucose renal threshold occurs when plasma glucose levels exceed 250 mg/dL (Fig. 21-1).

The glucose in the filtrate acts as an osmotic particle, impairing the reabsorption of water in the distal tubule and collecting duct. The origin of the term "diabetes" refers to the production of a large

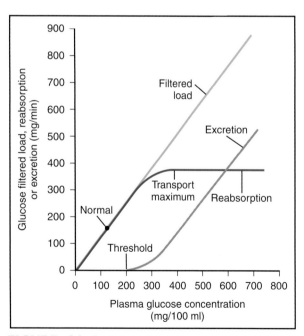

FIGURE 21–1 Relationships among the filtered load of glucose, the rate of glucose reabsorption by the renal tubules, and the rate of glucose secretion in the urine. The transport maximum is the maximum rate at which glucose can be reabsorbed from the tubules. The threshold for glucose refers to the filtered load of glucose at which glucose first begins to be excreted in the urine.

volume of urine, and "mellitus" indicates that the urine is sweet due to the presence of glucose. The osmotic diuresis accounts for two of the major symptoms of diabetes mellitus: polyuria and polydipsia.

Laboratory studies are consistent with both an acute and a chronic abnormality. The elevated glucose in the blood indicates that the diabetes is not being properly managed. The elevated HbA1c indicates a prolonged elevation in plasma glucose, sufficient to cause glucose residues to be attached to proteins. The normal lifespan of a red blood cell is 120 days, and the hemoglobin can become glycosylated during the entire lifespan. HbA1c levels are weighted and reflect more heavily plasma glucose levels during the prior 30 days.

Diabetes mellitus leads to damage to the glomerular basement membrane, characterized by glomerulosclerosis and thickening of the basement membrane. Glycosylation of the basement membrane proteins contributes to the ability of albumin to pass into Bowman's capsule and to be excreted in the urine. Because glomerular plasma oncotic pressure was a significant force slowing GFR, the removal of an oncotic force causes an increase in GFR. The elevation in GFR and renal plasma flow may initially cause a decrease in plasma urea and creatinine. In this patient's case, the disease has progressed to the point where there is a loss of renal function, indicated by an elevation in plasma urea and creatinine.

Microalbuminuria is an early indicator for diabetic nephropathy. The persistence of a small amount of albumin in the urine over multiple months contributes to the diagnosis of diabetic nephropathy.

Hypertension is both characteristic of renal damage and contributes to further renal damage. Approximately two thirds of adult diabetic patients have hypertension. The elevated blood pressure, along with glomerular sclerosis, causes damage and loss of some nephrons. The remaining nephrons increase their filtration rate, so that, acutely, whole kidney GFR is not diminished. The elevated glomerular capillary pressure in the remaining nephrons accelerates the glomerulosclerosis and loss of further nephrons, ultimately leading to complete loss of renal function (end-stage renal disease).

Peripheral edema is caused by the progressive loss of albumin in the urine. As albumin is excreted, plasma albumin levels fall and alter the balance of fluid exchange at the peripheral capillaries to favor net fluid movement into tissues, causing edema.

OUTCOME

Diabetic nephropathy is progressive and will culminate in end-stage renal disease. Approximately one third of all end-stage renal disease patients have diabetic nephropathy. While it is not reversible, the progression can be delayed by aggressive control of blood pressure and blood glucose levels, as well as protein restriction.

Once end-stage renal disease occurs, the only remaining options are dialysis or renal transplantation.

FURTHER READING

Web Sources
National Kidney and Urologic Diseases Information Clearinghouse. Proteinuria. NIH Publication No. 06–4732. Accessed September 2006. Available at http://kidney.niddk.nih.gov/kudiseases/pubs/proteinuria/
Medline Plus. Diabetic nephropathy. Accessed November 2006. Available at http://www.nlm.nih.gov/medlineplus/ency/article/000494.htm

Text Sources
Carroll RG: Elsevier's Integrated Physiology. Philadelphia, Elsevier, 2007.

Copstead L, Banasik J: Pathophysiology, 3rd ed. Philadelphia, Saunders, 2005.
Guyton AC, Hall JE: Textbook of Medical Physiology, 11th ed. Philadelphia, Saunders, 2006.
Kumar V: Robbins and Cotran: Pathologic Basis of Disease, 7th ed. Philadelphia, Saunders, 2005.
McPhee SJ, Papadakis MA, Tierney LM Jr: Current Medical Diagnosis and Treatment, 46th ed. New York, McGraw-Hill, 2007.
Rakel R: Textbook of Family Medicine, 7th ed. Philadelphia, Saunders, 2007.

A 70-year-old woman admitted 3 days earlier to the cardiac care unit after angioplasty has gone into renal failure.

The patient arrived in the emergency department complaining of chest pain and was diagnosed with an ongoing myocardial infarction. Imaging revealed a stenosis of three major coronary arteries, and the patient was immediately transferred to surgery for angioplasty. Subsequent imaging indicates that one of the three vessels is again stenosing, and the patient's progress is being monitored through serial radiologic imaging.

The patient was diagnosed 5 years ago with non–insulin-dependent diabetes mellitus (type 2), which has been managed with diet and exercise.

PHYSICAL EXAMINATION

VS: T 37°C, P 80/min, R 22/min, BP 100/70 mm Hg
PE: Incision scars on both legs, from the percutaneous angioplasty, are healing. No other notable findings.

LABORATORY STUDIES

Plasma analysis: Elevations in blood urea nitrogen and creatinine, increasing progressively with each daily measurement and reaching 50% above normal by day 3.

Urinalysis: Muddy brown epithelial cell casts and debris. Urine production is 300 mL/day (oliguria). Fractional excretion of sodium is 3%, and urine osmolarity is 200 mOsm/kg.

DIAGNOSIS

Acute tubular necrosis

PATHOPHYSIOLOGY OF KEY SYMPTOMS

Iodinated contrast media is toxic to renal tubular cells. In patients with underlying risk factors such as diabetes, or age and heart failure, contrast media containing more than 100 g of iodide will induce acute tubular necrosis.

The renal tubules are composed of epithelial cells, with the apical surface facing the lumen of the tubule. Tubular segments, particularly the proximal tubule and the thick ascending limb of the loop of Henle, have numerous mitochondria and are metabolically active. Transport proteins on both the apical and basolateral surfaces facilitate the selective reabsorption of nutrients and electrolytes across the tubular epithelium (Figs. 22-1 and 22-2).

Tubular fluid starts as an ultrafiltrate of plasma in Bowman's capsule and is modified as it passes through the different tubular segments (Fig. 22-3). Epithelia of the proximal tubule reabsorb essentially all of the filtered glucose, proteins, and amino acids that enter Bowman's capsule. The proximal tubule also reabsorbs 50% of the filtered load of urea and 66% of the filtered load of sodium. The thick ascending limb of loop of Henle reabsorbs sodium, potassium, and chloride. The distal tubule segments reabsorb sodium and chloride and secrete potassium. All of these transport processes require metabolic energy. Water and some other solutes are reabsorbed based on osmotic gradients or concentration gradients.

There is an immediate vasoconstriction and reduction in renal blood flow after administering a contrast agent. This results in damage and death of the tubular epithelial cells and impairment of renal function. The contrast media exert regional effects within the kidney, which results in the elimination of selective transport

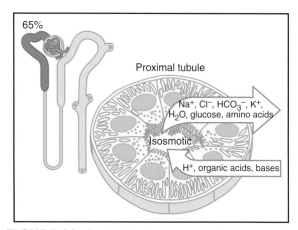

FIGURE 22–1 Cellular ultrastructure and primary transport characteristics of the proximal tubule. The proximal tubules reabsorb about 65% of the filtered sodium, chloride, bicarbonate, and potassium and essentially all the filtered glucose and amino acids. The proximal tubules also secrete organic acids, bases, and hydrogen ions into the tubular lumen.

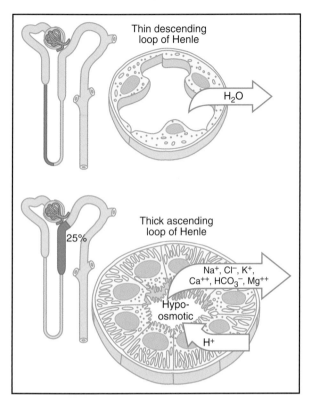

FIGURE 22–2 Cellular ultrastructure and transport characteristics of the thin descending loop of Henle *(top)* and the thick ascending segment of the loop of Henle *(bottom)*. The descending part of the thin segment of the loop of Henle is highly permeable to water and moderately permeable to most solutes but has few mitochondria and little or no active reabsorption. The thick ascending limb of the loop of Henle reabsorbs about 25% of the filtered loads of sodium, chloride, and potassium, as well as large amounts of calcium, bicarbonate, and magnesium. This segment also secretes hydrogen ions into the tubular lumen.

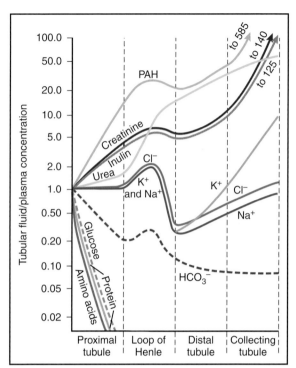

FIGURE 22–3 Changes in average concentrations of different substances at different points in the tubular system relative to the concentration of that substance in the plasma and in the glomerular filtrate. A value of 1.0 indicates that the concentration of the substance in the tubular fluid is the same as the concentration of that substance in the plasma. Values below 1.0 indicate that the substance is reabsorbed more avidly than water, whereas values above 1.0 indicate that the substance is reabsorbed to a lesser extent than water or is secreted into the tubules.

processes. The integrity of the epithelial cell tight junctions is disrupted, and the dead epithelial cells are sloughed into the lumen where they can occlude the lumen and disrupt the flow of filtrate. Epithelial cells from the later tubular segments will pass through the tubule and be excreted as "casts" and debris.

Impaired renal function leads to an increase in plasma creatinine and blood urea nitrogen (BUN). Creatinine and BUN remain elevated but begin to return toward normal as tubular function is reestablished. Normally, greater than 99% of the filtered sodium load is reabsorbed in the tubular segments. This means that the normal fractional excretion of sodium is less than 1%. Fractional excretion of greater than 2% of the filtered sodium load is characteristic of epithelial cell damage, as is the inability to produce a urine that has a higher osmolality than plasma.

In addition, hyperkalemia and hyperphosphatemia are commonly encountered (Fig. 22-4).

OUTCOME

Renal epithelial cells regenerate, and often the acute tubular necrosis resolves within 1 to 3 weeks in otherwise healthy individuals. The infusion of isotonic sodium bicarbonate or sodium chloride before and after administering a contrast agent helps to diminish the concentration of a contrast agent in the tubules and reduce the incidence of contrast-induced nephropathy. Loop diuretics can be used to induce adequate diuresis. In severe cases, dialysis can be used while waiting for renal function to recover.

Within 3 to 4 weeks, renal function usually returns to normal. If untreated, acute tubular necrosis can lead to renal failure and death.

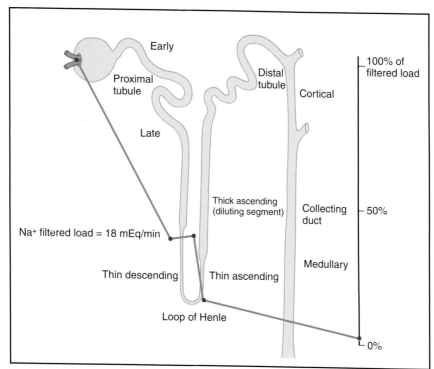

FIGURE 22-4 Ninety-nine percent of filtered Na^+ is reabsorbed as filtrate passes through the renal tubules. Reabsorption occurs primarily in the proximal tubule (66%) and loop of Henle (20%).

FURTHER READING

Web Sources

Lang EK, Foreman J, Schlegel JU, et al: The incidence of contrast medium induced acute tubular necrosis following arteriography. Radiology 138:203-206, 1981. Available at http://radiology.rsnajnls.org/cgi/reprint/138/1/203?eaf

Needham E: Management of acute renal failure. Am Fam Physician 72:9, 2005. Available at http://www.mdconsult.com/das/article/body/81736095-2/jorg=journal&source=MI&sp=15848990&sid=0/N/504089/1.html

Tumlin J, Stacuk F, Adam A, et al: Pathophysiology of contrast-induced nephropathy. Am J Cardiol 98(6A), 2006. Available at http://www.mdconsult.com/das/citation/body/81736095-2/jorg=journal&source=MI&sp=16437915&sid=0/N/16437915/1.html

Text Sources

Carroll RG: Elsevier's integrated physiology. Philadelphia, Elsevier, 2007.

Copstead L, Banasik J: Pathophysiology, 3rd ed. Philadelphia, Saunders, 2005.

Guyton AC, Hall JE: Textbook of Medical Physiology, 11th ed. Philadelphia, Saunders, 2006.

Kumar V, Abbas A, Fausto N: Robbins and Cotran Pathologic Basis of Disease, 7th ed. Philadelphia, Saunders, 2005.

McPhee SJ, Papadakis MA, Tierney LM Jr: Current Medical Diagnosis and Treatment, 46th ed. New York, McGraw-Hill, 2007.

Rakel R, Bope E: Conn's Current Therapy. Philadelphia, Saunders, 2008.

A 38-year-old man presents to his primary care physician complaining of difficulty in voiding for the past 6 months.

The patient was diagnosed with insulin-dependent diabetes mellitus at age 15. He has managed his diabetes with daily injections of insulin and has been able to achieve good plasma glucose control.

PHYSICAL EXAMINATION

VS: T 37°C, P 72/min, R 15/min, BP 120/80 mm Hg
PE: Unremarkable

LABORATORY STUDIES

Cystoscopy: No obstruction
Cystometry: Weak contraction of the detrusor muscle
Plasma analysis:

- Fasting glucose: 90 mg/dL (normal: 75-115 mg/dL)
- BUN: 12 mg/dL (normal: 7-18 mg/dL)
- Creatinine: 1.0 mg/dL (normal: 0.6-1.2 mg/dL)
- Plasma albumin: 3.8 mg/dL (normal: 3.5-5.5 mg/dL)
- Glycosylated hemoglobin: A1c (HbA1c) levels 4.2% (normal: 3.8% to 6.4%)

Urinalysis:

- Glucose: 0 (normal: 0)
- Albuminuria: 0 mg/24 hr (normal: 0)
- Urine cultures: Negative

DIAGNOSIS

Neurogenic bladder

PATHOPHYSIOLOGY OF KEY SYMPTOMS

Urine produced in the kidneys is transported through the ureter by peristalsis and is stored in the bladder until elimination from the body. The detrusor muscle is the major structural component of the bladder wall. The wall of the bladder is highly compliant and can accommodate an increase in volume of 300 mL with only a small increase in pressure.

When there is little urine in the bladder no pressure is exerted against the bladder wall. An increase in 50 to 300 mL of urine exerts a pressure against the wall, generating a force of 5 to 10 cm H_2O. Increases in volume above 300 mL cause pressure to rise; and above

400 mL, intrabladder pressure rises rapidly. Bladder cystometry measures the tension developed within the bladder (Fig. 23-1).

Normal micturition requires appropriate function of the brain, pons, spinal cord, sacral cord, and peripheral nerves. The micturition reflex is a spinal cord reflex involving sympathetic, parasympathetic, and somatic motor neurons (Fig. 23-2). The initiating event in the micturition reflex is an increase in tension in the detrusor muscle. The increased firing of stretch receptors in the bladder wall is transmitted to the spinal cord. The sensory information is transmitted to the brain stem, where it generates a sensation of urinary urgency. The sensory neurons also connect with spinal cord interneurons, leading to an increase in firing of parasympathetic nerves that supply the detrusor muscle. Parasympathetic activity causes further contraction of the detrusor muscle, and the reflex continues to build in strength.

The reflex ends with normal urination. There is an inhibition of the alpha-motor neuron that innervates the skeletal muscle of the external bladder sphincter. The increase in pressure within the bladder now propels

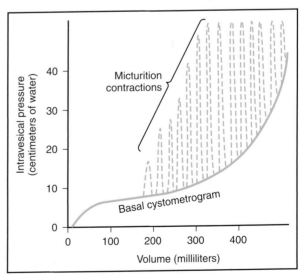

FIGURE 23–1 Normal cystometrogram also showing acute pressure waves *(dashed spikes)* caused by micturition reflexes.

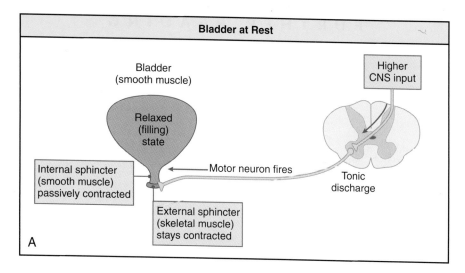

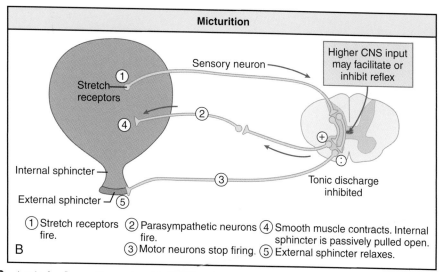

FIGURE 23–2   A spinal reflex mediates micturition. Filling the bladder increases bladder wall tension. Afferent sensory signals from the bladder cause a sympathetically mediated contraction of the bladder wall. This contraction further increases wall tension, until the tension plateaus, the reflex fatigues, or the bladder sphincters relax and micturition occurs.

urine through the relaxed bladder sphincters and out of the body through the urethra. If urination does not occur, the reflex fatigues and the bladder remains quiescent for a few minutes until the reflex begins again.

Diabetic neuropathy is a common complication of long-term diabetes. All nerves—sensory, autonomic, or motor—are susceptible to damage. The micturition reflex can be impaired by diabetic neuropathy.

Damage to the sensory nerves is often the first to manifest. This results in a decreased ability to sense when the bladder is distended, a loss of urinary urgency, and a decrease in the voiding frequency. The bladder continues to fill normally, and, consequently, distention of the bladder often occurs. As the peripheral neuropathy progresses, the contraction

of the detrusor muscle can also become diminished. Diminished effectiveness of the detrusor muscle results in an increase in the postvoid residual volume.

OUTCOME

No known therapies exist to allow regeneration of the nerve function. In the absence of normal nerve function, the micturition reflex will remain impaired. Augmented voiding techniques, such as double voiding and suprapubic pressure, may be useful. Alternatively, intermittent bladder catheterization can be used to empty the bladder, supplemented with suppressive antibiotics.

FURTHER READING

Web Sources

Rackley R: Neurogenic bladder. Accessed May 2006. Available at http://www.emedicine.com/med/topic3176.htm

University of Virginia Health System. Accessed September 2007. Available at http://www.healthsystem.virginia.edu/uvahealth/adult_urology/neurblad.cfm

Text Sources

Carroll RG: Elsevier's Integrated Physiology. Philadelphia, Elsevier, 2007.

Copstead L, Banasik J: Pathophysiology, 3rd ed. Philadelphia, Saunders, 2005.

Guyton AC, Hall JE: Textbook of Medical Physiology, 11th ed. Philadelphia, Saunders, 2006.

McCance KL, Huether SE: Pathophysiology: The Biologic Basis for Disease in Adults and Children, 3rd ed. St. Louis, Mosby, 1998.

McPhee SJ, Papadakis MA, Tierney LM Jr: Current Medical Diagnosis and Treatment, 46th ed. New York, McGraw-Hill, 2007.

A 48-year-old woman in an inpatient psychiatric hospital reports passing a high volume of urine and experiencing excessive thirst.

The patient was admitted to the hospital 1 year ago and was diagnosed with bipolar affective disorder. Lithium has been used successfully for the past year to control the psychiatric problems.

PHYSICAL EXAMINATION

VS: T 37°C, P 80/min, R 17/min, BP 100/70 mm Hg, BMI 22
PE: Patient appears dehydrated.

LABORATORY STUDIES

Plasma analysis:

- Sodium: 150 mEq/L (normal: 135 to 145 mEq/L)
- Potassium: 4.8 mEq/L (normal: 3.5 to 5 mEq/L)
- Chloride: 115 mEq/L (normal: 101 to 112 mEq/L)

pH: 7.48 (normal venous: 7.31 to 7.41)
Osmolality: 320 mOsm/kg (normal: 275 to 293 mOsm/kg)

Urinalysis:

- Urine osmolality: 200 mOsm/kg (normal: 100 to 900 mOsm/kg)
- 24-hour sample: 4.8 L (normal: <2 L/24 hr)

Water deprivation test: Little increase in urine osmolarity after 6 hours of water deprivation. Desmopressin injection had little effect.

DIAGNOSIS

Nephrogenic diabetes insipidus

PATHOPHYSIOLOGY OF KEY SYMPTOMS

Antidiuretic hormone (ADH, vasopressin) is synthesized in the hypothalamus and released in the posterior pituitary in response to an increase in plasma osmolarity. ADH binds to two subtypes of vasopressin receptors: (1) V_1 on the vasculature causing vasoconstriction and prostaglandin release and (2) V_2 in the collecting duct of the kidney that mediates the response to ADH.

The major biologic action of ADH is to stimulate water reabsorption in the distal tubule, which is why the term "antidiuretic hormone" is replacing "vasopressin" for this peptide. Binding of ADH to the V_2 receptor stimulates the production of cyclic adenosine monophosphate, leading to the insertion of aquaporin water channels into the apical surface of the collecting duct cells.

The renal glomerulus, proximal tubule, distal tubule, and cortical collecting duct are all in the cortex of the kidney. Only the loop of Henle, the medullary collecting duct, and the vasa recta pass through the renal medulla.

The osmolarity of the renal medullary interstitium is the driving force for the osmotic reabsorption of water from the collecting duct. Normal plasma osmolarity is 300 mOsm/L. Renal medullary interstitium osmolarity varies from a low of about 600 mOsm/L in a well-hydrated individual to a high of about 1400 mOsm/L in an individual who is dehydrated. About half of the renal medullary interstitium is due to urea accumulation, and the remainder is due to NaCl. ADH stimulates urea reabsorption from the medullary portions of the collecting duct, leading to its accumulation within the renal medulla. NaCl accumulation is the result of the $Na^+/K^+/2Cl^-$ transporter of the thick ascending limb of the loop of Henle.

The tight junctions of the ascending limb of the loop of Henle, the distal tubule, and the collecting duct are all impermeable to water. Consequently, tubular filtrate osmolarity can be different from that of the interstitial osmolarity. The filtrate of the ascending limb of the loop of Henle becomes dilute owing to the active transport of $Na^+/K^+/2Cl^-$. In the absence of ADH, there is little further water reabsorption and the body produces a large volume of dilute urine (see Fig. 19-2).

In the presence of ADH, aquaporin channels are inserted into the apical membrane, allowing the osmotically driven reabsorption of water. ADH increases filtrate osmolarity in the distal tubule to 300 mOsm/L, equal to the renal cortex interstitium osmolarity. In the medullary collecting duct, ADH increases filtrate osmolarity up to the level of the renal medullary interstitium osmolarity, up to 1400 mOsm/L in a dehydrated individual. ADH results in the production of a small volume of highly concentrated urine (see Fig. 19-2).

Lithium diminishes the ability of V_2 receptors to generate cyclic adenosine monophosphate. Consequently, the biologic action of ADH is diminished, resulting in an inability to reabsorb water and urea. Chronically, lithium may also diminish the transcription of aquaporin channels. If the disease is not too severe, this effect can be reversed if the patient is taken off of lithium. If lithium is necessary, the use of amiloride or thiazide and a low sodium diet is recommended. This combination allows a reduction in urinary volume and urinary dilution independent of ADH actions.

Impaired water reabsorption because of a defect in the kidney is termed "nephrogenic diabetes insipidus." "Nephrogenic" indicates the problem is the renal response to ADH, not the production of ADH. Plasma ADH levels are usually high, reflecting the ADH-releasing stimulus, high plasma osmolarity. "Diabetes" refers to the large volume of urine. "Insipidus" refers to the absence of glucose in this urine and is used to distinguish the disease from another polyuria, diabetes mellitus.

Excessive water loss leads to an increase in plasma osmolarity and an increase in plasma electrolyte concentration. The increase in osmolarity stimulates thirst, leading to a polydipsia. Excessive water ingestion is physiologically appropriate, allowing the patient to partially compensate for the inability of the kidney to conserve water. Over time, the body fluid osmolality stabilizes at a higher level, changing the osmotic threshold for thirst.

If the 24-hour urine collection shows a dilute urine, the diagnosis is confirmed with the water deprivation test. Because of the impairment of ADH, an individual can become severely dehydrated in a few hours, so the test must be carefully monitored. A normal individual should increase the urine osmolarity when water is withheld. The absence of an increase in urine osmolarity indicates impairment in water reabsorption. Injection of desmopressin should result in an increase in urine osmolarity if the kidneys are able to respond to ADH and is used to distinguish central diabetes insipidus from nephrogenic diabetes insipidus.

OUTCOME

If possible, lithium treatment should be stopped. If lithium is necessary, the use of amiloride or thiazide, combined with a low-sodium diet, will allow partial control of urinary volume and urinary dilution.

FURTHER READING

Web Source
Lederer L. Lithium Nephropathy. http://emedicine.com/med/topic1313.htm

Text Sources
Carroll RG: Elsevier's Integrated Physiology Philadelphia, Elsevier, 2007.

Copstead L, Banasik J: Pathophysiology, 3rd ed. Philadelphia, Saunders, 2005.

Garofeanu CG, et al: Causes of reversible nephrogenic diabetes insipidus: a systematic review. Am J Kidney Dis 45:626-637, 2005.

Goldman L, Ausiello D: Cecil Medicine, 23rd ed. Philadelphia, Saunders, 2008.

Guyton AC, Hall JE: Textbook of Medical Physiology, 11th ed. Philadelphia, Saunders, 2006.

Larsen PR, Kronenberg H, Melmed S, et al: Williams Textbook of Endocrinology, 10th ed. Philadelphia, Saunders, 2003.

McPhee SJ, Papadakis MA, Tierney LM Jr: Current Medical Diagnosis and Treatment, 46th ed. New York, McGraw-Hill, 2007.

SECTION IV

Hematology

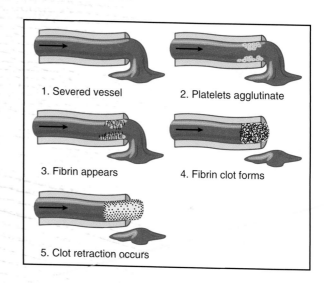

1. Severed vessel

2. Platelets agglutinate

3. Fibrin appears

4. Fibrin clot forms

5. Clot retraction occurs

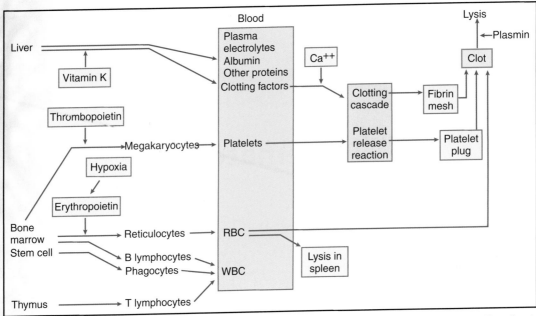

FIGURE IV–1   Blood and hemostasis map shows the convergence of clotting factors, platelets, and red blood cells in forming a clot. Blood components are synthesized in the liver, bone marrow, and thymus. A major functional role for blood is the formation of a platelet plug or a clot in response to vascular injury.

Blood is a complex suspension of cells and formed elements in plasma. The section on Cardiovascular Physiology describes the role of blood flow in the delivery of nutrients and the removal of metabolic wastes. The section on Respiration describes the function of red blood cells and, in particular, the protein hemoglobin, in the transport of oxygen and carbon dioxide. The focus of this section is on the role of the erythrocytes, platelets, and proteins involved in coagulation, emphasizing the complexity of platelet plug formation, clot formation, and clot lysis (Fig. IV-1).

The majority of proteins that circulate in the plasma are synthesized by the liver. Albumin accounts for almost half of the total plasma protein concentration. As a large molecular weight protein, albumin does not easily cross the capillary endothelial wall and, consequently, plays a large role in the exchange of fluid across the capillary. Most of the proteins involved in the clotting cascade are also synthesized in the liver. The hepatic synthesis of these proteins requires vitamin K as a cofactor and, therefore, drugs such as warfarin (Coumadin) can diminish the hepatic synthesis of the clotting factors (see Case 25). The clotting cascade is complex, and other agents, including herbal supplements, can interfere with the normal clotting process.

Diminished production of even a single component of the clotting cascade can lead to prolonged bleeding. Case 26 describes the hereditary defect in clotting factor VIII production described as hemophilia type A.

Formation of the platelet plug allows the repair of small areas of vascular damage independent of the clotting cascade. Platelets, also called thrombocytes, are fragments of megakaryocytes, and, when triggered by exposure to a damaged region of the vascular endothelium, undergo a reaction that allows them to adhere to other platelets. A decline in the platelet count, such as caused by an autoimmune disease (see Case 27), diminishes the ability to form clots and can lead to excessive bleeding at multiple sites in the body.

The concentration of red blood cells in the circulation reflects the balance between new red blood cell synthesis and red blood cell destruction. Normally, red blood cells have a life span of about 120 days and red blood cell synthesis replaces those red blood cells destroyed in the spleen and liver. Hemoglobin synthesis requires adequate stores of iron. Prolonged bleeding can deplete the body iron stores and impair the synthesis of new red blood cells (see Case 28). Iron deficiency results in the synthesis of cells that are smaller than normal and lack a sufficient amount of hemoglobin.

Blood circulating within the body has all of the factors necessary to form a clot. Clots formed within the vasculature flow through the vessels until they become trapped and occlude the vessel. The tendency for clot formation must be balanced by the ability to impede clot formation and by the ability to dissolve clots that are already formed. Anticoagulants can be used to diminish the likelihood of clot formation. The enzyme plasmin is responsible for the lysis of existing clots. Agents, such as tissue plasminogen activating factor, enhance the activity of plasmin and help to dissolve clots and restore blood flow (see Case 29).

CASE
25

A 58-year-old man comes to the emergency department complaining of bleeding in his mouth.

The bleeding began 24 hours ago and has been continuous in spite of compression. The patient suffered a myocardial infarction 18 months earlier and since that time has stopped smoking, has begun a moderate exercise program, and is on a low dose of warfarin (Coumadin) as a blood thinner. One month ago he began taking herbal supplements containing garlic and ginkgo biloba extract.

PHYSICAL EXAMINATION

VS: T 36.8°C, P 85/min, R 18/min, BP 95/65 mm Hg, BMI 29

PE: Patient has multiple small bleeding sites on the mucous membranes of the mouth and nose.

LABORATORY STUDIES

Hematocrit: 35% (normal: males 42%)
Stool sample test: Positive for blood
Prothrombin time (PT): 35 seconds (normal: 11-15 seconds)
Partial thromboplastin time (PTT): 48 seconds (normal: 26-35 seconds)

DIAGNOSIS

Coumadin-type herbal supplement toxicity

PATHOPHYSIOLOGY OF KEY SYMPTOMS

Blood lost from damaged blood vessels is limited by the process of hemostasis. Hemostasis has two major components: the formation of the platelet plug and the activation of the clotting cascade. The elevation of the clotting times, particularly the prothrombin time, indicates an impairment of the clotting cascade.

Hemostasis helps repair the vascular damage that accompanies daily living. For this patient, vascular damage is not being repaired, resulting in visible bleeding in the mucous membranes and likely more significant bleeding, particularly in the gastrointestinal tract and other internal organs. Cardiovascular signs consistent with a moderate hemorrhage include mild hypotension and a baroreceptor-mediated activation of the sympathetic nervous system resulting in an elevation of heart rate and respiratory rate.

The platelets, or thrombocytes, are fragments of megakaryocytes. Circulating platelets have a lifespan of approximately 10 days, and platelet formation is regulated by the hepatic hormone thrombopoietin. Platelets have three different types of granules. Dense granules contain adenosine triphosphate (ATP), adenosine diphosphate (ADP), and serotonin. Alpha granules contain proteins that enhance coagulation and platelet adhesion, such as fibrinogen, fibronectin, vitronectin, and von Willebrand factor. Platelets also contain lysosomal granules.

Exposure to a damaged section of the endothelial cell causes the platelets to adhere and to undergo a release reaction, secreting ADP, serotonin, and thromboxane A. ADP attracts additional platelets to aggregate and to seal the damaged area.

More extensive vascular damage is sealed by the formation of a blood clot. A series of plasma proteins called clotting factors result in the formation of fibrin. Fibrin is polymerized to form a mesh that traps red blood cells and platelets to help form a clot and seal the opening (Fig. 25-1).

This patient is on chronic anticoagulant therapy to reduce the likelihood of thrombus formation in the coronary circulation. Warfarin decreases the vitamin

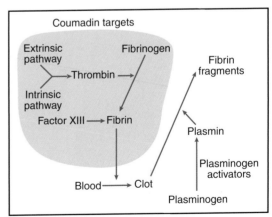

FIGURE 25–1 Effective circulation requires a balance between the ability to form clots to repair vascular injury and the need to maintain blood flow through vessels. The clotting cascade results in the formation of a fibrin mesh, which traps platelets and red blood cells to form a clot. Formation of the fibrin mesh is blocked by anticoagulants. Fibrinolytic agents, but not anticoagulants, can dissolve a clot after it is formed.

K–dependent hepatic synthesis of proteins, which includes a large number of the clotting factors. Consequently, chronic treatment with warfarin decreases the ability of the blood to form clots, reflected in the increased prothrombin time and partial thromboplastin time.

Herbal extracts can also interfere with hemostasis and amplify the anticoagulants and effects of warfarin. Garlic extracts diminish the platelet adhesion reaction, and ginkgo potentiates the action of warfarin through a mechanism that is not yet completely understood.

One of the possible effects of ginkgo is to improve blood flow in vessels through vasodilation.

OUTCOME

The patient was counseled to stop ingesting garlic and ginkgo. Fresh frozen plasma was infused to cause an immediate improvement in clotting times, because it will take weeks to reestablish normal hepatic synthesis of the clotting factors.

FURTHER READING

Web Source
Hawkins EB, Ehrlich SD: Ginkgo biloba. Accessed January 2007. Available at http://www.umm.edu/altmed/articles/ginkgo-biloba-000247.htm

Text Sources
Carroll RG: Elsevier's Integrated Physiology Philadelphia, Elsevier, 2007.

Copstead L, Banasik J: Pathophysiology, 3rd ed. Philadelphia, Saunders, 2005.
Guyton AC, Hall JE: Textbook of Medical Physiology, 11th ed. Philadelphia, Saunders, 2006.
McPhee SJ, Papadakis MA, Tierney LM Jr: Current Medical Diagnosis and Treatment, 46th ed. New York, McGraw-Hill, 2007.

A 3-year-old boy is brought to the pediatrician by his parents, who have noted excessive bleeding around the knees and elbows.

The parents have noted that the toddler bleeds very easily when the skin is scratched. Family history is significant for the presence of hemophilia in the mother's family.

PHYSICAL EXAMINATION

VS: T 37.2°C, P 60/min, R 20/min, BP 95/70 mm Hg, 45% for height and 50% weight on the growth charts
PE: Erythema is present particularly around the knees and elbows. Purpura is noted on the elbows.

LABORATORY STUDIES

Complete blood cell count:

- Hemoglobin: 10.9 g/dL (normal: 13.4-17.4 g/dL)
- Hematocrit: 32% (normal: 40%-54%)
- Platelets: 200,000/mm^3 (normal: 150,000-400,000/mm^3)

Coagulation Studies

- Platelets: 412 (normal: 150-440)
- Prothrombin time: 12.5 sec (normal: 11-15 sec)
- APTT (activated partial thromboplastin time): 42 sec (normal: 26.4-35 sec)
- Bleeding time: 6 min (normal: 2-8 min)

Factor VIII: C level: 5% (normal: 25%-100%)
von Willebrand factor antigen: 145% (normal: 71%-210%)

DIAGNOSIS

Hemophilia A

PATHOPHYSIOLOGY OF KEY SYMPTOMS

The patient's major symptoms are tied to a deficiency in the clotting process. Clot formation is a complex process, involving numerous plasma protein clotting factors, platelets, and red blood cells.

The clotting cascade results in the formation of a fibrin mesh that can trap platelets and red blood cells to form a blood clot. The 16 different blood clotting factors participate in either an extrinsic pathway and/or an intrinsic pathway. The extrinsic pathway requires an external stimulus, such as contact of the blood with the damaged portion of the vascular endothelial or blood contact with thromboplastin in the tissue spaces. The intrinsic pathway can be activated by vascular stasis, trauma to the blood, or contact with collagen. The ability to clot normally causes the loss of red blood cells from the circulation into both tissue spaces, joints, and the gastrointestinal tract.

Hemophilia A results from a hereditary deficiency in clotting factor VIII. The inheritance pattern is characterized as X-linked recessive, which means the disease is clinically significant in males but females can be carriers. Females, however, can exhibit the disease if they are the offspring of a hemophiliac father and a carrier mother.

Factor VIII is a key component in the intrinsic clotting pathway. In its absence, the clotting cascade is impaired. The coagulation panel confirms this, as the factor VIII:C level is abnormally low. The normal circulating levels of von Willebrand factor antigen rule out another common congenital bleeding disorder, von Willebrand's disease (Fig. 26-1).

The remaining measures of coagulation—prothrombin time, bleeding time, and fibrinogen level—are normal. This indicates that the clotting factor deficiency is limited only to factor VIII. The low hematocrit results from an increased loss of red blood cells through hemorrhage. The normal platelet levels indicate that platelet plug formation is likely normal.

OUTCOME

Treatment is centered on restoring normal levels of factor VIII. This can be done by intravenous infusion of recombinant factor VIII, particularly before events when bleeding is expected, such as surgery. For mild hemophiliacs, a vasopressin analogue (desmopressin) can be used to stimulate the release of factor VIII.

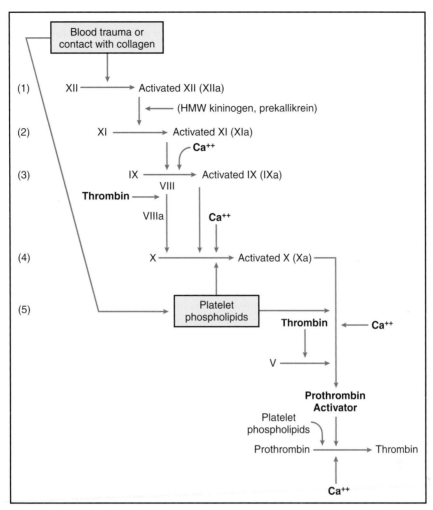

FIGURE 26–1   Intrinsic pathway for initiating blood clotting.

FURTHER READING

Text Sources

Abshire T: An approach to target joint bleeding in hemophilia: prophylaxis for all or individualized treatment? J Pediatr 145:581-583, 2004.

Carroll RG: Elsevier's Integrated Physiology. Philadelphia, Elsevier, 2007.

Copstead L, Banasik J: Pathophysiology, 3rd ed. Philadelphia, Saunders, 2005.

Dunn AL, Abshire T: Recent advances in the management of the child who has hemophilia. Hematol Oncol Clin North Am 18:1249, 2004.

Greer JP, Foerster J, Lukens JN, et al: Wintrobe's Clinical Hematology. Philadelphia, Lippincott Williams & Wilkins, 2004.

Guyton AC, Hall JE: Textbook of Medical Physiology, 11th ed. Philadelphia, Saunders, 2006.

Hillman RS, Ault KA, Rinder HM: Hematology in Clinical Practice, A Guide to Diagnosis and Management. New York, McGraw-Hill, 2005.

McPhee SJ, Papadakis MA, Tierney LM Jr: Current Medical Diagnosis and Treatment, 46th ed. New York, McGraw-Hill, 2007.

A 25-year-old woman comes to her primary care physician complaining of oral bleeding.

The patient has been on low molecular weight heparin for the past 2 years after the diagnosis of a pulmonary embolism.

PHYSICAL EXAMINATION

VS: T 37°C, P 70/min, R 18/min, BP 112/70 mm Hg, BMI 28

PE: Purpura, petechiae, and hemorrhagic bullae in the mouth

LABORATORY STUDIES

HIT (Heparin-induced thrombocytopenia): Positive antibody assay

DIAGNOSIS

Thrombocytopenia

PATHOPHYSIOLOGY OF KEY SYMPTOMS

The primary symptoms of this patient are all related to impaired platelet function. Platelets are usually capable of sealing small breaks in blood vessels without causing activation of the clotting cascade. When platelets encounter a damaged vascular endothelial cell, the platelets aggregate and form a platelet plug, sealing the damaged vessel. Impaired platelet function can cause prolonged bleeding, and the bleeding results in the appearance of small red dots on the skin and in the mouth (petechiae). It can also cause the appearance of somewhat larger or red purple dots (purpura) or even larger hemorrhagic bullae.

Platelets are fragments of megakaryocytes that play two roles in hemostasis. They form a platelet plug to seal small openings in blood vessels (temporary hemostasis) and contribute platelet factor III to the coagulation cascade. The formation of the fibrin clot helps to reinforce the platelet plug and to occlude larger areas of damage.

Damage to the endothelium of the blood vessel allows blood to come in contact with collagen. When a platelet contacts collagen, the platelet becomes activated and adheres to the damaged area. The platelets undergo a release reaction, secreting adenosine diphosphate (ADP), serotonin, and thromboxane. These substances cause the activation of adjacent platelets and allow the platelets to accumulate into a "platelet plug" (Fig. 27-1).

Heparin is used prophylactically to diminish blood clotting ability. Heparin is a sulfated protein that can stimulate the formation of antibodies that bind to antigens on the surface of the platelets. HIT is a result of the immune destruction of circulating platelets. In the absence of a sufficient number of platelets, hemostasis is impaired, resulting in the bleeding that can be seen on physical examination in the mouth and on the skin. HIT is mainly associated with unfractionated heparin. It can also occur with exposure to low molecular weight heparin.

OUTCOME

Discontinue the heparin therapy. Treat the HIT with alternative anticoagulant therapy, such as the direct thrombin inhibitors argatroban and lepirudin. Do not

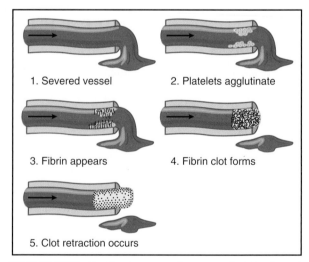

1. Severed vessel
2. Platelets agglutinate
3. Fibrin appears
4. Fibrin clot forms
5. Clot retraction occurs

FIGURE 27–1 Clotting process in a traumatized blood vessel. *(Modified from Seegers WH: Hemostatic Agents. Springfield, IL, Charles C Thomas, 1948.)*

give platelets to help with clotting, because existing antibodies will impair any new platelets added to the circulation. Ultrasonography should be used to screen the lower limbs to rule out deep vein thrombosis.

FURTHER READING

Text Sources

Carroll RG: Elsevier's Integrated Physiology. Philadelphia, Elsevier, 2007.

Copstead L, Banasik J: Pathophysiology, 3rd ed. Philadelphia, Saunders, 2005.

Guyton AC, Hall JE: Textbook of Medical Physiology, 11th ed. Philadelphia, Saunders, 2006.

Hillman RS, Ault KA, Rinder HM: Hematology in Clinical Practice, A Guide to Diagnosis and Management. New York, McGraw-Hill, 2005.

Levy JH: Heparin-induced thrombocytopenia; a prothrombotic disease. Hematol Oncol Clin North Am 21:65-88, 2007.

McPhee SJ, Papadakis MA, Tierney LM Jr: Current Medical Diagnosis and Treatment, 46th ed. New York, McGraw-Hill, 2007.

Menajovsky LB: Heparin-induced thrombocytopenia: clinical manifestations and management strategies. Am J Med 118(Suppl 8A):21S–30S, 2005.

Rodgers GP, Young NS: Bethesda Handbook of Clinical Hematology. Philadelphia, Lippincott Williams & Wilkins, 2005.

A 50-year-old man comes to his family physician complaining of fatigue.
  The patient indicates that climbing the stairs leaves him short of breath and that this has been getting progressively worse over the past month. He does not participate in any regular exercise. The patient works in a stressful job and to relieve stress the patient smokes, drinks 6 cups of coffee a day, and has two or three alcoholic drinks after work. He has been taking aspirin for the last 6 months for frequent stomach pain. The patient has decreased caloric intake for the past 3 months in an effort to lose weight, with moderate success.

PHYSICAL EXAMINATION

VS: T 36°C, P 105/min, R 24/min, BP 90/75 mm Hg, BMI 33
PE: Upper and lower endoscopy reveals a bleeding gastric ulcer.

LABORATORY STUDIES

Hematocrit: 30%
Red blood cell smear: Microcytic hypochromic cells
Serum iron values: 27 µg/dL
Transferrin saturation: 13%
Serum ferritin: 20 µg/L
Stool test: Positive for occult blood

DIAGNOSIS

Iron deficiency anemia

PATHOPHYSIOLOGY OF KEY SYMPTOMS

The patient's fatigue and shortness of breath when exercising are characteristic of anemia, confirmed by the finding of a low hematocrit. Gastrointestinal bleeding is the most common type of blood loss leading to an iron deficiency.

Hematocrit reflects the balance of red blood cell synthesis and red blood cell loss. Red blood cell synthesis occurs in the bone marrow and is stimulated by the renal hormone erythropoietin. Loss of red blood cells is usually due to destruction within the spleen and liver. Hemorrhage also results in a loss of red blood cells. If the red blood cell synthesis rate is not sufficient to keep up with the loss from hemorrhage, anemia will result.

Iron is essential for synthesis of hemoglobin. As body iron stores are depleted, hemoglobin synthesis is impaired, and, consequently, the red blood cells have diminished pigment and are termed "hypochromic." The iron deficiency also results in smaller than normal red blood cells, termed "microcytic." Severe iron deficiency is characterized by low hematocrit and the appearance of red blood cells as hypochromic and microcytic. It occurs when the hematocrit has fallen below 30%.

The normal lifespan of red blood cells is approximately 120 days. As red blood cells age, their membranes become more rigid, and thus the red blood cells rupture as they pass through the sinusoids of the spleen. The iron and hemoglobin released by the ruptured red blood cells are scavenged by transferrin and haptoglobin, respectively.

The remaining patient symptoms are also due to the hemorrhage. This includes the hypotension and the sympathetically mediated increase in heart rate and respiratory rate. Aspirin and alcohol intake increases the risk of gastrointestinal bleeding, and the presence of the gastrointestinal hemorrhage is indicated by the positive stool test for occult blood and confirmed by the endoscopy.

OUTCOME

The goal of treatment is to restore the patient's iron stores. Correction of the underlying hemorrhage, however, is necessary before this can occur. Once the bleeding is controlled, oral iron supplements such as ferrous sulfate may be prescribed. Vitamin C supplementation will assist both the absorption of the iron and the production of hemoglobin.

FURTHER READING

Web Sources

Feldman M, Friedman LS, Sleisenger MH: Sleisenger & Fordtran's Gastrointestinal and Liver Disease, Pathophysiology/Diagnosis/Management, 7th ed. Philadelphia, WB Saunders, 2002. Available at http://intl.elsevierhealth.com/feldman/downloads/preface.pdf

Medline Plus. Iron deficiency anemia. Accessed August 2007. Available at http://www.nlm.nih.gov/medlineplus/ency/article/000584.htm

Text Sources

Carroll RG: Elsevier's Integrated Physiology. Philadelphia, Elsevier, 2007.

Copstead L, Banasik J: Pathophysiology, 3rd ed. Philadelphia, Saunders, 2005.

Goldman L, Ausiello D: Gastrointestinal hemorrhage and occult gastrointestinal bleeding. In Cecil Medicine, 23rd ed. Philadelphia, Saunders, 2008.

Guyton AC, Hall JE: Textbook of Medical Physiology, 11th ed. Philadelphia, Saunders, 2006.

McPhee SJ, Papadakis MA, Tierney LM Jr: Current Medical Diagnosis and Treatment, 46th ed. New York, McGraw-Hill, 2007.

A 58-year-old man is transported to the emergency department after being awakened by a crushing pain in his chest that radiated down the left arm. The patient is immediately treated with morphine, nitroglycerin, and aspirin and placed on supplemental oxygen. Pulse oxymetry shows O_2 saturation of 95%. The patient is anxious and continues to complain of pain that was only partially relieved by the morphine.

The patient has a past history of hypertension, which has been controlled with diuretics.

PHYSICAL EXAMINATION

VS: T 36°C, P 118/min, R 28/min, BP 85/70 mm Hg, BMI 33

PE: The patient is pale and diaphoretic. Respirations are rapid and shallow, pulse is elevated, and blood pressure is low. Neurologic examination is normal.

LABORATORY STUDIES

ECG: Wide Q wave in leads I and aVL; ST segment elevation in leads I, aVL, and V_{2-5}

Blood tests (CBC, chem panel, cardiac markers): Elevated troponin I, elevated troponin T, and normal CK-MB

Lipid panel: Total cholesterol high, HDL low, LDL high

DIAGNOSIS

Myocardial infarction

COURSE

The electrocardiogram (ECG) and patient symptoms are consistent with a recent anteroapical infarction. Cardiac catheterization showed atherosclerosis in all major vessels with a 99% occlusion of the left anterior descending coronary artery. The patient is treated with tissue plasminogen activator (tPA), 15 mg initial bolus, followed by 50 mg over the next 30 minutes and 35 mg over the following 60 minutes. Angiography immediately after the end of the tPA treatment showed an increase in flow through the left anterior descending coronary artery to thrombolysis in myocardial infarction (TIMI) grade 3.

PATHOPHYSIOLOGY OF KEY SYMPTOMS

Damage to the vascular endothelium, such as caused by atherosclerotic plaques, can result in clot formation.

Blood clots can occlude the vessel at this site of formation (thrombus), or they may break free from the site and travel as an embolus until they occlude the lumen of the smaller vascular segment. Emboli formed on the venous side of the circulation generally are trapped in the pulmonary vasculature, and emboli formed on the arterial side of the circulation generally occlude blood flow to the region of an individual organ.

The cells of the brain and the heart are particularly susceptible to damage caused by the interruption of blood flow from an embolus. Occlusion of a region of the cerebral circulation results in a stroke, and occlusion of a region of the coronary circulation results in a myocardial infarction.

A blood clot consists of a fibrin mesh that traps platelets and red blood cells (see Fig. 27-1). The fibrin mesh results from the activation of the clotting cascade through either an intrinsic stimulus (vascular stasis) or an extrinsic pathway activation (contact with damaged vascular endothelium). Activated platelets contribute both to the clot and to the activation of the intrinsic pathway.

In this patient, a blood clot has resulted in occlusion of the coronary blood vessel and ischemic damage to the myocardium. Although the individual had coronary vascular stenosis, the sudden onset of severe pain in the absence of exercise is a common characteristic of a thrombus. Abnormalities noted during the physical examination are due to a strong sympathetic nervous system activation. This includes an elevated heart rate and elevated blood pressure from the increase in total peripheral resistance, sweating from the sympathetic cholinergic activation of the sweat glands, pale cold skin from sympathetic constriction of the cutaneous vasculature, and the sympathetically mediated increase in respiratory rate.

Laboratory studies are consistent with myocardial ischemia. The ischemic region of the myocardium causes an electrical abnormality called an "ST segment shift." The particular leads involved allow determination of the region of the heart that is ischemic. Myocardial enzymes that are normally intracellular begin to leak out from the damaged myocardial tissue. There is an early elevation in troponin and, after 24 hours, there is an elevation in the myocardial band isoform of creatine kinase (CK-MB). Because the infarct is relatively recent, the CK-MB levels are not yet elevated.

Acute resuscitation is centered on limiting ischemic damage, followed by reestablishment of blood flow. Chronic treatment is centered on diminishing the potential for future clot formation.

Ischemic damage is limited by the early administration of supplemental oxygen and the use of nitroglycerin as a coronary vasodilator. This ensures that any vascular segments that can be perfused are being supplied with oxygen-enriched blood.

tPA is used to stimulate the activity of the enzyme plasmin, which dissolves existing clots. Consequently, this class of drugs is often referred to as "clot busters." tPA is effective when administered early in the episode of ischemia, but its usefulness is diminished if the ischemia has persisted for more than 6 hours.

The tendency for future clot formation can be diminished acutely by treatment with heparin or chronically by treatment with dicumarol (see Fig. 25-1). Heparin potentiates the action of antithrombin 3 and diminishes formation of the fibrin mesh. Dicumarol blocks the vitamin K–dependent synthesis of plasma proteins, which includes almost all of the clotting factors. The delayed effectiveness of dicumarol as an anticoagulant is because the clotting factors already synthesized before beginning the dicumarol treatment remain in the circulation.

Platelets contribute to the formation of platelet plugs as well as clots. The tendency for platelets to adhere and to undergo a release reaction is diminished by aspirin. Consequently, aspirin is sometimes referred to as a "blood thinner."

OUTCOME

Following tPA treatment, heparin was administered and the dose adjusted to maintain an activated partial thromboplastin time of between 50 and 75 seconds. Aspirin treatment was continued.

Thrombolytic therapy reduced the pain within 15 minutes, and the ST segment shift returned to normal within 2 hours. The patient was transferred to the coronary care unit and monitored for 3 days before being discharged from the hospital.

FURTHER READING

Web Sources

Cannon C: Importance of TIMI 3 flow. Circulation 104:624-626, 2001. Available at http://circ.ahajournals.org/cgi/content/full/104/6/624

Klatt E: Myocardial infarction. University of Utah Medicine. Accessed October 2007. Available at http://library.med.utah.edu/WebPath/TUTORIAL/MYOCARD/MYOCARD.html

Ohman E, Harrington R, Cannon C, et al: Intravenous thrombolysis in acute myocardial infarction. Chest 119(1 Suppl):253S-277S, 2001. Available at http://www.chestjournal.org

Text Sources

Carroll RG: Elsevier's Integrated Physiology. Philadelphia, Elsevier, 2007.

Copstead L, Banasik J: Pathophysiology, 3rd ed. Philadelphia, Saunders, 2005.

Guyton AC, Hall JE: Textbook of Medical Physiology, 11th ed. Philadelphia, Saunders, 2006.

McPhee SJ, Papadakis MA, Tierney LM Jr: Current Medical Diagnosis and Treatment, 46th ed. New York, McGraw-Hill, 2007.

SECTION V

Respiration

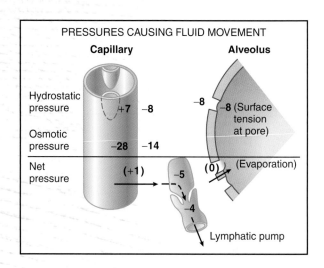

PRESSURES CAUSING FLUID MOVEMENT

Capillary   **Alveolus**

Hydrostatic pressure   +7   −8   −8   −8 (Surface tension at pore)

Osmotic pressure   −28   −14

Net pressure   (+1)   −5   (0)   (Evaporation)

−4

Lymphatic pump

Energy production by the mitochondria consumes oxygen and generates carbon dioxide as a metabolic waste product. Consequently, the body must absorb oxygen from the environment and eliminate carbon dioxide back into the environment. Respiratory physiology characterizes the movement of carbon dioxide and oxygen between the air and the mitochondria.

The exchange of gas between the body and the external environment occurs at the interface between the alveoli and the pulmonary capillaries. Diseases of the pulmonary system can be grouped as those resulting from a defect in exchange across the alveolar barrier, diseases resulting in abnormal alveolar gas composition, or diseases resulting in abnormal gas transport in the blood.

Air exchange between the alveoli and the pulmonary capillaries occurs by diffusion, described by Fick's law:

$$J = -DA(\Delta \text{Concentration}/\Delta \text{Distance})$$

The diffusion coefficient D includes the solubility of the gas. Although approximately equal amounts of oxygen and carbon dioxide cross the alveolar barrier, carbon dioxide is 10 times more diffusible across the alveolar barrier than is oxygen. This fact accounts for the low 6-mm Hg driving gradient (difference between alveolar gas composition and pulmonary arterial gas composition) for carbon dioxide compared with the 60-mm Hg driving gradient for oxygen. The low diffusion coefficient for oxygen also correctly predicts that defects in diffusion will impair oxygen exchange before impacting carbon dioxide exchange (see Case 35).

The partial pressure of gas within the alveoli is a function of three major factors: (1) the composition of the inspired gas; (2) the quantity of gas entering the alveoli each minute; and (3) the volume of gas already within the alveoli. The "concentration" of inspired gas is expressed as the partial pressure, determined by the atmospheric pressure × the percentage of gas in the inspired air. Air entering the body is humidified before it mixes with air already in the alveoli (Fig. V-1A).

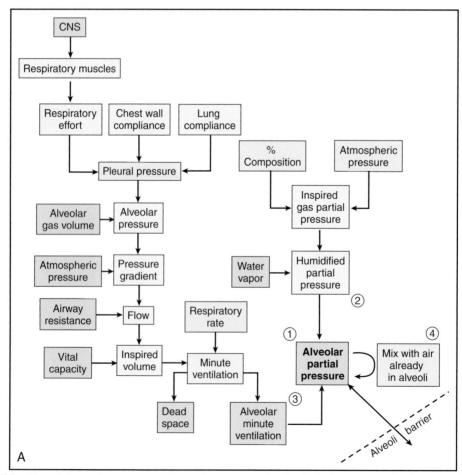

FIGURE V-1A   Map of the respiratory system. Gas exchange across the alveolar/pulmonary capillary barrier is the focal point for pulmonary function. Gas composition and the volume of air exchange determine the alveolar gas composition.

Minute ventilation is the amount of air that enters the body. However, alveolar minute ventilation is less than minute ventilation, because some air that enters the body remains in the trachea and bronchi, which are parts of the respiratory tree that do not participate in gas exchange. Minute ventilation is calculated as (respiratory rate) × (inspired volume). Air flow between the alveoli and the outside environment is determined by the pressure gradient between the alveoli and the outside air (see Cases 30 and 31) and the resistance to airflow as it moves through the respiratory passages (see Case 32).

Gas exchange in the lungs requires the balance of alveolar ventilation and pulmonary capillary perfusion. Hypoxic pulmonary vasoconstriction helps ensure that blood flow is directed preferentially to alveoli that are well ventilated (see Case 40). Hypocapnic bronchoconstriction helps ensure that ventilation is preferentially directed to alveoli that are well perfused (see Case 39).

Abnormal gas transport within the vascular system creates a different group of pulmonary pathophysiologies. The low solubility of oxygen is offset by the presence of oxygen carrying proteins, such as hemoglobin in the red blood cells and the myoglobins in skeletal muscle. Oxygen is first exchanged between the alveoli in the plasma, and, consequently, pulmonary venous plasma reflects the alveolar oxygen partial pressure. Arterial oxygen partial pressure is slightly lower than that in the pulmonary veins because of both ventilation/perfusion imbalances in some portions of the lung and admixture of blood draining a portion of the respiratory tree and the muscle of the left ventricle. Arterial oxygen partial pressure is sensed by the chemoreceptors of the carotid body aortic body (see Case 36) (Fig. V-1B).

Ninety-eight percent of the oxygen content of arterial blood is bound to hemoglobin. Consequently,

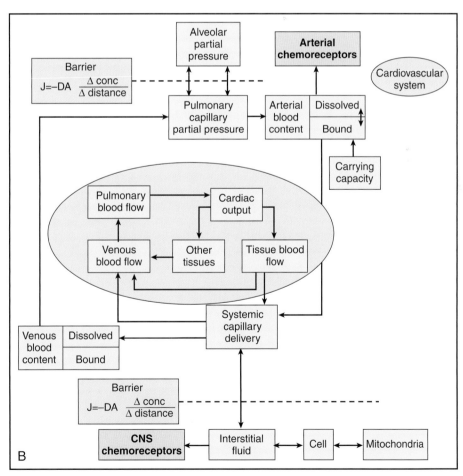

FIGURE V-1B Map of the respiratory system. Gas exchange across the alveolar/pulmonary capillary barrier is the focal point for pulmonary function. The focus shifts to blood flow (*pink shaded area*) and blood-carrying capacity. The two points of homeostatic regulation, the arterial chemoreceptors and the CNS chemoreceptors, are show in *shaded boxes*.

abnormalities in hematocrit or hemoglobin synthesis can result in hypoxia, the impaired oxygen delivery to the tissues (see Case 38). Hypoxia is different from ischemia in that ischemia results in impaired blood flow to the tissue, causing both hypoxia and hypercapnia, the accumulation of carbon dioxide.

Carbon dioxide is transported from the tissue activity in the lungs, primarily in the form of HCO_3^-. Thus, respiratory abnormalities rapidly result in alterations in acid-base balance within the body.

Acutely, control of pulmonary exchange is achieved by altering the rate and depth of respiration. The arterial blood normally reflects the gas composition of the alveoli. Hypercapnia, and, to a lesser degree, hypoxia, stimulate the chemoreceptors at the aortic body in the carotid body to increase minute ventilation. Medullary receptors within the central nervous system are sensitive only to the pH changes caused by alterations in carbon dioxide concentration.

Respiratory drive is controlled by nuclei in the medulla oblongata and the pons (see Case 33). Respiratory centers receive descending input from the cerebral cortex (see Case 37) and limbic system and ascending input from central and peripheral chemoreceptors (see Case 34), as well as mechanoreceptors in the lungs and in the airways. The output of the respiratory center is primarily through the phrenic nerve but also through the accessory muscles of respiration.

Chronic challenges to the pulmonary system, such as occurs in individuals living at extremely high altitudes, result in remodeling of the thoracic space to increase ventilation and an increase in red blood cell concentration mediated by increases in the production of the hormone erythropoietin.

A 55-year-old man comes to the clinic complaining of fatigue and persistent shortness of breath, which becomes worse during exercise.

The patient has a history of respiratory infections and has a chronic cough that is worse in the morning. He worked for 20 years in an automobile manufacturing plant and was laid off 5 years ago. The patient has smoked cigarettes since he was a teenager. Currently he estimates smoking one pack of cigarettes a day.

PHYSICAL EXAMINATION

VS: T 37°C, P 72/min, R 25/min, BP 120/80 mm Hg, BMI 28

PE: Patient is in mild respiratory distress with an elevated respiratory rate and shallow breaths. An end-expiratory wheeze is heard on auscultation. Otherwise, his lungs appear normal to auscultation and percussion. *tapping surface*

LABORATORY STUDIES

Pulmonary function tests: FEV_1 was 70% of predicted and peak expiratory flow was 60% of predicted. Forced vital capacity was 90% of predicted.

Chest radiograph: Normal

Arterial blood gases: Po_2 75, Pco_2 42, pH 7.32

*80-100   28-20?   7.4
35-45 mmHg*

DIAGNOSIS

Chronic obstructive pulmonary disease

COURSE

Chronic obstructive pulmonary disease (COPD) is a combination of loss of elastic tissue (emphysema) and airway obstruction (chronic bronchitis), usually caused by smoking. Cigarette smoke contains numerous particles and chemicals, some of which damage lung tissue. Cigarette smoke also paralyzes cilia that line the airways, eliminating the normal route for expulsion of mucus that helps clear inhaled particulate matter.

PATHOPHYSIOLOGY OF KEY SYMPTOMS

Absorption of O_2 and elimination of CO_2 occur by diffusion across the alveolar membrane. Pulmonary blood flow ensures the delivery of oxygen-depleted/CO_2-enriched (venous) blood to the lungs. Alveolar ventilation exchanges a portion of the air in the alveoli with the atmosphere during each breath. Alveolar ventilation requires (1) the development of a pressure gradient between the alveoli and the atmosphere and (2) an open airway. COPD, which is a combination of emphysema and chronic bronchitis, impairs both of those.

Emphysema results from the loss of elasticity in the respiratory bronchioles and alveoli of the lungs. Over time, alveoli become damaged and the multiple small alveoli are replaced by larger alveolar sacs, with the loss of surface area available for exchange. Eventually, the destruction of the alveoli results in a loss of elastic recoil of the lung, diminishing the effectiveness of the normally passive respiratory expiration. Both inspiration and expiration can require skeletal muscle effort.

Chronic bronchitis is an irritation of the bronchioles. The irritation results in a local inflammation and swelling, as well as increased mucus production, both of which act to narrow the bronchiole lumen. The reduced bronchiole diameter provides a high resistance to air flow, impeding the movement of air during breathing. The bronchitis results in the "obstructive" component of the COPD. Airway obstruction accounts for the diminished FEV_1 and diminished peak excitatory flow findings of the spirometry test.

The final respiratory impairment is a consequence of the loss of surface area available for diffusion. Both oxygen and carbon dioxide diffuse across the barrier separating the alveolar air in the blood in the pulmonary capillaries. Carbon dioxide is fairly soluble, and, consequently, diffuses easily from the blood into the alveolar air. Oxygen, in contrast, is poorly soluble, and the loss of the surface area available for exchange can result in an impairment of the absorption of oxygen.

Arterial blood gas determination can be used to monitor the effectiveness of gas exchange across the alveoli. Impairments and perfusion can cause a drop in the arterial Po_2 and an elevation in the arterial PCO_2. The larger proportional impairment in the diffusion of oxygen is reflected in the more significant drop in the arterial Po_2 than in elevation in the arterial Pco_2.

Normally, ventilation is controlled by CO_2 levels as sensed by the arterial chemoreceptors and the central nervous system chemoreceptors. The increase in ventilatory drive is a reflection in part of the elevation in P_{CO_2}. Over time, however, the respiratory acidosis is partially compensated by the renal retention of HCO_3^-. In addition, CO_2 drive in the central nervous system is also attenuated by HCO_3^- transport into the cerebrospinal fluid. These compensations blunt or completely remove the CO_2 stimulation of ventilation. As the disease progresses, arterial P_{O_2} levels fall below 60 mm Hg. Hypoxia, sensed by the arterial chemoreceptors, can become the primary ventilatory drive. In this instance, placing the patient on supplemental inspired oxygen can cause respiration to stop.

OUTCOME

Smoking cessation is critical to prevent further damage. The existing damage cannot be easily reversed. However, acute crises caused by infection can be treated with antibiotics and bronchoconstriction from inflammation can be reversed with corticosteroid treatment. Rehabilitation includes learning respiratory patterns to minimize energy expenditure and an exercise program. Breathing practices include exhaling through "pursed lips" to prevent collapse of the midsized airways. As alveolar surface area available for exchange is diminished, hypoxia will usually appear before hypercapnia. The hypoxia can be treated with supplemental oxygen.

The best case scenario is to stabilize the alveoli and limit further damage.

FURTHER READING

Text Sources

Carroll RG: Elsevier's Integrated Physiology. Philadelphia, Elsevier, 2007.

Copstead L, Banasik J: Pathophysiology, 3rd ed. Philadelphia, Saunders, 2005.

Doherty DE, Briggs DD Jr: Chronic obstructive pulmonary disease: epidemiology, pathogenesis, disease course, and prognosis, Clin Cornerstone 5:16, 2004.

Guyton AC, Hall JE: Textbook of Medical Physiology, 11th ed. Philadelphia, Saunders, 2006.

Mason RJ, Broadus V, Murray J, et al: Murray and Nadel's Textbook of Respiratory Medicine. Philadelphia, Saunders, 2005.

McPhee SJ, Papadakis MA, Tierney LM Jr: Current Medical Diagnosis and Treatment, 46th ed. New York, McGraw-Hill, 2007.

A 29-year-old man is transported by the rescue squad to the emergency department in acute respiratory distress after being stabbed in the left lateral chest.

The patient was involved in a domestic dispute. He has a 3-cm puncture wound on the left lateral chest between the third and fourth ribs. He is conscious, is able to speak, complains of chest pains associated with each breath, and has difficulty breathing. The puncture wound has minimal bleeding, and total blood loss is estimated at 100 mL. Air can be heard entering the thorax through the stab wound during inspiration, and bubbles formed at the stab wound during exhalation. This air movement was minimized by placing a compression bandage at the site of injury before transport.

PHYSICAL EXAMINATION

VS: T 36.7°C, P 105/min, R 28/min, BP 130/110 mm Hg

PE: Patient's breathing is labored and involving abdominal muscles. The thoracic cage is asymmetrical, with the left side protruding more than the right side. The left side shows much less movement than the right during breathing. Breath sounds are decreased on the left side, and the left side shows hyperresonance to percussion.

low raspitch

LABORATORY STUDIES

95-100

Pulse oximetry: 85% oxygen saturation

Chest radiograph: Confirms unilateral left-sided pneumothorax

Arterial blood gases: Po_2 90 mm Hg, Pco_2 44 mm Hg

80-100   35-45

DIAGNOSIS

Pneumothorax

COURSE

The patient is sedated, and an endotracheal tube is inserted. The wound is exposed and opened, and the patient is placed on positive-pressure ventilation (tidal volume 500 mL, rate 18, positive end-expiratory pressure 5 mL). The injury is surgically repaired, and a negative pressure is applied to the thoracostomy tube to reinflate lung. The patient is admitted to the intensive care unit for observation.

PATHOPHYSIOLOGY OF KEY SYMPTOMS

Breathing requires the creation of a pressure gradient between the alveoli and the atmospheric air. Normally, this pressure gradient is created by altering the volume of the thoracic cavity, which then expands or compresses the lungs. There is no direct passageway between the intrapleural thoracic space and the atmosphere. Consequently, the change in thoracic volume alters the size of the lungs.

Intrapleural pressure in the thorax is negative, created by the inward directed elastic recoil of the lung and the outward directed elastic recoil of the chest wall. During inspiration, contraction of the diaphragm creates a more negative intrapleural pressure and the consequent expansion of the lungs creates a negative alveolar pressure. Air flows into the lungs from outside the body in response to the pressure gradient between the alveoli and the atmospheric air (Fig. 31-1).

During expiration, the process is reversed. Relaxation of the diaphragm causes thoracic intrapleural

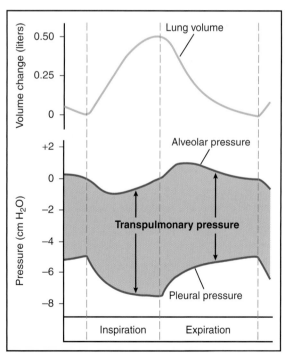

FIGURE 31-1 Changes in lung volume, alveolar pressure, pleural pressure, and transpulmonary pressure during normal breathing.

pressure to be less negative. The lungs decrease in size, creating a positive alveolar pressure. Air flows from the alveoli out of the body.

The opening of a passageway between the atmospheric air and the intrapleural space allows air to flow directly into the intrapleural space, bypassing the lungs. This opening can be created by damage to the trachea or bronchi, by rupture of alveoli on the surface of the lung, or by trauma to the chest wall. The presence of air in the intrapleural space disrupts the normal ventilation and is defined as a pneumothorax.

Air enters the intrapleural space through the opening in the thoracic wall created by the knife wound. The loss of the negative intrathoracic pressure results in the collapse of the left lung and the outward recoil of the left side of the thoracic cage (flail chest). The collapse is limited to one side of the lung because the complete mediastinum in humans isolates each lung into its own thoracic chamber. Loss of the negative intrapleural pressure on the left side of the chest causes the heart to be displaced toward the right side of the chest. All of these changes can be seen on a chest radiograph.

Contraction of the diaphragm and the muscles involved in inspiration acts to increase thoracic volume. As thoracic pressure becomes more negative, air moves through the knife wound instead of through the trachea and bronchi. Consequently, the left lung is not ventilated during inspiration.

The lack of ventilation of the left lung greatly diminishes the surface area available for gas exchange.

Hypoxia results in a vasoconstriction of the blood vessels in the left lung, both increasing pulmonary vascular resistance and shunting the majority of the cardiac output away from the left lung.

The shift in thoracic contents to the right side of the chest means that the right lung is not able to inflate to the same volume that it did before the injury. Impairment of right lung function, along with the loss of left lung function, causes inadequate gas exchange and the consequent arterial hypoxia, indicated by the diminished pulse oximetry reading. Inadequate gas exchange also causes an increase in carbon dioxide levels, resulting in an increased respiratory drive and the sensation of dyspnea. The increased ventilatory drive causes the patient to use the accessory muscles of breathing, such as the intercostals and abdominal muscles.

OUTCOME

Placing the patient on a positive-pressure ventilator restores ventilation to both lungs. The positive end-expiratory pressure enhances the opening of those alveoli in the left lung, which had collapsed. After surgical repair of the injury, negative intrathoracic pressure has to be created by suction in the left intrapleural space. The removal of the excess air in the left intrapleural space allows the visceral and parietal pleura to appose each other, restoring the normal coupling of the movement of the chest wall and the movement of lung tissue.

FURTHER READING

Web Sources
http://www.nlm.nih.gov/medlineplus/ency/article/000087.htm
http://www.intelihealth.com/IH/ihtIH/WSIHW000/9339/23667.html

Text Sources
Carroll RG: Elsevier's Integrated Physiology. Philadelphia, Elsevier, 2007.
Copstead L, Banasik J: Pathophysiology, 3rd ed. Philadelphia, Saunders, 2005.

Guyton AC, Hall JE: Textbook of Medical Physiology, 11th ed. Philadelphia, Saunders, 2006.
Lundgren C, Miller JN: The Lung at Depth. New York, Informa Healthcare, 1999.
Porth C: Pathophysiology, 7th ed. Philadelphia, Lippincott Williams & Wilkins, 2004.
McPhee SJ, Papadakis MA, Tierney LM Jr: Current Medical Diagnosis and Treatment, 46th ed. New York, McGraw-Hill, 2007.

A 10-year-old boy is brought to the emergency department because of difficulty breathing that developed during soccer practice.

The boy has a history of allergies, including a pollen allergy, but never previously showed this level of respiratory difficulty. He now complains of tightness in the chest. There is no family history of allergies or asthma. Both parents smoke cigarettes.

PHYSICAL EXAMINATION

VS: T 37°C, P 120/min, R 30/min and shallow, BP 110/95 mm Hg

PE: Patient is wheezing, anxious, and short of breath. The wheezing is more prominent on exhalation, and there is an extended forced expiratory phase. The chest anteroposterior diameter appears large for age and size. The nasal mucosa is edematous, and the pharynx is coated with a clear postnasal discharge. A beta$_2$-adrenergic agent was administered by an inhaler, and the symptoms quickly subsided. The patient's anxiety was relieved, and heart rate and breathing rate returned to normal. The patient was scheduled for pulmonary function tests.

LABORATORY STUDIES

Spirometry: Normal values. When challenged with methacholine, however, a hyperreactive bronchoconstriction occurred with decreased FEV$_1$, decreased forced vital capacity, and increased residual volume.

Forced spirometry flow/volume loop: Scooping, diminished peak flow.

DIAGNOSIS

Asthma

PATHOPHYSIOLOGY OF KEY SYMPTOMS

Asthma is characterized by a chronic inflammation of the pulmonary airways. The bronchiolar smooth muscle becomes hyperresponsive to allergens, irritants, or other agents. Exposure to these substances triggers a strong bronchoconstriction. The symptoms of an asthmatic attack result from the bronchoconstriction and are characteristic of an "obstructive" pulmonary disease. The bronchoconstriction, inflammation, and excess mucus all act to obstruct the lumen of the bronchioles.

The increased resistance to airflow in the bronchioles accounts for the wheezing, abnormal spirometry volumes, and shortness of breath.

Wheezing is due to the premature closing of airways during expiration. During inspiration, the negative intrapleural pressure helps to expand both the alveoli and the small pulmonary bronchioles. Consequently, inflation of the lungs is not diminished during an asthmatic attack. During exhalation, however, contraction of the accessory respiratory muscles acts to increase pleural pressure. This increased pleural pressure provides an external compression of the small bronchioles. Airflow past these narrowed airways can be heard as a wheeze that is more prominent during exhalation.

Increased resistance to airflow through the narrowed airways also causes a diminished peak expiratory flow rate. In spirometry, the same effect is indicated by a diminished FEV$_1$. During active exhalation, the increase in pleural pressure is acting to collapse the airways. Consequently, additional respiratory effort does not result in improved exhalation volumes (Fig. 32-1).

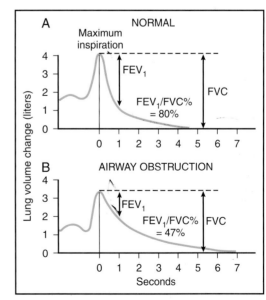

FIGURE 32–1 Recordings during the forced vital capacity maneuver in a healthy person (**A**) and in a person with partial airway obstruction (**B**). (The "zero" on the volume scale is residual volume.)

Airway resistance has its greatest impact at the moment of change between inspiration and expiration. Once air is moving, the influence of airway resistance is not as great. Therefore, the maximum respiratory efficiency (air exchange for the muscle effort) occurs with slower breathing rates and increased tidal volumes. Unfortunately, impaired ventilation during an asthmatic attack usually causes the sympathetic nervous system activation, with an increased respiratory rate and decreased tidal volume.

During an asthmatic attack, inhalation is slightly diminished by the bronchoconstriction but the exhalation is impaired because of the collapse of the small and mid-sized airways. The trachea and large bronchi remain open because of the structure from the cartilage. Consequently, a small additional volume is trapped in the lungs during each respiratory cycle. The cumulative effect is that the total lung volume is increased, but most of this increase occurs because of the increased residual volume. Increased total lung volume can be apparent in a physical examination by increased anteroposterior chest diameter and contributes to the sense of "tightness of the chest" during the attack.

Acute relief of symptoms is achieved by administering bronchodilators, such as beta$_2$-adrenergic agents. Chronic relief of symptoms involved diminishing the response to allergens or irritants. Generic anti-inflammatory agents, such as corticosteroids, reduce inflammation and consequently diminish the frequency and severity of future attacks. Corticosteroid treatment may be augmented with long-acting beta$_2$ agonists, leukotrienes inhibitors, or theophylline.

OUTCOME

Asthma can be managed and monitored. Management involves reducing the change of exposure to allergens or irritants and diminishing the airway constriction that occurs when exposures do occur. The degree of bronchoconstriction can be assessed on a chronic basis by monitoring the peak expiratory flow rate, a relatively easy assessment that the patient can do at home.

FURTHER READING

Web Sources

http://www.nhlbi.nih.gov/health/dci/Diseases/Asthma/Asthma_WhatIs.html

http://www.nlm.nih.gov/medlineplus/tutorials/asthma/htm/lesson.htm

Birnbaum S, Barreiro TJ: Methacholine challenge testing. Chest 131:1932-1935, 2007. Available at www.chestjournal.org/cgi/content/abstract/131/6/1932

Juniper EF, Johnston PR, Borkhoff CM, et al: Quality of life in asthma clinical trials: comparison of salmeterol and salbutamol. Am J Respir Crit Care Med 151:66-70, 1995. Available at www.ajrccm.atsjournals.org/cgi/content/abstract/151/1/66

Text Sources

Carroll RG: Elsevier's Integrated Physiology. Philadelphia, Elsevier, 2007.

Copstead L, Banasik J: Pathophysiology, 3rd ed. Philadelphia, Saunders, 2005.

Flores G, Abreu M, Tomany-Korman S, et al: Keeping children with asthma out of hospitals: parents' and physicians' perspectives on how pediatric asthma hospitalizations can be prevented. Pediatrics 116:957-965, 2005.

Garcia Garcia ML, Wahn U, Gilles L, et al: Montelukast, compared with fluticasone, for control of asthma among 6- to 14-year-old patients with mild asthma: The MOSAIC study. Pediatrics 116:360-369, 2005.

Guyton AC, Hall JE: Textbook of Medical Physiology, 11th ed. Philadelphia, Saunders, 2006.

McPhee SJ, Papadakis MA, Tierney LM Jr: Current Medical Diagnosis and Treatment, 46th ed. New York, McGraw-Hill, 2007.

A 38-year-old man is transported to the emergency department after being found unconscious and in respiratory depression in his apartment.

The paramedics intubate the patient and manually ventilate him with an Ambu bag. The patient is transported to the emergency department. On arrival, an arterial blood sample is obtained for blood gas analysis and for drug screen. The patient is placed on a ventilator with supplemental oxygen.

PHYSICAL EXAMINATION

VS: T 32.5°C, P 55/min, R 8/min, BP 80/50 mm Hg
PE: Patient is in a coma and does not respond to painful stimuli. Pupils are small and reactive. Muscle tone is flaccid, and the deep tendon reflexes are depressed. There is a positive Babinski sign (toes curled outward).

LABORATORY STUDIES

On arrival:

- Arterial blood gases: Po_2 60 mm Hg, Pco_2 80 mm Hg, HCO_3^- 26 mEq/L, pH 7.22
- Drug screen: Positive for short-acting barbiturate
- Pulse oximetry: 50% saturated

15 minutes after arrival (while being ventilated with supplemental oxygen):

- Arterial blood gases: Po_2 195 mm Hg, Pco_2 34 mm Hg, HCO_3^- 22 mEq/L, pH 7.48

DIAGNOSIS

Barbiturate overdose

PATHOPHYSIOLOGY OF KEY SYMPTOMS

The primary symptoms for this patient are due to the barbiturate-induced depression of the central nervous system. The brain stem, including the respiratory centers, along with the reticular activating system, the cerebellum, and the cerebral cortex are particularly sensitive to the depressant effects of barbiturates.

The rhythmic pattern of breathing is initiated in the pons and medulla of the brain stem. The dorsal respiratory neurons in the nucleus of the tractus solitarius generate a basic inspiratory respiratory rhythm. The pneumotaxic center of the pons controls the rate and the pattern of respiration. The brain stem control of breathing is modulated by ascending input from the carotid and aortic chemoreceptors, by input from the medullary chemoreceptors, and by descending input from the motor cortex, limbic system, and autonomic nervous system.

Central nervous system depression diminishes or completely abolishes ventilation. Hypoventilation impairs alveolar gas exchange, resulting in an increase in carbon dioxide levels and a decrease in oxygen levels. Normally, hypercapnia and hypoxia, working through the aortic and carotid chemoreceptors, should stimulate an increase in ventilation. Because of the central nervous system depression, this homeostatic control mechanism is not functioning.

Naloxone will help to block the action of opiates, which are commonly found in overdoses. There is no direct antidote to barbiturate overdose, so ventilation must be artificially maintained until the drugs are cleared from the body.

Advanced trauma life support (ATLS) guidelines, created by the American College of Surgeons, recommend the standard approach to assessing trauma victims based on the acronym ABCDE:

A = airway
B = breathing
C = circulation
D = neurologic disability
E = environment

The rescue squad initiated this sequence, first establishing a secure airway and then by beginning to bag-ventilate the patient.

On arriving at the hospital, the initial arterial blood gas values show a pronounced respiratory acidosis, indicated by the significantly elevated Pco_2 levels. As the patient is more appropriately ventilated, by 15 minutes the Pco_2 levels have fallen slightly below normal, indicating that the patient is now being hyperventilated.

The arterial blood oxygen levels on arrival also indicate an underventilation. The 15-minute blood gas level, however, now shows a greatly elevated Po_2. This elevation is due to supplementing inspired air with oxygen. The high Po_2 levels, however, do

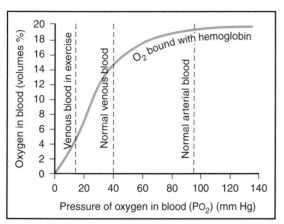

FIGURE 33–1 Effect of blood P_{O_2} on the quantity of oxygen bound with hemoglobin in each 100 mL of blood.

not represent much of an increase in arterial oxygen content, because the hemoglobin is fully saturated at a P_{O_2} about 100 mm Hg (Fig. 33-1).

The patient also shows neurologic and neuromuscular signs consistent with depression of neuronal function. This includes flaccid muscle tone and the depression of the deep tendon reflexes. The Babinski sign indicates the loss of motor cortex control of the muscles of the foot, usually indicating damage or depression of the pyramidal tract. After 2 years of age, maturation of central nervous system control results in the loss of the Babinski sign, so that stroking of the foot causes the toes to curl inward. Prior to 2 years of age, or in an individual with impaired motor cortex control, stroking of the foot will cause the toes to fan outward.

OUTCOME

The patient was administered 50% dextrose and naloxone (Narcan).

FURTHER READING

Web Sources

http://www.facs.org/trauma/atls/index.html
Barbiturate overdose. Available at National Institutes of Health. www.nlm.nih.gov.
http://www.nlm.nih.gov/medlineplus/ency/article/000951.htm
University of Maryland Medical Center. Barbiturate intoxication and overdose. Available at http://www.umm.edu/ency/article/000951trt.htm

Text Sources

Barile FA: Clinical Toxicology. New York, Informa Healthcare, 2004.

Carroll RG: Elsevier's Integrated Physiology. Philadelphia, Elsevier, 2007.
Copstead L, Banasik J: Pathophysiology, 3rd ed. Philadelphia, Saunders, 2005.
Guyton AC, Hall JE: Textbook of Medical Physiology, 11th ed. Philadelphia, Saunders, 2006.
Hall JB, Schmidt GA, Wood LDH: Principles of Critical Care, 3rd ed. New York, McGraw-Hill, 2005.
McPhee SJ, Papadakis MA, Tierney LM Jr: Current Medical Diagnosis and Treatment, 46th ed. New York, McGraw-Hill, 2007.

A 62-year-old man comes to the ski resort clinic on a mountain peak (14,000 ft) complaining of dyspnea, headache, dizziness, and inability to sleep. He was short of breath while climbing the stairs at the lodge and noticed that he was breathing rapidly even when sitting down.

The patient arrived at the resort yesterday from a sea-level town and reports no current health issues or medications. He plans to remain at the resort for a week.

PHYSICAL EXAMINATION

VS: T 37°C, P 80/min, R 42/min, BP 110/80 mm Hg, BMI 26
PE: Patient has a rapid, shallow breathing pattern. Pulse is slightly elevated. Fingernails show slight cyanosis.

LABORATORY STUDIES

End-tidal gases: P_{O_2} 60 mm Hg, P_{CO_2} 30 mm Hg
Pulse oximetry: 70% saturated

DIAGNOSIS

Acute mountain sickness

COURSE

Severe cases of acute mountain sickness can lead to high-altitude pulmonary edema (HAPE), characterized by crackles in the lungs and further impaired oxygen uptake. In addition, high-altitude cerebral edema (HACE) can develop and become life threatening.

PATHOPHYSIOLOGY OF KEY SYMPTOMS

The initiating event is the arterial hypoxia caused by the decline in inspired O_2 due to the drop in barometric pressure. At 14,000 ft, inspired air has a P_{O_2} of approximately 93 mm Hg and alveolar air has a P_{O_2} of around 55 mm Hg (Table 34-1).

Ventilation is controlled by respiratory centers in the pons and the medulla. The intrinsic activity of the respiratory centers is altered by both descending input from the higher brain areas and negative feedback control from peripheral and central chemoreceptors. The central chemoreceptors respond only to CO_2/pH, and the peripheral chemoreceptors respond both to CO_2/pH and to O_2. At rest, negative feedback control of ventilation is tied to CO_2 levels. Hypoxia only becomes a significant ventilatory stimulus when P_{O_2} levels drop below 60 mm Hg.

An end-tidal gas measurement indicates that the alveolar P_{O_2} in this patient is 60 mm Hg. Arterial blood gas values will be even lower because of venous admixture. This level of hypoxia is sufficient to stimulate the arterial chemoreceptors and cause an increase in ventilation. Hyperventilation leads to a drop in CO_2 levels, and the patient will have a mild respiratory alkalosis. The hypocapnia removes some of the normal

			Breathing Air			Breathing Pure Oxygen		
Altitude (ft)	Barometric Pressure (mm Hg)	P_{O_2} in Air (mm Hg)	P_{CO_2} in Alveoli (mm Hg)	P_{O_2} in Alveoli (mm Hg)	Arterial Oxygen Saturation (%)	P_{CO_2} in Alveoli (mm Hg)	P_{O_2} in Alveoli (mm Hg)	Arterial Oxygen Saturation (%)
0	760	159	40 (40)	104 (104)	97 (97)	40	673	100
10,000	523	110	36 (23)	67 (77)	90 (92)	40	436	100
20,000	349	73	24 (10)	40 (53)	73 (85)	40	262	100
30,000	226	47	24 (7)	18 (30)	24 (38)	40	139	99
40,000	141	29				36	58	84
50,000	87	18				24	16	15

TABLE 34-1 Effects of Acute Exposure to Low Atmospheric Pressures on Alveolar Gas Concentrations and Arterial Oxygen Saturation*

*Numbers in parentheses are acclimatized values.

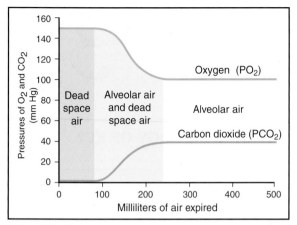

FIGURE 34–1 Partial pressures of oxygen and carbon dioxide in the various portions of normal expired air.

respiratory drive from CO_2, and the increase in ventilation is attenuated but remains elevated compared with sea level (Fig. 34-1).

The headache is chiefly the result of changes in cerebral blood flow and dehydration. Hypocapnia normally causes cerebral vasoconstriction. When arterial Po_2 falls below 60 mm Hg, however, the cerebral vasculature remains dilated. This produces an increase in intracranial pressure that, if left unchecked, causes high-altitude cerebral edema. Ascent to altitude causes an increase in urinary excretion of water and sodium. This natriuresis and diuresis causes a loss of body fluid volume, accentuating the headache.

The dizziness is a result of the hypoxia and is compounded by cerebral vasodilation caused by the drop in CO_2. Diminished cerebral blood flow contributes to the headache.

The difficulty sleeping can be a result of hypoxia causing the patient to awaken intermittently or possibly from a Cheyne-Stokes breathing pattern. In this pattern, there is a 1- to 5-minute cycling of deep and shallow breathing. Respirations gradually increase in intensity and then diminish to a very low level, before beginning the cycle again. The major cause of this breathing is a time delay between when the blood passes through the alveoli and when it reaches the chemoreceptors. This breathing pattern is common at very high altitudes and is also characteristic of low cardiac output states.

If altitude sickness is life threatening, immediate action must be taken. The simplest treatment is to return to lower altitudes or simulate lower altitudes in a hyperbaric chamber. Supplemental inspired oxygen should be provided. If that is not an option, a carbonic anhydrase inhibitor (acetazolamide) may be used to correct the respiratory acidosis and may relieve some symptoms. Acetazolamide is also a diuretic, and increased fluid intake may be necessary to prevent dehydration.

OUTCOME

Acetazolamide (250 mg bid, PO) was started along with a recommended increase in fluid intake, and the symptoms gradually subsided. After 2 days of rest, the patient was able to resume his vacation.

FURTHER READING

Web Source
Honig A: Peripheral arterial chemoreceptors and reflex control of sodium and water homeostasis. Am J Physiol Reg Integ Comp Physiol 257(6): 1282-1302, 1989. Available at http://ajpregu. physiology.org/cgi/content/abstract/257/6/R1282

Text Sources
Auerbach PS: Wilderness Medicine, 5th ed. St. Louis, Mosby, 2007.
Carroll RG: Elsevier's Integrated Physiology. Philadelphia, Elsevier, 2007.
Copstead L, Banasik J: Pathophysiology, 3rd ed. Philadelphia, Saunders, 2005.
Feddersen B, et al: Right temporal cerebral dysfunctions herald symptoms of acute mountain sickness. J Neurol 254:359-363.
Guyton AC, Hall JE: Textbook of Medical Physiology, 11th ed. Philadelphia, Saunders, 2006.
Marx JA, Hockberger RS, Walls RM: Rosen's Emergency Medicine: Concepts and Clinical Practice, 6th ed. St. Louis, Mosby, 2006.
McPhee SJ, Papadakis MA, Tierney LM Jr: Current Medical Diagnosis and Treatment, 46th ed. New York, McGraw-Hill, 2007.

A 68-year-old man comes to the clinic complaining of difficulty in breathing.

The patient suffered a myocardial infarction involving the anterior wall of the left ventricle 6 months earlier. Myocardial injury reduced the ventricular ejection fraction to 40%. During the past month, the patient has gained 8 pounds. He indicates that he has difficulty sleeping when lying down, which has been getting worse over the past month.

55–70%

test determines how well heart beats pumps w/

PHYSICAL EXAMINATION *12–20*

VS: T 37°C, P 80/min, R 26/min and shallow, BP 100/65 mm Hg

PE: Inspiratory crackles are present, particularly at the base of the lungs. The patient's fingernails have a slight cyanotic color. Supplemental O$_2$ was initiated.

LABORATORY STUDIES

ECG: Normal sinus rhythm, evidence of past myocardial infarction

Ultrasonography: Enlarged left atrium and pulmonary vein *95–100%*

Pulse oximetry: 70% at arrival, 97% after beginning supplemental O$_2$

Chest radiography: Blurry fluid build-up in the lung space appearing in a typical "butterfly" shape

DIAGNOSIS

Pulmonary edema

PATHOPHYSIOLOGY OF KEY SYMPTOMS

Pulmonary edema occurs when the net volume of plasma filtered through the pulmonary capillaries exceeds the ability of the pulmonary lymphatic vessels to transport the fluid back to the vascular system. Accumulation of fluid in the pulmonary interstitium increases the distance between the alveoli and the pulmonary capillaries and, consequently, impairs gas diffusion.

Fluid exchange across the pulmonary capillaries is governed by the same balance of hydrostatic pressures and protein-mediated oncotic pressure as occurs in other capillary beds. The relatively low pulmonary capillary pressure (normally 10 to 15 mm Hg) results in the net balance for fluid exchange across the pulmonary capillaries favoring reabsorption. Consequently,

there is normally very little free fluid in the pulmonary interstitial space (Fig. 35-1).

Events that result in an increase in pulmonary capillary pressure, however, shift this balance. An increase in pulmonary capillary pressure above 25 mm Hg results in the formation of pulmonary edema. The most common cause of increased pulmonary capillary pressure is impaired pumping of the left ventricle, such as occurs after a myocardial infarction. Impaired pumping of the left ventricle decreases renal perfusion pressure, resulting in the renal retention of sodium and water. This increase in body fluid volume contributes to the progression of pulmonary edema. The resultant accumulation of fluid in the lungs is sometimes called pulmonary congestion, and the heart failure is characterized as congestive heart failure. *renal failure*

The major symptom of pulmonary edema is difficulty in breathing. Fluid accumulation in the lungs stimulates pulmonary "J receptors," contributing to the sensation of dyspnea. Fluid distribution within the thoracic space is influenced by gravity and the body position. When upright, fluid tends to

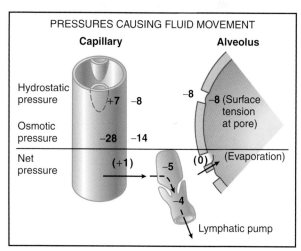

FIGURE 35–1 Hydrostatic and osmotic forces at the capillary *(left)* and alveolar membrane *(right)* of the lungs. Also shown is the tip end of a lymphatic vessel *(center)* that pumps fluid from the pulmonary interstitial spaces. *(Modified from Guyton AC, Taylor AE, Granger HJ: Circulatory Physiology II: Dynamics and Control of the Body Fluids. Philadelphia, WB Saunders, 1975.)*

accumulate predominantly in the basal portions of the lungs, allowing relatively unimpeded air exchange in the apical areas of the lungs. In a recumbent position, the edema fluid distributes more evenly through the lung tissue, resulting in a greater impairment of gas exchange. Consequently, individuals with pulmonary edema often report difficulty in sleeping because of dyspnea and rely on pillows or sleeping in chairs to maintain an upright position.

Impaired diffusion impacts oxygen exchange more than carbon dioxide exchange. Patients with pulmonary edema become hypoxic but not hypercapnic. This is because oxygen is much less soluble in water than is carbon dioxide. In this patient, the hypoxia is indicated by the low pulse oximetry reading. Provision of supplemental oxygen increases alveolar P_{O_2} sufficiently to overcome the diffusion impairment caused by the increased distance.

CO₂ is more easily diffused

OUTCOME

Treatment is started by administering oxygen via nasal mask or nasal cannula. Additional treatment involves the use of diuretics (preload reducers) to lower body fluid volume and, consequently, pulmonary capillary pressure. Diminished body fluid volume, however, also results in a lower arterial blood pressure. Treatment of patients with impaired left ventricular function requires balancing the risks of pulmonary edema if body fluid volume becomes too high or of hypotension and myocardial ischemia if body fluid volume becomes too low. Afterload reducers (Vasotec, Capoten) may also help by dilating the peripheral vessels and reducing the arterial blood pressure.

FURTHER READING

Web Sources
http://www.mayoclinic.com/health/pulmonary-edema/DS00412/DSECTION=1
http://www.nlm.nih.gov/medlineplus/ency/article/000140.htm

Text Sources
Blanchard R, Loeb SE: Heart Failure in Pulmonary Edema. Clifton Park, NY, Delmar, 2000.
Carroll RG: Elsevier's Integrated Physiology. Philadelphia, Elsevier, 2007.

Copstead L, Banasik J: Pathophysiology, 3rd ed. Philadelphia, Saunders, 2005.
Guyton AC, Hall JE: Textbook of Medical Physiology, 11th ed. Philadelphia, Saunders, 2006.
McPhee SJ, Papadakis MA, Tierney LM Jr: Current Medical Diagnosis and Treatment, 46th ed. New York, McGraw-Hill, 2007.
West JB: Pulmonary Pathophysiology: The Essentials, 7th ed. Philadelphia, Lippincott Williams & Wilkins, 2007.

A 28-year-old man is brought to the emergency department complaining of headache, vertigo, dizziness, and confusion.

It was a cold winter evening. The patient lives alone in a rural area and was using a kerosene heater to heat his house. He was found by a neighbor walking outside the house without a jacket. There was an odor of kerosene and some smoke in the house.

PHYSICAL EXAMINATION

VS: T 35°C, P 90/min, R 22/min, BP 120/90 mm Hg
PE: The patient remains confused and complains of chest pain and weakness.

LABORATORY STUDIES

Arterial blood gases: Po_2 95 mm Hg, Pco_2 40 mm Hg, pH 7.4
Mixed venous blood gases: Po_2 22 mm Hg, Pco_2 43 mm Hg, pH 7.37
Carboxyhemoglobin level: 40%
Hematocrit: 42%
Arterial O_2 content: Estimated at 12 mL O_2/dL blood

DIAGNOSIS

Carbon monoxide poisoning

PATHOPHYSIOLOGY OF KEY SYMPTOMS

The major symptoms for this patient are due to central nervous system hypoxia. The hypoxia is caused by the defect in oxygen delivery to the brain from the low arterial blood oxygen content.

Oxygen is transported in the blood through two separate mechanisms. Oxygen dissolves in the plasma of the blood in proportion to the oxygen partial pressure. Normal alveolar Po_2 is around 100 mm Hg, and, assuming no abnormalities in diffusion, the Po_2 of the blood in the pulmonary capillary is also around 100 mm Hg. Blood in the pulmonary vein has a slightly lower Po_2 because of venous admixture from relatively oxygen depleted blood from the bronchial circulation. Therefore, normal arterial Po_2 is 95 to 100 mm Hg.

The amount of oxygen that can be dissolved in the plasma is not sufficient to support life.

Hemoglobin contained within the red blood cells is the primary oxygen transport mechanism, accounting

for approximately 98% of the oxygen dissolved in arterial blood. Each hemoglobin protein can bind up to four oxygen molecules. The shape of the oxygen-hemoglobin dissociation curve reflects the very high affinity of hemoglobin for oxygen. At a normal arterial Po_2 of 100 mm Hg, the oxygen binding sites on hemoglobin are 98% saturated. At a normal venous Po_2 of 40 mm Hg, the oxygen binding sites on hemoglobin are still 75% saturated (see Fig. 33-1).

The arterial oxygen content, therefore, is a function primarily of the amount of oxygen bound to hemoglobin. A drop in hematocrit, or a chemical change in hemoglobin that interferes with oxygen binding, can result in a decrease in the amount of oxygen bound to hemoglobin without interfering with the amount of oxygen dissolved in the plasma. Carbon monoxide binds to hemoglobin with an affinity 200 times greater than that of oxygen. Carboxyhemoglobin can no longer bind oxygen and, consequently, diminishes the total blood oxygen content.

The arterial Po_2 in this patient is normal, because the dissolved oxygen content came into equilibrium with the oxygen partial pressure of the alveoli. The aortic body and carotid body chemoreceptors sense the dissolved oxygen content, and, consequently, there is no ventilatory stimulus from hypoxia in this patient.

Mixed venous blood gas, however, shows a marked hypoxia. A small amount of dissolved oxygen in the plasma is not sufficient to support metabolism. In the systemic capillaries, oxygen is extracted from the plasma and then from the oxygen stores' remaining functional hemoglobin molecules. The hypoxia in the mixed venous blood gas sample indicates that the tissues, including the central nervous system, are hypoxic. Central nervous system chemoreceptors only respond to CO_2/pH, and, consequently, there is no central chemoreceptor stimulation of ventilation in this patient. The defect in oxygen delivery also impairs oxygen utilization in the mitochondria and, thus, the body does not generate as much CO_2 from metabolism as is normal.

Because the defect is in the hemoglobin-carrying capacity and not hemoglobin percent saturation, an increase in ventilation would not lead to an increase in arterial blood oxygen content. The hemoglobin that is capable of binding oxygen is close to 100% saturated at a normal alveolar minute ventilation rate.

Restoration of oxygen delivery to the brain will result in a diminishing of this patient's symptoms. The defect in oxygen-carrying capacity, however, represents a significant barrier. Breathing 100% oxygen would increase fivefold the amount of oxygen dissolved in the plasma. This increase alone, however, would not be sufficient to support metabolism. Patients with severe carbon monoxide poisoning, where carboxyhemoglobin levels exceed 70%, are treated in a hyperbaric oxygen chamber. At the higher total barometric pressure, the dissolved oxygen can be sufficient to support basal metabolism.

Given time, carbon monoxide will disassociate from hemoglobin and hemoglobin-carrying capability can be restored. Alternatively, transfusion can be used to introduce normal hemoglobin into the patient to enhance the blood oxygen-carrying capacity.

FURTHER READING

Web Sources

Kao L, Nañagas K: Carbon monoxide poisoning. Med Clin North Am 89(6), 2005. Available at http://www.mdconsult.com.jproxy.lib.ecu.edu/das/article/body/79904162-7/jorg=clinics&source=MI&sp=17624236&sid=633469065/N/497894/1.html

McAuley D: Arterial oxygen content, 2005. Available at http://www.globalrph.com/arterial_oxygen_content.htm

Perez E: U.S. National Library of Medicine. Carbon monoxide. Accessed January 2007. Available at http://www.nlm.nih.gov/medlineplus/ency/article/002804.htm

Rutherford D: Carbon monoxide poisoning. Accessed February 2005. Available at http://www.netdoctor.co.uk/health_advice/facts/carbonmonoxide.htm

Text Sources

Carroll RG: Elsevier's Integrated Physiology. Philadelphia, Elsevier, 2007.

Copstead L, Banasik J: Pathophysiology, 3rd ed. Philadelphia, Saunders, 2005.

Guyton AC, Hall JE: Textbook of Medical Physiology, 11th ed. Philadelphia, Saunders, 2006.

McPhee SJ, Papadakis MA, Tierney LM Jr: Current Medical Diagnosis and Treatment, 46th ed. New York, McGraw-Hill, 2007.

A 57-year-old man comes to the cardiovascular rehabilitation clinic to begin an exercise program.

The patient suffered a myocardial infarction 3 months earlier and had a drug-eluting stent inserted into a branch of the left anterior descending coronary artery. Imaging indicates a recovery of myocardial blood flow, and the patient is counseled to begin an exercise program to strengthen his heart. The patient is able to walk at a brisk pace for 20 minutes. In contrast, jogging or climbing stairs causes him to become short of breath.

PHYSICAL EXAMINATION

VS: T 37°C, P 80/min, R 17/min, BP 130/90 mm Hg, BMI 33

PE: Scars on the leg from catheters used to guide the placement of the stent are healed. There are some crackles heard at the base of both lungs on inspiration.

Chest radiograph: Fluid accumulation in the base of the lungs

LABORATORY STUDIES

The patient begins a cardiovascular stress test on a treadmill during which the speed and inclination of the treadmill are increased every 10 minutes. Heart rate is monitored through an electrocardiogram, arterial oxygen saturation is monitored through a pulse oximeter, and blood pressure is taken at regular intervals.

At low exercise intensity, arterial pressure increases to 140/85 mm Hg, heart rate increases to 120 beats/min, and respiratory rate increases to 30/min. Pulse oximetry decreased to 95%. After 10 minutes, an increase in exercise intensity causes little change in arterial pressure but pulse oximetry fell to 91%. Ten minutes later, intensity level was again increased, and the exercise was stopped after 2 additional minutes. Respiratory rate was 30/min and pulse oximetry was 89% when the patient was stopped from exercising. The patient was monitored for an additional 20 minutes during the recovery phase from exercise.

DIAGNOSIS

Exercise intolerance

PATHOPHYSIOLOGY OF KEY SYMPTOMS

Exercise results in an increase in alveolar minute ventilation, usually from an increase both in frequency and depth of breathing.

Arterial blood gas values do not normally change during exercise. Consequently, the increasing ventilation during exercise is not mediated by the peripheral or central chemoreceptors. The majority of the increasing ventilation during exercise is mediated by the higher centers of the central nervous system, including the motor cortex (Fig. 37-1).

Alveolar minute ventilation is proportional to the intensity of the exercise. The increase in alveolar ventilation is not hyperventilation but rather is physiologically appropriate and is matched with the increase in carbon dioxide production by the exercising muscles.

Normally, blood passing through the pulmonary capillaries requires 0.25 second to come in equilibrium with alveolar gas. Even during strenuous exercise, blood remains in the pulmonary capillaries long enough to come into equilibrium.

The inspiratory crackles heard at the base of both lungs on inspiration in this patient is most likely due to pulmonary edema resulting from a myocardial

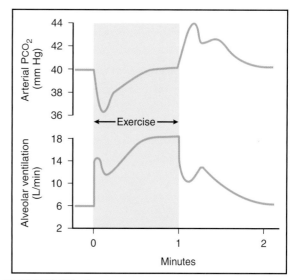

FIGURE 37–1 Changes in alveolar ventilation *(bottom curve)* and arterial Pco₂ *(top curve)* during a 1-minute period of exercise and also after termination of exercise. *(Extrapolated to the human being from data in dogs in Bainton CR: Effect of speed vs. grade and shivering on ventilation in dogs during active exercise. J Appl Physiol 33:778, 1972.)*

infarction. The patient should be given a diuretic to reduce body fluid volume as a first step in treating the edema.

In individuals with impaired diffusion capability, however, the blood in the pulmonary capillaries may not reach equilibrium with alveolar gas. Exercise increases the velocity of blood flow to the pulmonary circulation and, consequently, diminishes time for diffusion to occur. Thus, exercise may exacerbate the diffusion-limited gas exchange characteristic of early stages of pulmonary edema. The impairment of oxygen exchange is more apparent than that of carbon dioxide exchange, because oxygen is much less soluble in water than is carbon dioxide.

The impairment in oxygen exchange is reflected by the fall in the pulse oximetry values. During an exercise test, arterial oxygen saturation is closely monitored, and the exercise session is terminated once the patient's SaO_2 falls below 90%. Supplemental oxygen is provided to assist recovery in the postexercise period.

Impaired oxygen delivery to the tissues results in exercise intolerance. Consequently, an individual with either impaired cardiac function and/or impaired pulmonary function will not be able to exercise at a normal workload. When oxygen delivery is inadequate to support metabolic need, the tissues shift to an anaerobic metabolism for a short period of time, which generates an oxygen debt that must be repaid on cessation of exercise.

FURTHER READING

Text Sources

ACSM's Guidelines for Exercise Testing and Prescription, 7th ed. Philadelphia, Lippincott Williams & Wilkins, 2006.

Carroll RG: Elsevier's Integrated Physiology. Philadelphia, Elsevier, 2007.

Copstead L, Banasik J: Pathophysiology, 3rd ed. Philadelphia, Saunders, 2005.

Goldman L, Ausiello D: Cecil Medicine, 23rd ed. Philadelphia, Saunders, 2007.

Guyton AC, Hall JE: Textbook of Medical Physiology, 11th ed. Philadelphia, Saunders, 2006.

McPhee SJ, Papadakis MA, Tierney LM Jr: Current Medical Diagnosis and Treatment, 46th ed. New York, McGraw-Hill, 2007.

Silverman HM: The Pill Book, 12th ed. New York, Bantam, 2006.

A 17-year-old man is brought to the emergency department by his coworkers because of "abnormal behavior."

The patient is working for the summer in a plastics factory. He has been working there for 1 month, but today he appeared confused, sleepy, and complained of dizziness and headaches.

PHYSICAL EXAMINATION

VS: T 37°C, P 120/min, R 30/min and shallow, BP 100/90 mm Hg

PE: Skin appears unusually pink. Retinal arteries and veins both appear pink. Patient's mental status is confused and lethargic. He appears weak from a loss of muscle strength. A bitter almond smell is detected on the patient's breath.

LABORATORY STUDIES

Arterial blood gases: Po_2 105 mm Hg, Pco_2 18 mm Hg, pH 7.32, wide anion gap

Pulse oximetry: 98%

Mixed venous blood gases: Po_2 60 mm Hg, Pco_2 20 mm Hg, pH 7.30

Plasma lactate concentration: Elevated 18 mmol/L

Plasma analysis: Cyanide

DIAGNOSIS

Cyanide poisoning

PATHOPHYSIOLOGY OF KEY SYMPTOMS

Cyanide is used in the manufacture of plastics, pesticides, and photographic materials and, therefore, cyanide poisoning can occur in the factory setting. Cyanide poisons the mitochondria by binding to cytochrome oxidase, uncoupling the oxidative phosphorylation pathway by preventing electron transport. The mitochondria can no longer produce adenosine triphosphate (ATP), and the symptoms match those characteristic of other forms of hypoxia. One difference is the arterial blood gases in this case will show elevated Po_2 (because the body in not using it for metabolism) and diminished Pco_2 (because little is being produced). The mixed venous blood gases show an elevated O_2 because tissue extraction of O_2 is greatly diminished.

The diminished ATP production affects all organ systems, but the central nervous system is the primary target of cyanide toxicity. The impaired neuronal function results in altered mental status, including confusion, lethargy, dizziness, and headache. Higher concentrations of cyanide can result in convulsion, coma, and death. Diminished ATP availability to the skeletal muscle also results in muscle weakness.

Mixed venous blood Po_2 is elevated, and Pco_2 is low, owing to the lack of aerobic metabolism in the tissues. Arterial blood gas values show slightly elevated Po_2, reflecting a slight increase in alveolar Po_2 due to the fall in Pco_2. The arterial blood gas sample also shows diminished Pco_2, reflecting both the low Pco_2 of the blood entering the lungs and the small CO_2 exchange at the lungs.

The patient has a high respiratory rate from hypoxic stimulation of the arterial chemoreceptors. The arterial Po_2 is elevated, but the arterial chemoreceptors have to metabolize oxygen to sense Po_2 levels. Consequently, the cyanide disruption in chemoreceptor metabolism results in the chemoreceptor determination of hypoxia. Arterial CO_2 levels are low and thus do not contribute to the ventilatory drive that occurs after cyanide poisoning.

The patient exhibits a mild acidosis because anaerobic metabolism (lactic acidosis) is used as the remaining route for ATP production.

OUTCOME

Initial treatment is to supplement inspired O_2 to ensure any remaining functional mitochndria have O_2 available and to administer $NaHCO_3$ to correct the acidosis.

After confirmation of the presence of cyanide, a cyanide antidote kit is administered. This treatment consists of amyl nitrate inhalation, intravenous sodium nitrate, and intravenous sodium thiosulfate. The sodium nitrite reduces hemoglobin to form methemoglobin, and the methemoglobin has a higher affinity for cyanide than do the mitochondrial enzymes. Consequently, the cyanide is displaced from the cytochrome oxidase. The thiosulfate binds cyanide in a complex that is more easily excreted by the kidneys in the urine.

The U.S. Food and Drug Administration approved a new "Cyanokit" to treat cyanide poisoning in 2006. The kit contains the drug hydroxycobalamin, intravenous tubing, and a sterile spike for reconstituting the drug with saline. When cyanide is present, the drug in "Cyanokit" is converted to vitamin B_{12}. A side effect from this drug is red urine and skin. This new approach has the advantage in that methemoglobin is not formed and thus normal oxygen transport by the red blood cells is not impaired.

The patient was admitted to the hospital.

FURTHER READING

Web Sources

Martin C: Emergency Medicine 34(7):11, 2002. Available at http://www.emedmag.com/html/pre/ter/CT0702.asp

Treatment for cyanide poisoning receives FDA approval. 12/19/2006. http://www.fda.gov/bbs/topic/NEWS/2006/NEW01531.html

Text Sources

Carroll RG: Elsevier's Integrated Physiology. Philadelphia, Elsevier, 2007.

Copstead L, Banasik J: Pathophysiology, 3rd ed. Philadelphia, Saunders, 2005.

Guyton AC, Hall JE: Textbook of Medical Physiology, 11th ed. Philadelphia, Saunders, 2006.

McPhee SJ, Papadakis MA, Tierney LM Jr: Current Medical Diagnosis and Treatment, 46th ed. New York, McGraw-Hill, 2007.

Smith C, Marks A, Lieberman MA: Marks' Basic Medical Biochemistry: A Clinical Approach, 2nd ed. Philadelphia, Lippincott Williams & Wilkins, 2004.

A 66-year-old woman is brought into the clinic by her husband after she began to complain of severe chest pain exacerbated with inspiration.

The patient states that she began feeling pain in her chest and thought she was having a heart attack. She states that the pain was increased when she inhaled. She feels like she can't breathe and complains that her heart won't stop racing. Prior medical history reveals that she had been treated for clots in her legs 6 months ago. She states that she got better and stopped taking the warfarin she was prescribed because she didn't like the way it made her feel. She admits to having bouts of calf pain over the past few weeks but thought it was a result of her recent attempts to improve her health by taking evening walks.

PHYSICAL EXAMINATION

VS: T 37.2°C, P 95/min, R 26/min, BP 128/92 mm Hg, BMI 33

PE: Patient shows dyspnea with intermittent bouts of coughing. Grimacing is evident on inspiration with guarding action of holding chest. Auscultation of the lungs reveals significant rales. There is localized wheezing and a pleural friction rub.

LABORATORY STUDIES

Pulse oximetry: 85% oxygen saturation

ECG: Sinus tachycardia rhythm, S1Q3T3 (cor pulmonale) T-wave inversion in V_1 to V_4, and right ventricular strain

Chest radiograph: Elevated diaphragm, pleural effusion, atelectasis, and dilation of the pulmonary artery

Arterial blood gases: Po_2 95 mm Hg, Pco_2 40 mm Hg, pH 7.48

Expiratory end-tidal respiratory gases: Po_2 105 mm Hg and Pco_2 38 mm Hg

Ventilation/perfusion lung scan: Positive if more than two segmental perfusion defects in the presence of normal ventilation

Spiral CT: Positive for medium-sized pulmonary embolism

D-Dimer test: Positive (ELISA) if > 500 ng/mL D-dimer fragments present

Pulmonary angiography: Positive for medium-sized pulmonary embolism on the left side of chest

DIAGNOSIS

Pulmonary embolism

PATHOPHYSIOLOGY OF KEY SYMPTOMS

Pulmonary embolism forms in the venous side of the circulation and is the result of a blood clot becoming trapped in one of the branches of the pulmonary artery. Venous clots often lodge in the pulmonary blood vessels because the diameter of pulmonary blood vessels becomes progressively smaller in the pulmonary artery down to the alveolar capillaries. In contrast, clots formed on the left side of the heart or in the arterial circulation become lodged in a branch of the systemic circulation, occluding blood flow distal to the clot. For this patient, blockade of a region of the pulmonary vasculature creates a ventilation/perfusion mismatch.

The lack of gas exchange in the affected portions of the lung creates a physiologic dead space, an area that is ventilated but not perfused. Consequently, the end-tidal CO_2 levels are lower than the arterial CO_2 levels and the end tidal Po_2 levels are higher than the arterial Po_2. This is because the air in the physiologic dead space did not participate in gas exchange with blood flowing through the pulmonary vasculature.

The electrocardiogram findings are consistent with the pressure overload on the right side of the heart, often called right ventricular strain or cor pulmonale.

Obstruction of a region of the pulmonary vasculature does cause an increase in total pulmonary vascular resistance. Consequently, pulmonary artery blood pressure is elevated, and the chest radiographic shows dilation of the pulmonary artery. The elevation in pulmonary capillary blood pressure also increases fluid movement into the alveoli, resulting in atelectasis as well as the appearance of a small amount of blood in the sputum. The elevated pulmonary vascular pressure also leads to fluid accumulation in the pulmonary pleural space, known as a pleural effusion.

The blood that successfully transits the lungs does participate in normal gas exchange. Therefore, the arterial blood gas values and the pulse oximetry are within normal limits.

Imaging techniques confirm the diagnosis of pulmonary embolism. The spiral computed tomography (CT), in combination with intravenous contrast injection, provides a clear image of the area of reduced pulmonary perfusion. The most reliable test for ruling out pulmonary embolism is pulmonary angiography.

FURTHER READING

Web Sources

Feied C, Handler JA: Pulmonary Embolism. E Medicine. Accessed June 2006. Available at http://www.emedicine.com/emerg/topic490.htm

Pulmonary embolism. Mayo Foundation for Medical Education and Research. Accessed September 2007. Available at http://www.mayoclinic.com/health/pulmonary-embolism/DS00429

Text Sources

Carroll RG: Elsevier's Integrated Physiology. Philadelphia, Elsevier, 2007.

Copstead L, Banasik J: Pathophysiology, 3rd ed. Philadelphia, Saunders, 2005.

Dudek RW, Louis TM: High-Yield Gross Anatomy, 3rd ed. Philadelphia, Lippincott Williams & Wilkins, 2007.

Guyton AC, Hall JE: Textbook of Medical Physiology, 11th ed. Philadelphia, Saunders, 2006.

McPhee SJ, Papadakis MA, Tierney LM Jr: Current Medical Diagnosis and Treatment, 46th ed. New York, McGraw-Hill, 2007.

Silverthorn DU: Human Physiology: An Integrated Approach, 4th ed. Upper Saddle River, NJ, Pearson/Benjamin Cummings, 2007.

A 24-year-old man presents to his primary care physician complaining of fever and chills that have persisted for 1 week.

During this time, the patient has had an unproductive cough and shortness of breath when he exerts himself. His chest now hurts when he coughs, and the sputum has a greenish tint. He has a general feeling of malaise and has noticed a decrease in appetite. He has been using an over-the-counter cold medicine for symptom relief, but symptoms return when the medication wears off. The patient has been working outside on a construction job this winter and is under a lot of stress with the recent move into a new apartment with his pregnant wife.

PHYSICAL EXAMINATION

VS: T 40°C, P 90/min, R 25/min, BP 112/70 mm Hg
PE: Physical appearance includes a pale sunken face. Breathing pattern is rapid and shallow, with some dyspnea during deep breaths. There are altered breath sounds and rales in the upper right lobe noted during chest auscultation. The upper right lobe is also dull to percussion. An increase in fremitus is evident. Cough produces green/yellow sputum.

LABORATORY STUDIES

Pulse oximetry: 90% saturation on room air
Chest radiograph: Segmented lobe infiltrate
Gram stain: Numerous gram-positive diplococci along with polymorphonuclear leukocytes suggesting infection with *Streptococcus pneumoniae*

DIAGNOSIS

Pneumonia

PATHOPHYSIOLOGY OF KEY SYMPTOMS

Bacteria can be transported into the alveoli during inhalation. Once the bacteria colonize the alveoli, bacteria cross the alveoli and enter the body, triggering an immune system response, particularly among the neutrophils. The neutrophils phagocytize the bacteria and destroy them. Neutrophils damaged during this process also rupture and set up an inflammatory response. Cytokines released from the neutrophils cause the fever and chills.

The inflammatory response leads to fluid accumulation within the alveoli. Filling of the alveolar space with fluid results in the altered breath sounds and the dullness to percussion and is visible on the radiograph. Mucous fluid in the airways contributes to the rales.

Gas exchange requires air to enter the alveolar space. Air cannot enter the fluid-filled alveoli, and thus air exchange is limited. This is reflected by a drop in arterial P_{O_2} and an increase in arterial P_{CO_2}. The drop in arterial P_{O_2} is also indicated by the decreased pulse oximetry reading.

Hypoxia and hypercapnia provide a ventilatory stimulus at both the peripheral chemoreceptors, augmented by the hypercapnic response in the central nervous system chemoreceptors. Consolidation of the lungs, however, impairs chest wall expansion, creating a restrictive lung disease. The most characteristic breathing pattern for an individual with a restrictive lung disease is rapid shallow breathing, along with an impaired ability to inspire or with pain associated with deep inspiration. Spirometry if measured would show low tidal volume and low vital capacity, but the FEV_1 (as a percent of forced vital capacity) would be normal. The individual can only move a portion of his predicted vital capacity, but the portion that he is able to move can be moved quickly, because there is no airway restriction.

OUTCOME

Acute bacterial pneumonia in an otherwise healthy 24-year-old man can be treated with oral antibiotics, rest, fluid, and home care.

FURTHER READING

Web Sources

www.nlm.nih.gov/medlineplus/pneumonia.html
www.mayoclinic.com/health/pneumonia/DS00135

Text Sources

Carroll RG: Elsevier's Integrated Physiology. Philadelphia, Elsevier, 2007.
Copstead L, Banasik J: Pathophysiology, 3rd ed. Philadelphia, Saunders, 2005.

Guyton AC, Hall JE: Textbook of Medical Physiology, 11th ed. Philadelphia, Saunders, 2006.
McPhee SJ, Papadakis MA, Tierney LM Jr: Current Medical Diagnosis and Treatment, 46th ed. New York, McGraw-Hill, 2007.

Section VI

Neurology

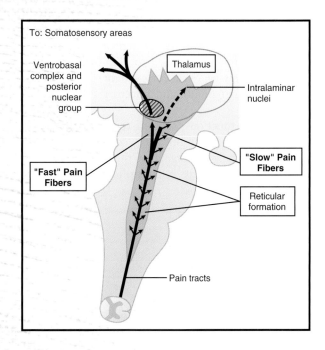

The nervous system is the dominant controller of physiologic function and, along with the endocrine system, regulates the activity of all other organ systems. The peripheral nervous system consists of the specialized sensory receptors, the afferent nerves that lead to the spinal cord, and the alpha motor and autonomic efferent nerves that innervate skeletal muscle, the vasculature, and most other organs. The central nervous system consists of the neurons and supporting cells of the spinal cord and brain.

Specialized receptors transduce inputs of light, sound, touch, proprioception, taste, pain, and temperature. This sensory information is transmitted by action potentials along afferent nerves through the dorsal roots to the spinal cord (see Case 51). In the spinal cord, the sensory information is integrated and either acted on (spinal reflexes) or transmitted to the brain in specialized nerve tracts (see Case 49) (Fig VI-1). The majority of sensory information is filtered before it ascends to the somatosensory cortex (pain, touch); visual cortex (light) (see Case 42); auditory cortex (sound); and olfactory cortex (smell, taste).

Vegetative functions, such as regulation of blood pressure and respiration, are controlled in the pons and medulla oblongata of the brain stem (see Case 41). Temperature is controlled by clusters of neurons within the hypothalamus. The efferent arm of the control is the sympathetic and parasympathetic branches of the autonomic nervous system.

Voluntary movement involves a complex interaction of numerous brain regions, stimulation of the primary motor cortex, and outflow along the corticospinal and corticorubrospinal pathways to the alpha-motor neurons (see Case 50). Case 41 contains additional details of the outflow along the alpha-motor neurons to the muscle cells.

An early step in voluntary movement is activation of the somatosensory cortex. The planning centers of the premotor cortex need information about where the body is in space to plan movement efficiently (see Case 47). The cortical association areas also interact with the basal ganglia nuclei (see Case 44) and the cerebellum, all of which contribute to the output to the primary motor cortex. During movement, the cerebellum is primarily responsible for continuous modulation of the activity (see Case 43), integrating input from the visual cortex, somatosensory cortex, vestibular system (see Case 48), and motor cortex.

Learning and memory involve the amygdala, cerebellum, basal ganglia, and medial temporal lobe of the cortex (see Cases 45 and 46). The complex traits of personality involve large areas of the brain but, in particular, the prefrontal cortex.

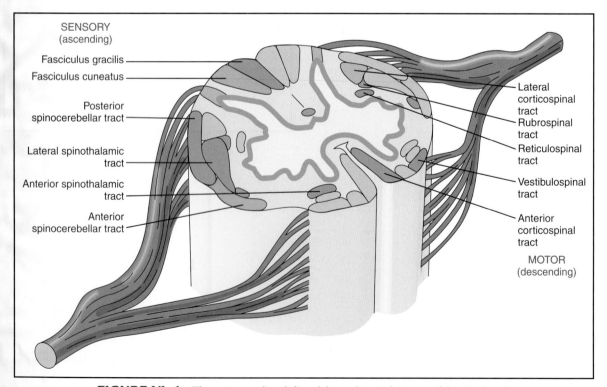

FIGURE VI–1 The main ascending (left) and descending (right) tracts of the spinal cord.

A 19-year-old male college student is transported to the emergency department by ambulance after hitting his head in a fall from a balcony.

The student had been leaning over the balcony and fell approximately 12 feet to a carpeted floor. Witnesses indicate that he landed on his head and shoulder and immediately lost consciousness. The paramedics were called at once and, when they arrived, found the student not breathing and unresponsive to verbal commands. The patient was intubated and ventilated. His head and neck were immobilized and he was transported to the emergency department. The patient is not on any medications and has no known health problems.

PHYSICAL EXAMINATION

VS: T 34°C, P 15/min, R 10/min, BP 60/30 mm Hg
PE: Patient unresponsive, and in decerebrate posture, extension and adduction of the arms, legs and feet extended. Pupils fixed and dilated bilaterally. Glasgow Coma Scale score: 3 (severe) (normal: 15)

LABORATORY STUDIES

Radiographs of head and cervical spine: Compression fracture of the skull overlying the temporal lobe

DIAGNOSIS

Traumatic injury (coma)

PATHOPHYSIOLOGY OF KEY SYMPTOMS

Traumatic brain injury incapacitates neuronal function at all levels. In this case, fracture of the temporal bone likely produced a tear in the middle meningeal artery of the dura. This arterial hemorrhage can produce an epidural hematoma that expands rapidly.

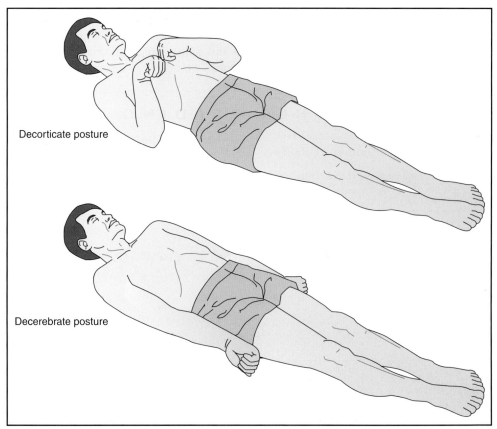

Decorticate posture

Decerebrate posture

FIGURE 41–1 Abnormal motor activity with coma. Decorticate posturing is indicated by flexed wrist and arm and extended legs and feet. Decerebrate posturing is indicated by arm and leg extension.

This emergent situation, if not treated immediately, can result in herniation of the temporal lobes through the tentorial notch of the dura, resulting in pressure on the brain stem and its arterial supply and in damage to the brain stem. The lack of consciousness indicates malfunction of the cerebral cortex; the lack of breathing and the lack of eye reflexes indicates disruption of brain stem activities.

The brain stem controls the normal homeostatic functions of the body. Anatomically, it is continuous with the spinal cord and consists of the medulla oblongata, the pons, and the midbrain. The brain stem serves as a conduit for both afferent and efferent nerves that connect the spinal cord to the cortex and cerebellum. The medulla oblongata integrates many reflex activities, including coughing, gagging, swallowing, and vomiting. Nuclei in the medulla oblongata regulate autonomic nervous system output to the cardiovascular system and, along with nuclei in the pons, control respiration. The midbrain contains auditory and visual reflex centers. Interspersed among the tracts and nuclei of the brain stem are neurons that collectively are known as the ascending reticular activating system (ARAS). The function of the ARAS is to control the level of arousal and attentiveness. It participates in sleep-wake cycling. Damage to the ARAS or its blood supply will impair consciousness, and bilateral damage to this structure will result in coma. Cranial nerves III through XII exit the central nervous system at the brain stem.

Coma is a prolonged period of consciousness during which an individual does not react to external stimuli. The Glasgow Coma Scale assesses function of the eyes, response to verbal commands, and motor function as indices of neurologic function. Normal function is characterized by a Glasgow Coma Scale score of 15, and a complete lack of function is indicated by a score of 3.

Decerebrate posture indicates damage to the brain stem and results from the removal of all inhibitory descending inputs onto the spinal cord alpha-motor neurons (Fig. 41-1).

The optic nerve (cranial nerve II) primarily projects visual information via the thalamus to visual cortical areas. It also sends afferent fibers to the midbrain for control of the papillary light reflex. The nuclei involved in processing the reflex are located in the midbrain, and the efferent limb of the reflex is carried by the oculomotor nerve (cranial nerve III), which exits the brain stem at that level. The absence of a pupillary reaction to light (pupils fixed) and dilation indicate loss of function of the optic nerve, the oculomotor nerve, or the brain stem. The combination of a Glasgow Coma Scale score of 3 and pupils fixed and dilated is indicative of brain death.

FURTHER READING

Text Sources

Carroll RG: Elsevier's Integrated Physiology. Philadelphia, Elsevier, 2007.

Copstead LC, Banasik J: Pathophysiology, 3rd ed. Philadelphia, Saunders, 2005.

Guyton AC, Hall JE: Textbook of Medical Physiology, 11th ed. Philadelphia, Saunders, 2006.

McPhee SJ, Papadakis MA, Tierney LM Jr: Current Medical Diagnosis and Treatment, 46th ed. New York, McGraw-Hill, 2007.

A 27-year-old man is brought to the emergency department after having been involved in a motor vehicle collision.

The patient indicates that he was stopped at a stop sign and pulled into an intersection before he was hit broadside by another car that had the right of way. There is no prior history for seizures. The patient does not wear prescriptive lenses nor does he have a history of visual problems. He is currently taking topiramate (Topamax) for migraines and eszopiclone (Lunesta) for insomnia brought on because of stress.

PHYSICAL EXAMINATION

VS: T 37°C, P 90/min, R 28/min, BP 135/85 mm Hg
PE: No apparent head trauma from the collision. Reflexes were normal. Goldmann field examination shows that central vision is intact but peripheral vision is missing bilaterally.

LABORATORY STUDIES

MRI: Intracranial tumor near the optic chiasm

DIAGNOSIS

Bitemporal hemianopsia

PATHOPHYSIOLOGY OF KEY SYMPTOMS

Visual field deficits accompany many neurologic disorders. Localization of the deficit to the visual field of only one eye indicates a problem with the retinal receptors or the optic nerve of that eye. Localization of the deficit to homologous (comparable) portions of the visual fields of both eyes indicates a problem after the inputs have joined after the optic chiasm (optic tract, optic radiations, or visual cortex). Loss of vision on the temporal sides of the visual fields of both eyes (bitemporal hemianopsia) is indicative of a problem at the optic chiasm.

Lateral representation within the visual system is complex and depends on the location in the visual pathway. As an individual looks straight ahead in the environment, objects to the left of midline are in the left visual space and objects to the right of midline are in right visual space. Objects in left visual space are sensed by the receptors located on the nasal side of the left eye and also by receptors on the temporal side of the right eye. A similar pattern holds for objects in the right visual space, which are refracted by the lens

of the eye on the nasal side of the right eye and the temporal side of the left eye (Fig. 42-1).

Visual sensory information from the rods and cones of the retina exits the eye by way of the optic nerve. At the optic chiasm, nerves from the nasal side of the retina cross to the contralateral optic tract whereas nerves from the temporal side of the retina remain in the ipsilateral optic tract. The fibers from the optic tract then synapse in the thalamus (in the lateral geniculate nucleus) and pass by way of the optic radiations to the primary visual cortex

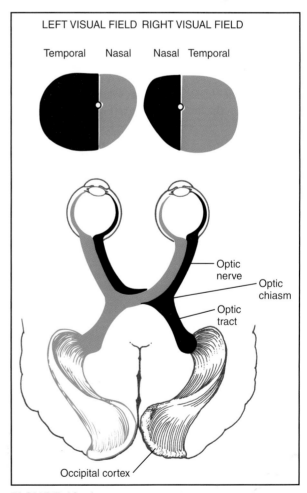

FIGURE 42–1 Visual pathways. (*From Jarvis C: Physical Examination and Health Assessment, 4th ed. Philadelphia, Saunders, 2004.*)

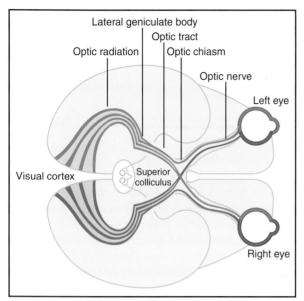

FIGURE 42–2 Principal visual pathways from the eyes to the visual cortex. *(Modified from Polyak SL: The Retina. Chicago, University of Chicago, 1941.)*

of the medial occipital lobe. This complex anatomic arrangement ensures that objects in the left side of visual space (for both eyes) are represented in the right visual cortex and that objects in the right side of visual space are represented in the left visual cortex (Fig. 42-2).

The anatomy of the visual pathways allows visual field deficits to indicate specific regions where the abnormality will be located. A defect in both the nasal and temporal visual fields of one eye indicates that the damage occurred in the optic nerve before the optic chiasm, because that is the only time those fibers travel in the same structure. Damage to the optic chiasm results in a defect of only those optic nerves that cross at the chiasm, from those neurons that originate from rods and cones on the nasal side of each retina. The nasal side of the retinas senses temporal visual space, and the defect is called bitemporal hemianopsia. Complete defects in the left or right visual space indicate damage to the nerves between the optic chiasm and the visual cortex. These defects can be in the optic tract, in the lateral geniculate body of the thalamus, in the optic radiation, or within the visual cortex.

The most common cause of bitemporal hemianopsia is compression of the optic chiasm by tumor, often of the pituitary gland. In this patient, presence of a tumor is confirmed by magnetic resonance imaging. Pituitary adenomas are usually clonal in origin and cause hypersecretion of one of the anterior pituitary hormones. Prolactin-secreting tumors are the most common. Treatment depends on the cellular origin of the tumor and the tumor size.

FURTHER READING

Text Sources
Carroll RG: Elsevier's Integrated Physiology. Philadelphia, Elsevier, 2007.
Copstead LC, Banasik J: Pathophysiology, 3rd ed. Philadelphia, Saunders, 2005.

Guyton AC, Hall JE: Textbook of Medical Physiology, 11th ed. Philadelphia, Saunders, 2006.
McPhee SJ, Papadakis MA, Tierney LM Jr: Current Medical Diagnosis and Treatment, 46th ed. New York, McGraw-Hill, 2007.

An 8-year-old boy is brought by his parents to the pediatrician because of an increasing pattern of clumsiness and headaches.

The parents have noted that the child is having difficulty in grabbing or picking up objects, such as crayons, with his right hand. His ability to draw lines is greatly diminished. The child's teacher first brought this to the parents' attention 3 weeks ago, and it has been getting progressively worse. During the past 4 days, the child has been complaining of headaches. The child has been properly immunized and has reached all developmental milestones.

PHYSICAL EXAMINATION

VS: T 37°C, P 85/min, R 20/min, BP 95/80 mm Hg
PE: Some swelling of the optic nerve observed by funduscope but no visual disturbances. An intention tremor is present when moving the right hand to pick up an object. There is no tremor at rest, and moving the left hand to pick up an object does not generate an intention tremor. Muscle strength is not diminished. Romberg test is negative.

LABORATORY STUDIES

MRI: Laterally located cyst at the junction of the vermis and hemisphere of the middle lobe of the right cerebellum

DIAGNOSIS

Astrocytoma of the vermis of the cerebellum

PATHOPHYSIOLOGY OF KEY SYMPTOMS

The patient shows a deterioration of both fine and gross motor skills. This observation, combined with a headache, suggests a defect within the central nervous system areas involved in motor control. The primary regions controlling motor activity are the motor areas of the cortex, the basal ganglia, and the cerebellum.

Cerebellum, or "little brain," is a large collection of nuclei that coordinate and control motor activity.

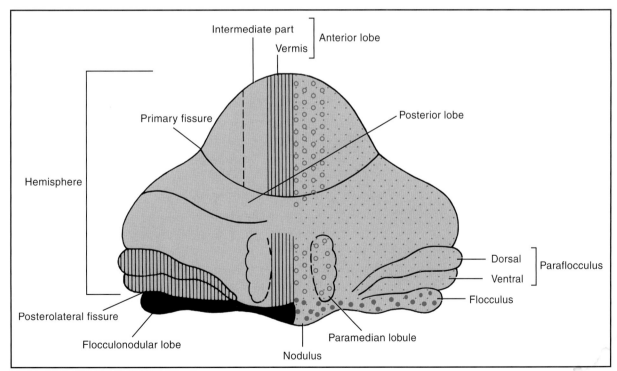

FIGURE 43–1 The subdivision of the cerebellum into archicerebellum, paleocerebellum, and neocerebellum is shown by the *black, hatched, and gray areas*. Terminations of vestibulocerebellar fibers are indicated by the *large dots*, spinocerebellar fibers by the *open circles*, and pontocerebellar fibers by the *small dots*. (*Redrawn from Brodal A: Neurological Anatomy, 3rd ed. New York, Oxford University Press, 1981.*)

Functionally, the cerebellum can be divided into three regions: the vestibulocerebellum, the spinocerebellum, and the cerebrocerebellum (Fig. 43-1).

The vestibulocerebellum is located primarily in the flocculonodular lobe. The primary function of this region is to control balance and eye movements. Consequently, the vestibulocerebellum receives input from the semicircular canals and otolith organs, vestibular nuclei, visual cortex, and superior colliculi and sends output to the motor cortex, the brain stem nuclei giving rise to the vestibulospinal and reticulospinal motor pathways, and the ocular muscles. Lesions in this area cause disturbance in balance and gait and may produce nystagmus.

The spinocerebellum is located in the vermis and intermediate parts of the hemispheres of the anterior lobe and posterior lobe. The primary function of this region is to coordinate body and limb movements. The major inputs are from proprioceptors of the visual and auditory systems. Efferent nerves modulate descending motor systems. Although not as detailed as the sensory and motor cortex, the spinocerebellum does contain a rudimentary somatotopic organization.

The cerebrocerebellum is located in the lateral parts of the hemispheres of the anterior and posterior lobe. The primary function of this area is planning movement and evaluating sensory information. The major inputs are from the parietal lobe, and output is to the ventral lateral thalamus that projects to the motor areas of cortex and the red nucleus.

The cerebellum, pons, and medulla oblongata are encased in the posterior fossa of the skull. Any increase in tissue mass in this area generates an increase in pressure, compressing the brain stem and cerebellum. Headaches are from the increase in intracranial pressure; and as the tumor grows, additional symptoms related to brain stem compression may develop.

The Romberg test distinguishes between a sensory defect and a cerebellar defect. In this test, the subject is asked to stand erect with the feet together and the eyes closed. If the person becomes unsteady, this is an indication that the loss of balance is due to a defect in proprioception. An individual with a cerebellar ataxia will be unable to balance even with the eyes open.

Surgery to remove the tumor reduced pressure on the brain stem. Histologic identification indicates a nonmalignant pilocytic astrocytoma.

FURTHER READING

Web Source
Posterior Fossa Tumors. http://www.emedicine.com/med/topic2907.htm

Text Sources
Berne RM, Levy MN, Koeppen BM, et al: Physiology, 5th ed. St. Louis, Mosby, 2003.
Carroll RG: Elsevier's Integrated Physiology. Philadelphia, Elsevier, 2007.
Copstead LC, Banasik J: Pathophysiology, 3rd ed. Philadelphia, Saunders, 2005.
Guyton AC, Hall JE: Textbook of Medical Physiology, 11th ed. Philadelphia, Saunders, 2006.
McPhee SJ, Papadakis MA, Tierney LM Jr: Current Medical Diagnosis and Treatment, 46th ed. New York, McGraw-Hill, 2007.

A 68-year-old man visits his physician's office complaining of trembling hands and difficulty in walking.

The patient is married and lives at home with his wife of 40 years. Their three children have left home but still live in the same town. The patient had kidney stones 12 years ago but has not had any other significant health problems.

PHYSICAL EXAMINATION

VS: T 37°C, P 72/min, R 15/min, BP 120/80 mm Hg
PE: Neurologic examination: Resting tremor of the left hand that diminishes when performing a task. During passive movement of the left arm, the muscles are rigid, causing "cogwheel" motion during stretching. The patient's facial expressions are reduced. When walking, the patient has difficulty taking the first step but then is able to walk smoothly with a shuffling gait. Unified Parkinson's Disease Rating Scale (UPDRS) score: 95% (normal 100%).

LABORATORY STUDIES

MRI: Normal

DIAGNOSIS

Parkinson's disease

PATHOPHYSIOLOGY OF KEY SYMPTOMS

The patient's primary symptoms revolve around movement. Whereas a decline in balance and coordination are part of the normal aging process, rapid deterioration of movements potentially represents a disturbance in the cerebrum, cerebellum, or basal ganglia.

The basal ganglia are a group of interconnected nuclei that modulate movement (Fig. 44-1). The striatum consists of γ-aminobutyric acid (GABA)ergic neurons that innervate the globus pallidus and the pars reticularis of the substantia nigra. Damage to the striatum causes Huntington's disease. The major output of the substantia nigra is through dopaminergic neurons to the striatum. Damage to the neurons of the substantia nigra causes Parkinson's disease. The globus pallidus projects to the thalamus and subthalamic nuclei using GABA as a neurotransmitter. Damage to the globus pallidus causes Tourette's syndrome.

The subthalamic nucleus uses glutamate as a neurotransmitter to stimulate the internal globus pallidus. Damage to the subthalamic nucleus results in hemiballismus.

Parkinson's disease is a progressive degenerative motor disease that results from damage to the substantia nigra of the basal ganglia. Neuronal damage is accompanied by a disruption of post-translational trafficking of proteins. The protein alpha-synuclein binds to ubiquitin, which cannot be transported into the Golgi apparatus for secretion. The combined alpha-synuclein and ubiquitin complex accumulates within the cell as histologically identifiable Lewy bodies.

The dopamine-secreting neurons of the substantia nigra modulate the normal output of the putamen

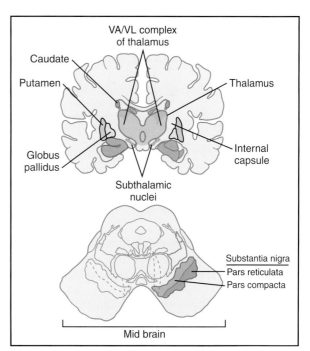

FIGURE 44–1 Components of the basal ganglia and other closely associated brain regions. The main components of the basal ganglia are the caudate, putamen, globus pallidus, and substantia nigra pars reticulata. The motor loop of the basal ganglia connects with motor areas in the frontal cortex, the ventroanterior and ventrolateral (VA and VL) thalamic nuclei, and the superior colliculus. Input from the substantia nigra pars compacta is critical for normal basal ganglia function.

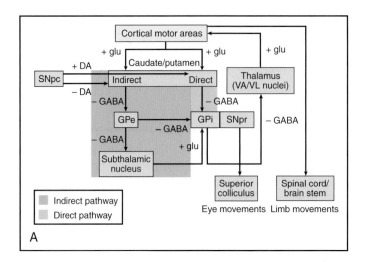

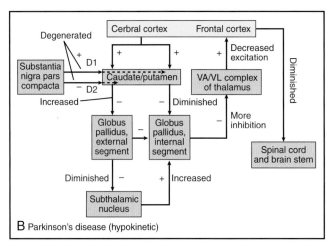

FIGURE 44–2 Functional connectivity of the basal ganglia for motor control. **A,** Connections between various basal ganglia components and other associated motor areas. The excitatory cortical input to the caudate and putamen influences output from the internal segment of Globus Pallidus (GPi) and substantia nigra pars reticularis (SNpr) via a direct and an indirect pathway. Note that the two inhibitory steps in the indirect pathway mean that activity through this pathway has an effect on basal ganglia output to the thalamus and superior colliculus opposite that of the direct pathway. Note that dopamine is a neuromodulator that acts on D_1 and D_2 receptors on striatal neurons participating in the direct and indirect pathways, respectively. **B,** Changes in activity flow that occur in Parkinson's disease in which the substantia nigra pars compacta (SNpc) is degenerated.

(via connections to the globus pallidus) to the thalamus. The lack of dopamine causes an increased inhibition of the ventral lateral nucleus of the thalamus, diminishing the stimulation of the motor cortex (Fig. 44-2).

Parkinson's disease has a gradual onset, often beginning with mild tremor of the hands or feet while at rest. This tremor is different than the intention tremor characteristic of cerebellar diseases. As the disease progresses, the tremor can become more pronounced and additional symptoms of bradykinesia, slowness of movement, postural instability, and impaired balance may develop. In advanced states there are emotional changes as well as difficulty with swallowing and speaking.

The disease is difficult to diagnose because there are biomarkers or imaging defects characteristic to Parkinson's disease. An extensive neurologic workup is often done to rule out other causes for the motor disorder. The Unified Parkinson's Disease Rating Scale assesses mentation, activities of daily living, and motor function as a mechanism to assist the diagnosis and to track the progression of the disease.

The symptoms of Parkinson's disease can be diminished by restoring central nervous system dopamine levels. The combination of levodopa and carbidopa is effective, because carbidopa delays the conversion of levodopa to dopamine until after it has reached the central nervous system. Neurons in the substantia nigra can converse levodopa into dopamine, replenishing their stores. Alternatively, other dopamine mimetic drugs provide relief by similar mechanisms. Anticholinergics may also help diminish symptoms by blocking activity of other basal ganglia nuclei.

Deep brain stimulation is an approved therapy for patients who do not show symptomatic relief from the drugs. This approach uses a programmable pulse generator and stimulator to activate the basal ganglia.

FURTHER READING

Web Sources

http://www.mayoclinic.com/health/parkinsons-disease/DS00295
http://www.ninds.nih.gov/disorders/parkinsons_disease/parkinsons_disease.htm
http://www.parkinson.org

Text Sources

Berne RM, Levy MN, Koeppen BM, et al: Physiology, 5th ed. St. Louis, Mosby, 2003.

Carroll RG: Elsevier's Integrated Physiology. Philadelphia, Elsevier, 2007.
Copstead LC, Banasik J: Pathophysiology, 3rd ed. Philadelphia, Saunders, 2005.
Guyton AC, Hall JE: Textbook of Medical Physiology, 11th ed. Philadelphia, WB Saunders, 2006.
McPhee SJ, Papadakis MA, Tierney LM Jr: Current Medical Diagnosis and Treatment, 46th ed. New York, McGraw-Hill, 2007.

A 19-year-old college student comes to student health services complaining of sporadic loss of memory.

The periods of amnesia occur while the student is awake and occasionally in class. During those times, his classmates report that he begins smacking his lips and fumbling around, disrupting the class. When confronted by his teacher, the student has no recollection of those events and was confused and disoriented. He rests for about 30 minutes and then feels fine. There is no family history of seizures. The student did suffer a head injury while playing sports 6 months earlier, but he does not indicate any cognitive defects.

PHYSICAL EXAMINATION

VS: T 37°C, P 76/min, R 18/min, BP 118/76 mm Hg
PE: No abnormalities noted

LABORATORY STUDIES

EEG: Normal
MRI: Normal

DIAGNOSIS

Symptomatic epilepsy

PATHOPHYSIOLOGY OF KEY SYMPTOMS

This patient's symptoms are tied to abnormal function of the central nervous system. Inability to remember activities (amnesia), disorientation, and confusion indicate a disruption of the higher cognitive processes.

Synchronized activity of neurons of the brain generates waves of electrical activity that can be recorded as an electroencephalogram (EEG) by surface electrodes on the scalp. The frequency of these brain waves varies based on the level of coordinated neuronal activity (Fig. 45-1).

The slowest of the brain waves are the high-amplitude delta waves, occurring at frequencies of less than 3.5 cycles/sec. Delta waves occur during slow-wave sleep, reflecting a time when ascending input from the thalamus is suppressed and the cortical neurons can generate their own rhythm. Theta waves have a lower amplitude and occur at frequencies of 4 to 7 cycles/sec. Theta waves are associated with emotional stress. Alpha waves have a still lower amplitude (an oscillation of 8 to 13 cycles/sec) and appear to be due to a rhythmic feedback oscillation in the thalamic cortical system. In adults, alpha waves are associated with a quiet and awake period. Beta waves have the highest frequency (14 to 80 cycles/sec) and a very low amplitude and represent asynchronous neuronal activity when the brain is alert and processing sensory input.

Epilepsy results from the excessive activity in clusters of neurons. The abnormal neuronal activity

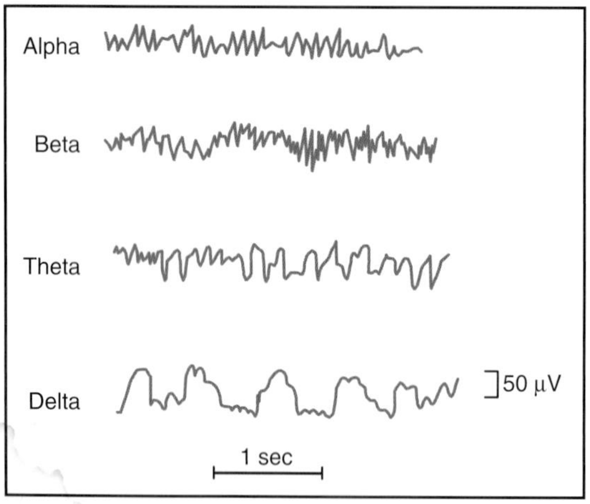

FIGURE 45–1 Different types of brain waves in the normal electroencephalogram.

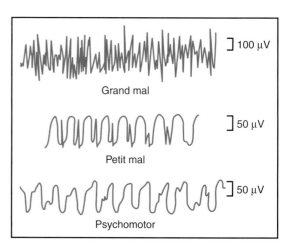

FIGURE 45–2 Electroencephalograms in different types of epilepsy.

causes strange sensations, emotions, and behaviors, possibly causing muscle spasms and loss of consciousness. Epilepsy can be induced by damage to the brain, illness, abnormal brain development, or neurotransmitter imbalances.

Seizures are classified based on the number of areas of the brain involved. Partial seizures are localized to just one area the brain; and although they may alter conscious perception, they rarely result in the loss of consciousness. Generalized seizures involve all areas of the brain, creating large-amplitude and often repetitive brain wave activity. The EEG in this patient is normal because the abnormal brain wave activity only occurs during seizures and not during the interval between seizures (Fig. 45-2).

The mechanisms underlying the inability to remember events during the seizure (transient epileptic amnesia) are poorly understood. The major structures involved in memory—the hippocampus, limbic system, and temporal lobe—are most likely involved.

Treatments can be used to diminish or completely eliminate seizures. There are a wide variety of antiepileptic drugs, the efficacy of which varies by the type and the severity of epilepsy. Surgery may be an option when the seizures originate from a well-defined area of damaged neurons. Vagal nerve stimulation diminishes the frequency and intensity of seizures in some patients. Finally, a ketogenic diet can be used to treat epilepsy, particularly in children.

FURTHER READING

Text Sources

Carroll RG: Elsevier's Integrated Physiology. Philadelphia, Elsevier, 2007.

Copstead LC, Banasik J: Pathophysiology, 3rd ed. Philadelphia, Saunders, 2005.

Guyton AC, Hall JE: Textbook of Medical Physiology, 11th ed. Philadelphia, Saunders, 2006.

Kapur N: Transient epileptic amnesia, a clinical update and a reformulation. J Neurol Neurosurg Psychiatry 56:1184–1190, 1993.

McPhee SJ, Papadakis MA, Tierney LM Jr: Current Medical Diagnosis and Treatment, 46th ed. New York, McGraw-Hill, 2007.

A 74-year-old woman is brought to her physician's office by her daughter, who complains that her mother is behaving oddly.

The woman lives in a house in a small town and has lived alone for the 5 years since her husband died. She admits to forgetting about food while its cooking on the stove but says it is because she is so busy. The woman can remember events 20 years ago but has difficulty recalling recent events. She has begun to call her grandchildren by her children's names. The patient is healthy and is not on any current medications.

PHYSICAL EXAMINATION

VS: T 37°C, P 72/min, R 15/min, BP 118/65 mm Hg, BMI 22
PE: No significant findings

LABORATORY STUDIES

CT: Significant atrophy of the parietal, temporal, and frontal lobes of the cerebral cortex and degeneration of the cingulate gyrus (Fig. 46-1)

DIAGNOSIS

Alzheimer's disease

PATHOPHYSIOLOGY OF KEY SYMPTOMS

The patient's presenting symptoms indicate a gradual cognitive decline. Cognition requires interaction of numerous brain structures, and, consequently, cognitive decline is characteristic of a wide variety of diseases. Specific testing helps to identify potential pathologic processes underlying the cognitive decline.

Memory is the ability to retain and recall information. Physiologically, memories are stored in the brain by enhancing specific patterns of synaptic activity. Memories are stored throughout the cerebral cortex by these preferential neuronal activity patterns. At one extreme, short-term memory persists for only a few seconds and is likely due to synaptic facilitation. At the other extreme, long-term memory persists for years and involves remodeling of synapses as well as long-term potentiation and inhibition. The hippocampus of the limbic system is a key structure involved in the conversion of short-term memory to long-term memory.

Long-term memories can be characterized as either declarative or nondeclarative memory. Declarative memory is explicit and includes complex associations including the event, the surroundings, and the significance of the event. Declarative memory is frequently stored in the temporal lobes. In contrast, nondeclarative memory is associated with complex motor abilities, such as being able to eat with a fork, habits, or emotional responses. The components of nondeclarative memories can be stored throughout the brain, including the cerebellum, basal ganglia, or amygdala (Fig. 46-2).

Alzheimer's disease is a progressive neurodegenerative disorder characterized initially by impaired memory. Over time, the disease progresses to dementia, cognitive decline, and decline in major body functions, and finally death. The diagnosis of Alzheimer's disease is confirmed at autopsy by the presence of insoluble amyloid β plaques in the extracellular spaces and neurofibrillary tangles of the tau protein within the neurons. Risk factors for the development of Alzheimer's disease include the presence of the ε4 allele of apolipoprotein E, hypercholesterolemia and being female, elderly, and having a relative with the disease (Fig. 46-3).

Currently there is no cure for Alzheimer's disease. Symptoms of the disease can be diminished by treatment with acetylcholinesterase inhibitors and NMDA receptor antagonists. These treatments do not, however, diminish the overproduction of the amyloid-β protein or the neurofibrillary tangles.

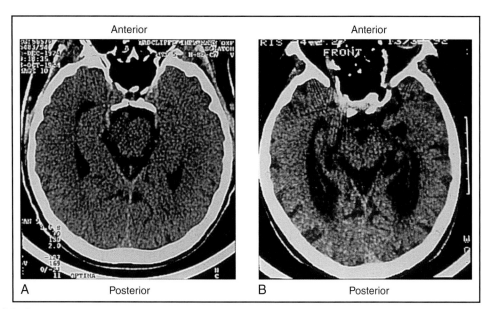

FIGURE 46–1   Axial (horizontal) CT section through the temporal lobes. **A,** Normal. **B,** Alzheimer's disease. *(Courtesy of James King-Holmes and Science Photo Library.)*

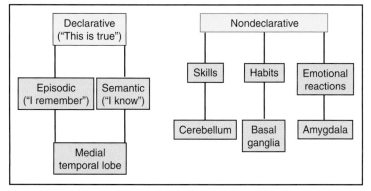

FIGURE 46–2   Major categories of memory. Although the locations of all the altered synapses that underlie each is not known with certainty, the indicated anatomic structures are prominently involved in the synaptic alterations.

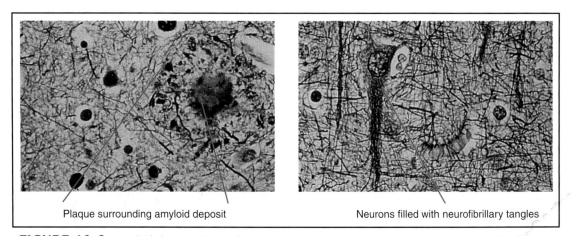

Plaque surrounding amyloid deposit   Neurons filled with neurofibrillary tangles

FIGURE 46–3   Amyloid plaques and neurofibrillary tangles. *(Courtesy of James King-Holmes and Science Photo Library.)*

FURTHER READING

Web Source

http://www.nia.nih.gov/Alzheimers/Publications/adfact.htm

Text Sources

Carroll RG: Elsevier's Integrated Physiology. Philadelphia, Elsevier, 2007.

Copstead LC, Banasik J: Pathophysiology, 3rd ed. Philadelphia, Saunders, 2005.

Guyton AC, Hall JE: Textbook of Medical Physiology, 11th ed. Philadelphia, Saunders, 2006.

McPhee SJ, Papadakis MA, Tierney LM Jr: Current Medical Diagnosis and Treatment, 46th ed. New York, McGraw-Hill, 2007.

Nolte J: Elsevier's Integrated Neuroscience. Philadelphia, Elsevier, 2007.

A 53-year-old man is brought to the emergency department by ambulance because he is having difficulty speaking.

The patient tried to explain to his wife that something was wrong, but he was unable to speak clearly. He is, however, able to communicate in writing. He has been on beta blockers to control hypertension and has type 2 diabetes that is being managed with diet and exercise.

PHYSICAL EXAMINATION

VS: T 36.5°C, P 85/min, R 18/min, BP 134/88 mm Hg, BMI 31

PE: The patient is anxious but able to respond to spoken commands. Reflexes are intact.

LABORATORY STUDIES

CT: Occlusion in the left hemisphere of a branch of the anterior main division of the middle cerebral artery supplying the frontal cortex.

DIAGNOSIS

Expressive aphasia after a stroke

PATHOPHYSIOLOGY OF KEY SYMPTOMS

The patient's primary symptom is difficulty in speaking (expressive aphasia). Speech is a complex activity requiring correct function of premotor areas (especially Broca's area) and motor areas of the cortex, as well as upper and lower motor neurons innervating the vocal cords and diaphragm. The abrupt loss of speech suggests a neurologic cause, such as inadequate perfusion.

A cerebrovascular accident (CVA, stroke) results from impairment of a vascular supply to the brain. Ischemic stroke can be caused by a thrombus or embolus that lodges in a small branch of cerebral blood vessels. Hemorrhagic stroke is caused by the rupture of a blood vessel, usually at the site of an aneurysm. In both cases, blood supply to neurons distal to the injury is interrupted. Neurons have a very low tolerance for ischemia,

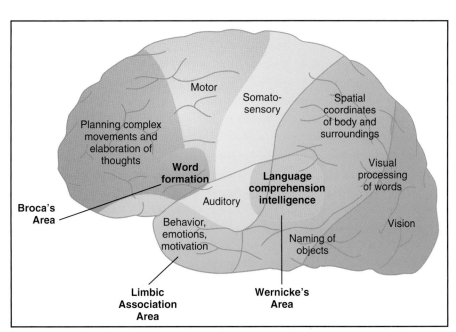

FIGURE 47–1 Map of specific functional areas in the cerebral cortex, showing especially Wernicke's and Broca's areas for language comprehension and speech production, which in 95% of all people are located in the left hemisphere.

and neuronal death occurs within minutes. Prompt restoration of blood flow limits the size of neurologic damage and enhances recovery. Consequently, treatment involves rapid identification of the site of blockage and restoration of blood flow by stenting or treatment with thrombolytics. Permanent neurologic damage cannot currently be reversed, but physical therapy and occupational therapy can help restore function.

Risk factors for stroke include advanced age, hypertension, diabetes, enhanced coagulation, and atrial fibrillation. Approximately one in four individuals who recover from their stroke will have another stroke within 5 years. The incidence of future strokes can be prevented by treatment with antiplatelet agents and anticoagulants.

Broca's area is a region of the posterior lateral prefrontal cortex and the premotor area. This region of the brain controls the motor patterns for expressing individual words. It is located adjacent to the prefrontal cortex, auditory cortex, and motor cortex and receives extensive innervation from all three. Broca's area also interacts with the language comprehension region of the temporal lobe, Wernicke's area. In contrast to most motor and sensory cortical regions, Broca's area and Wernicke's area are not bilaterally represented and are usually only found in the left hemisphere (Fig. 47-1).

Because the stroke was identified early, prompt treatment with thrombolytics should greatly diminish the region of damage. The patient was admitted to the catheterization laboratory, and treatment with tissue plasminogen activator dissolved the clot and restored flow through the blocked blood vessel. The patient recovered fully and now is on anticoagulants.

FURTHER READING

Web Source
http://www.ninds.nih.gov/disorders/stroke/stroke.htm

Text Sources
Carroll RG: Elsevier's Integrated Physiology. Philadelphia, Elsevier, 2007.

Copstead LC, Banasik J: Pathophysiology, 3rd ed. Philadelphia, Saunders, 2005.
Guyton AC, Hall JE: Textbook of Medical Physiology, 11th ed. Philadelphia, Saunders, 2006.
McPhee SJ, Papadakis MA, Tierney LM Jr: Current Medical Diagnosis and Treatment, 46th ed. New York, McGraw-Hill, 2007.

A 50-year-old man comes to the physician's office complaining of a persistent and disabling sense that he is spinning even while he is sitting still.

The sensation has become progressively worse since it was first noted about 5 months ago. He has stopped social drinking but with no sign of improvement. He also indicates his left ear is problematic, with mild ear pain, a gradual decrease in hearing, and often a constant ringing (tinnitus).

PHYSICAL EXAMINATION

VS: T 37°C, P 72/min, R 15/min, BP 126/80 mm Hg
PE: The patient appears confused and has a mild slurred speech. During the examination, the patient exhibits a positive Romberg test and ataxia, along with vertical nystagmus.

LABORATORY STUDIES

Audiogram: 35 dB (normal: 0-25 dB)
Electronystagmography (ENG):

- Calibration: Positive, spontaneous vertical nystagmus
- Tracking test: Positive, left-sided horizontal nystagmus
- Positional test: Positive, dizziness associated with all head positions
- Caloric test: Negative (normal) to both cold and warm water

Visual evoked potential: 5 beats of nystagmus (normal: < 3 beats of nystagmus)
MRI: Eighth cranial nerve schwannoma arising within the internal auditory canal and involving the cerebellopontine angle

DIAGNOSIS

Vertigo from acoustic neuroma

PATHOPHYSIOLOGY OF KEY SYMPTOMS

The patient's symptoms are generally tied to the function of the vestibulocochlear nerve (cranial nerve VIII), which carries the afferent signals from the cochlea (hearing) and vestibular system (balance). Vestibular system disorders manifest as vertigo, often accompanied by nystagmus. This simultaneous occurrence of both of these deficits indicates a problem tied to the eighth cranial nerve.

The vestibular system is a complex sensory organ that determines both acceleration and position relative to gravity. There are three semicircular canals oriented at right angles to each other so that movement in all three planes in space can be detected. The hair cells of the crista ampullaris detect movement of the fluid within the semicircular canal and transmit this information along the sensory nerves of the vestibular system. The macula of the utricle and saccule contains small calcium carbonate stones that activate hair cells

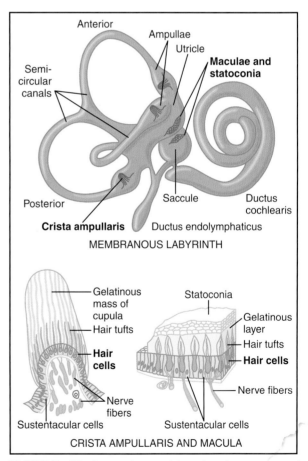

MEMBRANOUS LABYRINTH

CRISTA AMPULLARIS AND MACULA

FIGURE 48–1 Membranous labyrinth and organization of the crista ampullaris and the macula.

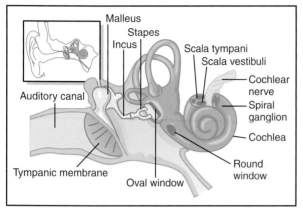

FIGURE 48–2 Tympanic membrane, ossicular system of the middle ear, and inner ear.

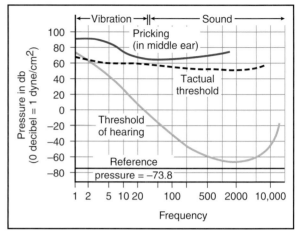

FIGURE 48–3 Relation of the threshold of hearing and of somesthetic perception (pricking and tactual threshold) to the sound energy level at each sound frequency.

and thus detect the orientation of the head with respect to gravity as well as linear acceleration (Fig. 48-1).

Hearing is also transmitted along a branch of the eighth cranial nerve. Sound information is transmitted through the outer and middle ear and is transduced in the cochlea of the inner ear (Fig. 48-2). Sound intensity is measured in decibels (dB), and hearing acuity varies with the frequency of the sound. Hearing acuity can be assessed with an audiogram (Fig. 48-3).

Balance is a result of the complex interplay between the vestibular system, vision, proprioceptors in the body, and the cerebellum. Disruption of any component of the balance systems can result in a number of symptoms, including loss of balance, vertigo, visual blurring, nausea, and disorientation.

Vertigo is a common symptom of vestibular disorders. Objective vertigo is a sensation of motion without any actual change in body position. Vertigo results from inconsistent input from the two vestibular apparatuses. In this patient, input from the left vestibular apparatus is disrupted while input from the right vestibular apparatus, along with the remainder of the positional senses, is normal. Because the patient is unable to reach a consistent interpretation, an abnormal sensation of movement is perceived.

Nystagmus is an involuntary rhythmic eye movement caused by disruption of the vestibulo-ocular reflex. Normally, the vestibular system allows the eyes to track objects while the head is moving. Abnormal or inconsistent input from the multiple sense organs of the vestibular apparatus disrupts the control of eye movement, generating nystagmus. Electronystagmography evaluates the stimulus function by detecting nystagmus while stressing balance.

An acoustic neuroma is a slowly growing benign tumor of the Schwann cells of the eighth cranial nerve. The tumors most often originate in the vestibular branch of the nerve and, as they grow, compress and disrupt function of the auditory branch of the nerve. Large tumors may compress the brain stem, resulting in headaches and mental confusion. Large tumors can also compress the facial nerve, causing numbness and motor problems in areas of the face. Magnetic resonance imaging (MRI) allows imaging of the tumor and can be used to assess growth of the tumor over time.

If the tumor is not symptomatic, observation through regular imaging and hearing tests may be the best option. Destruction of the tumor can be accomplished by irradiation or by invasive surgery.

FURTHER READING

Web Sources

http://www.mayoclinic.com/health/acoustic-neuroma/DS00803
http://www.nidcd.nih.gov/health/hearing/acoustic_neuroma.asp

Text Sources

Carroll RG: Elsevier's Integrated Physiology. Philadelphia, Elsevier, 2007.

Copstead LC, Banasik J: Pathophysiology, 3rd ed. Philadelphia, Saunders, 2005.

Guyton AC, Hall JE: Textbook of Medical Physiology, 11th ed. Philadelphia, Saunders, 2006.

McPhee SJ, Papadakis MA, Tierney LM Jr: Current Medical Diagnosis and Treatment, 46th ed. New York, McGraw-Hill, 2007.

A 37-year-old man comes to the physician's office complaining of chronic pain in the upper and middle back, headaches, muscle weakness in the hands, and loss of sensitivity to hot and cold temperatures.

About 2 years ago, the patient began to feel fatigued and found it hard to perform everyday tasks. Recently, he accidentally scalded his young daughter at bath time when he didn't realize the water was hot. This prompted him to seek medical attention.

PHYSICAL EXAMINATION

VS: T 37°C, P 60/min, R 14/min, BP 120/80 mm Hg
PE: Loss of sensitivity, especially to hot and cold; muscle weakness and spasticity; headaches; a thoracic kyphoscoliosis. The loss of pain and temperature sensitivity is bilateral and symmetrically distributed in the upper extremities and thorax in a "cape-like" pattern.

LABORATORY STUDIES

Skull and cervical spine radiographs: Thoracic scoliosis and osteoporosis
MRI: Focal cord enlargement due to an intramedullary neoplasm

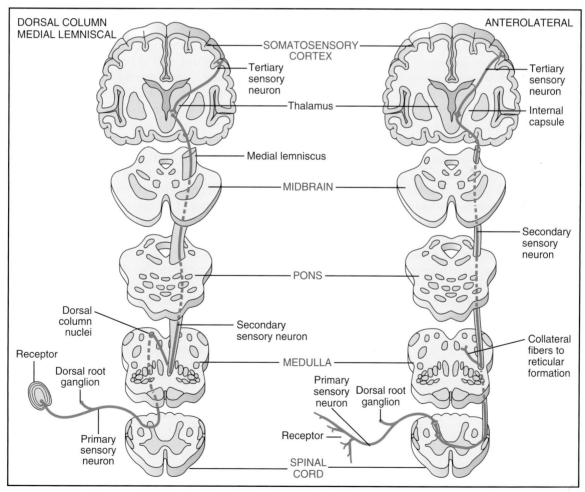

FIGURE 49–1   Comparison of the two major ascending somatosensory tracts. **Left,** Dorsal column-medial lemniscal tract. **Right,** Anterolateral tract. Note that the dorsal column tracts do not cross the midline until the level of the medulla, whereas the anterolateral tracts cross at the spinal cord level.

DIAGNOSIS

Syringomyelia

PATHOPHYSIOLOGY OF KEY SYMPTOMS

The patient's symptoms are a combination of defects in afferent sensory transmission and efferent motor transmission, indicating a defect within the nerves or spinal cord. Unilateral symptoms would be indicative of a nerve problem. This patient's symptoms are bilateral and are most likely due to a problem within the spinal cord.

Spinal cord sensory transmission ascends predominantly in the dorsal columns and the anterolateral tracts. Sensory nerves that transmit the modalities of fine touch, vibration, and proprioception enter the spinal cord at the dorsal root and ascend ipsilaterally to the medulla. A second-order sensory neuron crosses the midline forming the medial lemniscus and carries the information to the thalamus. The tertiary sensory neuron ascends from the thalamus to the somatosensory cortex. In contrast, pain and temperature sensory inputs travel through the anterolateral pathway. Sensory neurons enter the dorsal root and synapse in the dorsal horn of the gray matter of the ipsilateral cord. Second-order neurons send their axons across the midline to the contralateral anterolateral tract in which they ascend to make synaptic connection in the thalamus. The third neuron in the pathway projects to the somatosensory cortex. The anterolateral system is highly divergent; and as the pathway ascends, collaterals relay information to many targets, including the reticular formation and periaqueductal gray matter of the brain stem. Within the spinal cord, somatotopic organization is maintained, because nerve fibers originating from the upper parts of the body are carried in the more medial portions of the tract and nerve fibers originating from the lower parts of the body are carried in the more lateral portions of the tract (Fig. 49-1).

Cerebrospinal fluid (CSF) is formed in the choroid plexuses of the lateral ventricles at a rate of 500 mL/day. From there, CSF flows into the third ventricle,

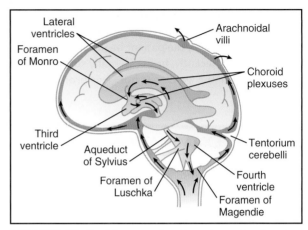

FIGURE 49–2   The *arrows* show the pathway of cerebrospinal fluid flow from the choroid plexuses in the lateral ventricles to the arachnoidal villi protruding into the dural sinuses.

through the aqueduct of Sylvius into the fourth ventricle, and out through a foramen into the cisterna magna. The fluid space of the cisterna magna is continuous with the subarachnoid space that surrounds the brain and the spinal cord. CSF is absorbed by the villi of the arachnoid membrane, creating a flow of CSF through the brain and spinal cord (Fig. 49-2).

Syringomyelia results from a cyst forming within the center of the spinal cord. The cyst, called a syrinx, expands over time, disrupting the nerve fibers near the center of the spinal cord. This often involves the loss of pain in temperature at this site of the syrinx, as the anterolateral tracts cross the midline at the level of spinal cord entry. This accounts for the bilateral and symmetrical pattern of loss in dermatomes related to the location of the syrinx. Lower dermatomes are not affected because the lesion does not affect the anterolateral white matter of the cord. The syrinx can also obstruct the canal, preventing the flow of CSF.

Treatment involves releasing the increased pressure on the cord, both the direct compression from the tumor and pressure from the buildup of CSF. The CSF outflow can be restored by direct surgical drainage or by shunt placement or, as in this case, by surgical removal of the tumor.

FURTHER READING

Web Source
http://www.ninds.nih.gov/disorders/syringomyelia/syringomyelia.htm

Text Sources
Carroll RG: Elsevier's Integrated Physiology, Philadelphia, Elsevier, 2007.

Copstead LC, Banasik J: Pathophysiology, 3rd ed. Philadelphia, Saunders, 2005.

Guyton AC, Hall JE: Textbook of Medical Physiology, 11th ed. Philadelphia, Saunders, 2006.

McPhee SJ, Papadakis MA, Tierney LM Jr.: Current Medical Diagnosis and Treatment, 46th ed. New York, McGraw-Hill, 2007.

...ld man comes to his physician complaining of a drooping eyelid and facial
...itching on the left side of his face.

The patient first noticed the symptoms about 6 hours ago, but they have continued
to worsen. He is now having trouble tasting and is drooling from the left corner of his
mouth. The patient has not had any neurologic problems in the past, although he did
have the flu 3 weeks ago.

PHYSICAL EXAMINATION

VS: T 38.2°C, P 80/min, R 18/min, BP 120/76 mm Hg
PE: The patient has extreme left-sided facial weakness
and paralysis. He is unable to blink his left eye. All
right-sided facial function is normal.

LABORATORY STUDIES

Radiograph: Negative, no sign of tumor
MRI: Normal, no indication of stroke, brain lesion, or
tumor
EMG: Abnormal; shows damage to the left facial
nerve

DIAGNOSIS

Bell's palsy

PATHOPHYSIOLOGY OF KEY SYMPTOMS

The patient's symptoms are a combination of motor
and sensory defects. The motor defects are indicated
by partial paralysis of muscles associated with the facial
nerve. The sensory defects are also specific to modalities carried by the facial nerve. The symptoms are limited to one side of the face, indicating damage only to
that nerve.

The cortical regions involved in muscle control are
the primary motor cortex, the premotor area, and the
supplemental motor areas. The premotor area coordi-
nates patterns of movement and is interconnected with
the basal ganglia, cerebellum, somatosensory areas,
thalamus, and primary motor cortex (Fig. 50-1).

The primary motor cortex exerts executive control
of voluntary movement. It is located in the frontal
lobes anterior to the central sulcus (precentral gyrus).
The neurons of the primary motor cortex have a somatotopic organization, with the feet and legs located
midline and the head and face extending toward the

lateral (Sylvian) fissure. Axons from the neurons of the
primary motor cortex (upper motor neurons) descend
and synapse within the spinal cord (corticospinal tract)
or synapse within the motor nuclei of the brain stem
(corticobulbar tract). Corticorubral fibers project to the
red nucleus of the mesencephalon, which then sends a
projection into the spinal cord as the rubrospinal tract.
Motor signals are also transmitted to the basal ganglia
and cerebellum. Lower motor neurons are the final
common pathway to skeletal muscles. They are the
motor neurons of the cranial nerve nuclei that innervate skeletal muscles as well as the motor neurons of
the ventral horn of the spinal cord that innervate the
rest of the body's musculature (Fig. 50-2).

Paralysis results from disruption at any level of
normal motor control. A stroke or tumor can damage
neurons in the primary motor cortex. Lesions,
compression, or demyelination can damage the upper
motor neurons. Similar processes can disrupt action
potentials transmitted along the alpha-motor neurons
(lower motor neurons) that exit the spinal cord and pass
to the muscle. Neuromuscular junction transmission
can be impaired or the muscle cell itself damaged.

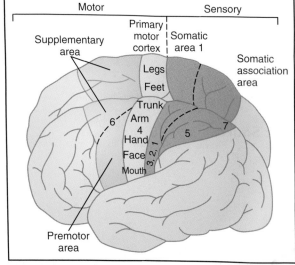

FIGURE 50–1 Motor and somatosensory functional areas
of the cerebral cortex. The numbers 4, 5, 6, and 7 are Brodmann's
cortical areas.

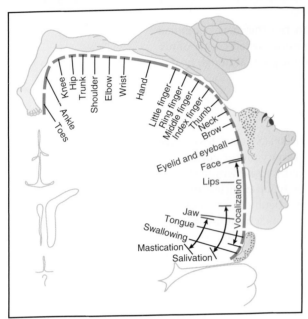

FIGURE 50–2 Degree of representation of the different muscles of the body in the motor cortex. (*Redrawn from Penfield W, Rasmussen T: The Cerebral Cortex of Man: A Clinical Study of Localization of Function. New York, Hafner, 1968.*)

Systemic defects, such as multiple sclerosis or amyotrophic lateral sclerosis, cause widespread symptoms. In this patient, the defect involves regions innervated by a single cranial nerve, suggesting a local involvement. The nuclei of the facial nerve are located in the pons. The pattern of innervation of the nucleus by the descending upper motor neurons is different for the region projecting to the muscles of the upper face and the region projecting to the muscles of the lower face.

The neurons projecting [...] receive input only from the co[...] whereas the neurons projecting to [...] upper face receive bilateral input. This [...] lesion of the upper motor neurons will spare [...] cles of the upper face. If a lesion occurs in the nuc[...] or the cranial nerve, the pattern of weakness differs; the entire ipsilateral side of the face is affected.

Bell's palsy is a unilateral paralysis of muscles and innervated by cranial nerve VII, the facial nerve. There are five major branches of the facial nerve. The muscles of face and neck are innervated by the efferent facial nerves, as are the stapedius muscles of the middle ear that modulate sound intensity. Efferent parasympathetic fibers innervate the lacrimal gland of the eye and the salivary glands. The afferent component of the facial nerve transmits taste and a small amount of cutaneous sensory input. The facial nerve travels through the fallopian canal when exiting the skull before branching. Inflammation can compress the nerve within the canal and consequently disrupts some or all aspects of facial nerve function.

Initial treatment is centered on ameliorating the symptoms, particularly protecting the cornea from drying owing to the lack of tear production. The pathophysiology of Bell's palsy is not completely known, and it is likely that multiple different mechanisms can cause the disease. Research suggests the involvement of inflammation and swelling of the facial nerve or of herpes simplex type 1 infection. Consequently, treatments involve anti-inflammatory or antiviral drugs. If the disorder is left untreated, most individuals spontaneously recover and return to normal function within 1 year.

FURTHER READING

Web Source

http://www.ninds.nih.gov/disorders/bells/bells.htm

Text Sources

Carroll RG: Elsevier's Integrated Physiology. Philadelphia, Elsevier, 2007.

Copstead LC, Banasik J: Pathophysiology, 3rd ed. Philadelphia, Saunders, 2005.
Guyton AC, Hall JE: Textbook of Medical Physiology, 11th ed. Philadelphia, Saunders, 2006.
McPhee SJ, Papadakis MA, Tierney LM Jr: Current Medical Diagnosis and Treatment, 46th ed. New York, McGraw-Hill, 2007.

A 22-year-old woman presents to the university health clinic complaining of weakness, tingling, and intense pain in her right hand.

The tingling and numbness is particularly intense on the palmar side of the thumb, upper right hand, and wrist. The pain is increased in intensity and is now waking the patient at night. She describes the pain as a burning sensation that can be diminished by moderate movement and stretching of the wrist.

PHYSICAL EXAMINATION

VS: T 37°C, P 66/min, R 15/min, BP 118/76 mm Hg
PE: The patient appears healthy and is not in acute distress. There is pain when assessing range of motion of the right wrist. There is visible atrophy of the right thenar eminence compared with the left.

LABORATORY STUDIES

Bilateral hand radiographs: Negative for fracture or arthritis
Phalen's maneuver: Positive (symptoms reappear)
Tinel's test: Positive (symptoms radiate along the medial nerve)

DIAGNOSIS

Carpal tunnel syndrome

PATHOPHYSIOLOGY OF KEY SYMPTOMS

The patient's complaint is primarily due to pain in the hand, accompanied by minor sensory and motor defects. The simultaneous appearances of both sensory and motor defects that are limited to a discrete dermatome suggest damage to one of the spinal nerves.

Pain receptors are free nerve endings distributed throughout the skin and, to a lesser degree, in visceral organs and spaces. Pain receptors are activated by mechanical, thermal, and chemical stimuli. Mechanical activation is generally sensed as fast pain, and thermal and chemical activation is generally sensed as slow pain.

Fast pain is carried along myelinated Aδ fibers that synapse in the dorsal horn and ascend through the neospinothalamic tract to the thalamus and then on to the somatosensory cortex (Fig. 51-1). Within the spinal cord, glutamate is a neurotransmitter secreted at Aδ synapses. Slow pain is carried along the unmyelinated C fibers, which make polysynaptic connections

in the spinal cord and ascend through the paleospinothalamic tract to the brain stem and thalamus. Within the spinal cord, substance P is the neurotransmitter released at C fiber synapses. The multiple synaptic connections transmitting slow pain mean that slow pain is very poorly localized on a somatotopic map.

The median nerve is a mixed nerve with both sensory and motor components. Compression of the median nerve generates action potentials within the axons, resulting in activation of sensory neurons (tingling), slow pain fibers (burning), and fast pain nerve fibers (localized intense pain). Disruption of alpha-motor neurons leads to muscle weakness in the hand.

Carpal tunnel syndrome results from the compression of the median nerve as it passes through the carpal tunnel. The carpal tunnel is a narrow pathway at the base of the hand bordered by ligaments and bones. The median nerve carries sensory afferent information from the palm side of the thumb and fingers.

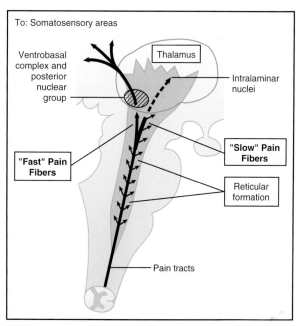

FIGURE 51-1 Transmission of pain signals into the brain stem, thalamus, and cerebral cortex by way of the fast pricking pain pathway and slow burning pain pathway.

Evocative testing is used to confirm the carpal tunnel as the site of the defect. The Phalen, or wrist-flexion, test involves pressing the backs of the hands together while holding the forearms upright and the fingers pointed down. The Tinel test is direct compression or tapping on the carpal tunnel. A positive response is the appearance of symptoms within 1 minute.

Treatment options involve analgesia, immobilization, and diminishing the swelling. If the swelling is due to an underlying pathologic process, treating this problem can diminish the symptoms. Alternatively, any inflammation may be reduced by treatment with nonsteroidal anti-inflammatory drugs (NSAIDs) or corticosteroids. If symptoms persist, surgery can be done to expand the carpal tunnel.

FURTHER READING

Web Source

http://www.ninds.nih.gov/disorders/carpal_tunnel/detail_carpal_tunnel.htm

Text Sources

Carroll RG: Elsevier's Integrated Physiology. Philadelphia, Elsevier, 2007.

Copstead LC, Banasik J: Pathophysiology, 3rd ed. Philadelphia, Saunders, 2005.
Guyton AC, Hall JE: Textbook of Medical Physiology, 11th ed. Philadelphia, Saunders, 2006.
McPhee SJ, Papadakis MA, Tierney LM Jr: Current Medical Diagnosis and Treatment, 46th ed. New York, McGraw-Hill, 2007.

SECTION VII

Gastroenterology

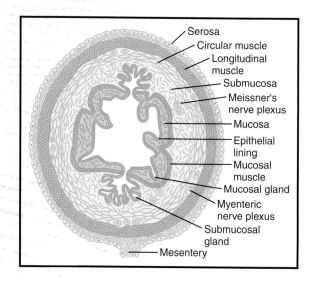

The gastrointestinal system isolates ingested food for digestion of the complex molecules and absorption of nutrients. It is lined with a continuous layer of epithelial cells. Consequently, the lumen of the gastrointestinal system is functionally outside the body and can provide a very different environment from that of the body. For example, the lumen of the large intestine has an extensive bacterial microflora. Perforation of the large intestine allows this microflora to enter the blood, creating septic shock.

The major functions governing the gastrointestinal tract are (1) motility, (2) secretion, (3) digestion, and (4) absorption. Figure VII-1 illustrates these functions and specific diseases presented in this section. The pathophysiology of the diseases affecting the gastrointestinal system is best understood when characterized against these major functions.

Motility is controlled predominantly by smooth muscle, with skeletal muscle involvement at the entry and the exit of the gastrointestinal tract. The oral component of swallowing is initiated voluntarily by the skeletal muscle of the mouth and the tongue. The esophagus begins as skeletal muscle but transitions to layers of circular and longitudinal smooth muscle that extend through the length of the gastrointestinal tract. Food exiting the esophagus moves by peristalsis sequentially through the stomach, small intestine, and large intestine. Sphincters impede the movement of the gastrointestinal contents (see Case 54). Entry to the esophagus requires a relaxation of the upper esophageal sphincter, and passage from the esophagus to the stomach requires relaxation of a lower esophageal sphincter (see Case 52). Movement from the stomach into the small intestine requires relaxation of the pyloric sphincter, and movement from the small intestine into the large intestine requires relaxation of the ileocecal valve. Passage of feces or intestinal gas requires relaxation of the smooth muscle internal anal sphincter and also relaxation of the voluntary skeletal muscle of the external anal sphincter (see Case 60).

The water and mucus of gastric secretions facilitate the movement of food through the gastrointestinal tract, and other gastrointestinal secretions mediate the digestion of complex macromolecules. The gastrointestinal system secretes 7 to 9 L of water each day and reabsorbs all but 100 to 200 mL (see Case 59). Gastrointestinal secretions determine the luminal environment, including the alkaline environment of the mouth, the acidic environment of the stomach (see Case 53), and the alkaline environment of the intestines.

Digestive enzymes degrade macromolecules into smaller molecules to facilitate their absorption. The majority of the digestive enzymes are secreted by the pancreas into the duodenum (see Case 56). In addition, saliva contains amylase, the gastric chief cells secrete pepsinogen, and the liver secretes bile acids. Duodenal contents modulate gastric emptying, so that the chyme entering the duodenum can be digested and absorbed before the pyloric sphincter relaxes and allows more chyme to enter.

Absorption across the intestinal epithelia occurs predominantly in the small intestine (see Case 55). Apical transport proteins mediate this sodium-coupled absorption of amino acids, di- and tri-peptides, simple sugars, and fatty acids (see Case 57). The absorption of fructose and some basic and most neutral amino acids occurs by a sodium-independent process.

Most absorbed compounds enter the hepatic portal vein circulation and pass through the liver before entering the vena cava. One exception to this is lipids, which are converted into chylomicrons after absorption and are absorbed by the lymphatic system rather than the hepatic portal vascular system (see Case 58).

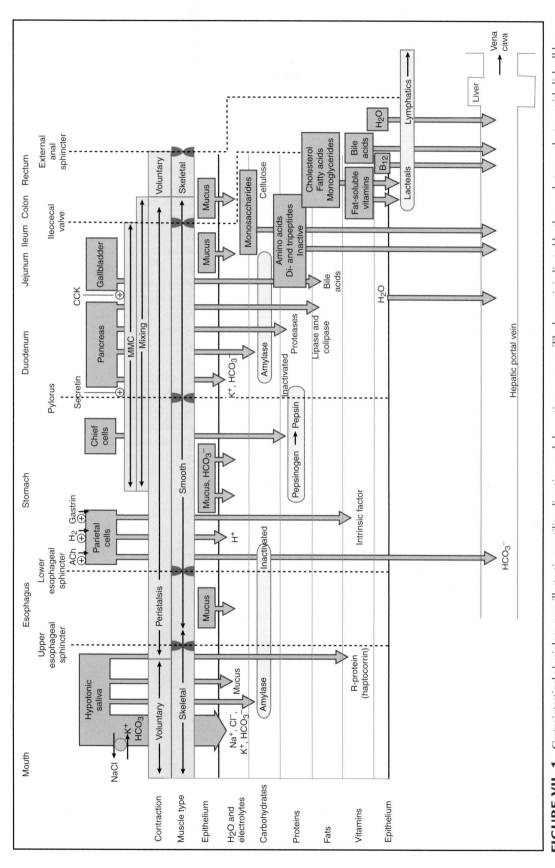

FIGURE VII–1 Gastrointestinal physiology map illustrating motility, digestion, and absorptive processes. The dietary components are identified on the left. The top of the diagram shows the anatomic structures with *vertical dashed lines* marking the sphincters. The top part also shows the main secretions that enter the limit of the gastrointestinal tract and the locations of skeletal and smooth muscle that propel the diet through the tract. Absorption of dietary components into the hepatic portal vein or the lacteals is shown at the bottom.

An 80-year-old woman is brought to her primary care physician by her adult daughter because the woman is losing weight and unable to keep food down.

During the past several months the patient has lost weight and has had difficulty in swallowing both solid and liquid food. She frequently regurgitates undigested food both during the day and at night while sleeping. The patient describes a feeling of "fullness" and discomfort in her chest. She also frequently coughs and aspirates while eating.

PHYSICAL EXAMINATION

VS: T 37°C, P 74/min, R 15/min, BP 130/75 mm Hg
PE: Normal

LABORATORY STUDIES

Chest radiograph: Shows an air-fluid interface in an enlarged, fluid-filled esophagus

Barium esophagography: Esophageal dilation, a loss of esophageal peristalsis, poor esophageal emptying, and a smooth symmetrical "bird's beak" tapering of the distal esophagus.

Endoscopy: Normal with no sign of distal stricture or carcinoma

Esophageal manometry: Confirms complete absence of peristalsis in the lower third of the esophagus and elevated lower esophageal sphincter pressure with incomplete relaxation during swallowing

DIAGNOSIS

Achalasia

PATHOPHYSIOLOGY OF KEY SYMPTOMS

Achalasia results from the failure to move food from the esophagus into the proximal portion of the stomach. Consequently, the food can accumulate in the esophagus, where it can putrefy, and possibly move from the esophagus back upward through the upper esophageal sphincter and be aspirated.

The esophagus connects the pharynx and the stomach. Entry into the esophagus from the pharynx is limited by the tonic contracture of the upper esophageal sphincter. Retrograde entry into the esophagus from the stomach is similarly limited by the tonic contraction of the lower esophageal sphincter.

The musculature of the esophagus is a mixture of skeletal muscle and smooth muscle innervated by the enteric nervous system. The upper portions of the esophagus are predominantly skeletal muscle, the middle third of the esophagus a mixture of skeletal and smooth muscle, and the lower portion of the esophagus predominantly smooth muscle.

Movement of swallowed food through the esophagus occurs by peristalsis and is coordinated by the enteric nervous system. The stimulation of stretch receptors in the pharynx initiates the reflex. During swallowing reflex, contraction of the vocal cords and the neck muscles position the epiglottis to prevent food entry into the respiratory passages.

The swallowing reflex begins as a voluntary action in the mouth and continues as an involuntary reflex through the pharynx and the esophagus (Fig. 52-1). Esophageal peristalsis results from two muscular actions: a contraction of the muscle proximal to the bolus of food and a relaxation of the muscle distal to the bolus of food. As the wave of relaxation progresses down the esophagus, the bolus of food is moved down

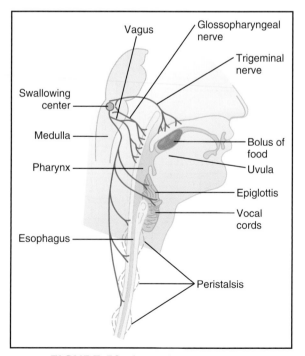

FIGURE 52–1 Swallowing mechanism.

the esophagus by the wave of contraction proximal to the bolus.

Peristalsis requires the relaxation of the tonically contracted esophageal sphincters. It is coordinated by the actions of the enteric nervous system, and the relaxation of the lower esophageal sphincter is mediated by the neurotransmitters nitric oxide and vasoactive intestinal peptide. In achalasia, enteric nervous system is disrupted and the lower esophageal sphincter does not relax. This traps swallowed food in the distal portions of the esophagus. In this patient, the achalasia is sufficiently severe to prevent the movement of fluids from the esophagus into the stomach. Consequently, an air-fluid interface is seen on the chest radiograph, along with fluid in the lower portion of the esophagus.

OUTCOME

Treatment of achalasia is based on disrupting the contraction of the lower esophageal sphincter. Mechanically, it is possible to inflate a balloon to tear the muscles of the lower esophageal sphincter or surgically to cut the muscles. Pharmacologically, calcium channel blockers can be used to relax the smooth muscle, because smooth muscle contraction is dependent on the entry of extracellular calcium. Alternatively, repeated injections of botulinum toxin into the lower esophageal sphincter can provide improvement for about 6 months.

The consequence of disruption of the lower esophageal sphincter is that gastric contents now have access to the distal portions of the esophagus. The reflux of gastric acids can result in irritation and damage to the esophageal epithelia. Successful treatment of achalasia, therefore, can result in gastroesophageal reflux disease.

FURTHER READING

Text Sources
Carroll RG: Elsevier's Integrated Physiology. Philadelphia, Elsevier, 2007.
Copstead L, Banasik J: Pathophysiology, 3rd ed. Philadelphia, Saunders, 2005.
Dudek RW, Louis TM: High-Yield Gross Anatomy, 3rd ed. Philadelphia, Lippincott Williams & Wilkins, 2007.

Guyton AC, Hall JE: Textbook of Medical Physiology, 11th ed. Philadelphia, Saunders, 2006.
McPhee SJ, Papadakis MA, Tierney LM Jr: Current Medical Diagnosis and Treatment, 46th ed. New York, McGraw-Hill, 2007.

53

A 55-year-old man visits his primary care physician complaining of burning abdominal pain that begins shortly after eating.

The patient has experienced pain associated with eating for the past few months. Sometimes the pain diminishes after eating and recurs 2 hours later. In the past, the pain had been relieved by antacids but not by nonsteroidal anti-inflammatory drugs (NSAIDs). The patient has smoked one pack of cigarettes a day for 40 years and drinks 4 cups of coffee a day. He reports an 8-pound weight loss over the past 3 months without intentional diet or exercise.

PHYSICAL EXAMINATION

VS: T 37 °C, P 78/min, R 22/min, BP 145/90 mm Hg, BMI 25

PE: The patient appears generally healthy. During physical examination, the patient reports epigastric tenderness to deep palpation.

LABORATORY STUDIES

Fecal analysis: Positive for occult blood and positive fecal antigen assay for *Helicobacter pylori*

Endoscopy with gastric mucosal biopsy: Ulcer detected; biopsy positive for *H. pylori* infection

DIAGNOSIS

Peptic ulcer

PATHOPHYSIOLOGY OF KEY SYMPTOMS

Acid-base balance of the stomach and small intestine results from acid secretion in the stomach (Fig. 53-1) that is neutralized by the bicarbonate secretion of the small intestine (Fig. 53-2). The gastric and duodenal mucosa is protected from damage by the luminal pH by a layer of mucus. Damage to the mucosal layer causes pain and can cause bleeding into the intestinal lumen. The presence of blood in the stool indicates that the mucosal layer has been damaged.

A peptic ulcer results from the simultaneous imbalance of acid secretion and the disruption of the barrier that normally protects the gastric and duodenal mucosa (Fig. 53-3). Once the mucosal barrier is damaged, the pain associated with peptic ulcers is associated with gastric acid secretion. Gastric mucus secretion is stimulated by certain prostaglandins. NSAIDs and other drugs that inhibit cyclooxygenase block prostaglandin

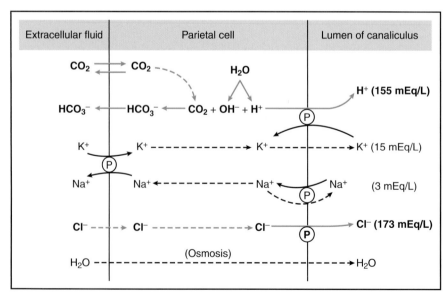

FIGURE 53–1   Postulated mechanism for secretion of hydrochloric acid. (The points labeled "P" indicate active pumps, and the *dashed lines* represent free diffusion and osmosis.)

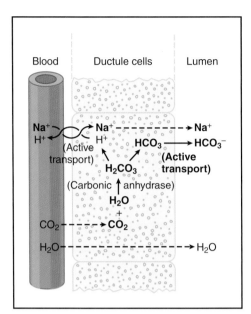

FIGURE 53–2 Secretion of isosmotic sodium bicarbonate solution by the pancreatic ductules and ducts.

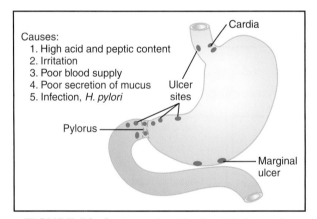

FIGURE 53–3 Peptic ulcer. *H. pylori, Helicobacter pylori.*

production and, consequently, can damage the gastric mucosal barrier. Therefore, patients taking aspirin or other NSAIDs for pain relief often experience exacerbation of the ulcer.

Ingestion of food increases gastric acid production by multiple mechanisms, including vagal activation (the cephalic phase), the presence of food in the stomach (the gastric phase), and the presence of food in the duodenum (the intestinal phase) (Fig. 53-4). The major mediators of gastric acid secretion are vagal nerve activity, gastrin produced by gastric G cells, and histamine produced by the enterochromaffin-like (ECL) cells. Gastric acid production is diminished by a drop in the gastric luminal pH, mediated by somatostatin.

Gastric acidity is initially neutralized by the buffering action of food. Consequently, ingestion of food causes some acute symptomatic relief. The same food ingestion, however, is a stimulus for additional acid production. Thus, the pain can recur as gastric acidity again falls owing to the higher acid secretion.

Gastric acid is neutralized when the chyme enters the duodenum. Acidity in the duodenal lumen is a potent stimulus for pancreatic bicarbonate secretion, mediated by the hormone secretin. Duodenal acidity is also a strong inhibitor of gastric emptying. Consequently, movement of gastric acid into the duodenum is normally limited to a volume that can be neutralized.

H. pylori is a gram-negative bacillus often found in the stomach. *H. pylori* produces urease enzymes that metabolize urea to ammonia and CO_2. The ammonia neutralizes the gastric acid and protects the bacillus. The ammonia also damages the gastric epithelial cells, contributing to the formation of an ulcer.

Many individuals with gastric *H. pylori* never develop any symptoms of peptic ulcer disease. However, in individuals who do develop peptic ulcer disease, *H. pylori* is almost always present.

OUTCOME

The most effective treatment of peptic ulcers is to use antibiotics directed against *H. pylori.* After the *H. pylori* infection is removed, the gastric mucosal barrier can be reestablished, isolating the gastric and intestinal mucosa from the luminal acidity. The pain associated with peptic ulcer disease can be managed by diminishing luminal pH. Ingestion of antacids (primarily bicarbonate) buffer the gastric luminal pH and provide rapid relief. Alternatively, symptoms can be relieved by diminishing acid secretion by the gastric parietal cells. Parietal cell acid secretion is stimulated by vagal nerve activity, gastrin, and locally released histamine. H_2 antagonists such as cimetidine diminish the rate of acid production and provide short-term relief. Proton pump inhibitors inactivate the H^+/K^+ ATPase protein, providing longer-term relief.

Source	Substance Secreted	Stimulus for Release	Function
Mucous neck cells	Mucus	Tonic secretion; also irritation of mucosa	Physical barrier between lumen and epithelium
	Bicarbonate	Secreted with mucus	Buffers gastric acid to prevent damage to epithelium
Parietal cells	Gastric acid (HCl)	Acetylcholine, gastrin, histamine	Activates pepsin; kills bacteria
	Intrinsic factor		Complexes with vitamin B_{12} to permit absorption
Enterochromaffin-like (ECL) cells	Histamine	Acetylcholine, gastrin	Stimulates gastric acid secretion
Chief cells	Pepsin(ogen)	Acetylcholine, acid, secretin	Digests proteins
	Gastric lipase		Digests fats
D cells	Somatostatin	Acid in the stomach	Inhibits gastric acid secretion
G cells	Gastrin	Acetylcholine, peptides, and amino acids	Stimulates gastric acid secretion

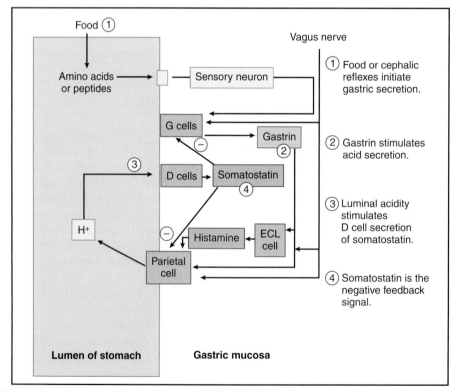

FIGURE 53–4 Gastric acid secretion is regulated by neural, endocrine, and paracrine agents. Gastric acid secretion by the parietal cell is under complex regulation. The enterochromaffin-like (ECL) cell releases histamine that stimulates acid secretion. Both the hormone gastrin and the neurotransmitter acetylcholine can stimulate the ECL cell to release histamine and can directly stimulate the parietal cell to secrete acid. Gastrin is released by amino acids or peptides in the lumen of the stomach, and acetylcholine is released by nervous system reflexes. Excess acid in the lumen of the stomach causes D cells to release somatostatin, which inhibits both gastrin release and parietal cell acid secretion.

FURTHER READING

Text Sources

Carroll RG: Elsevier's Integrated Physiology. Philadelphia, Elsevier, 2007.

Copstead L, Banasik J: Pathophysiology, 3rd ed. Philadelphia, Saunders, 2005.

Dudek R, Louis T: High-Yield Gross Anatomy. Philadelphia, Lippincott Williams & Wilkins, 2008.

Guyton AC, Hall JE: Textbook of Medical Physiology, 11th ed. Philadelphia, Saunders, 2006.

McPhee SJ, Papadakis MA, Tierney LM Jr: Current Medical Diagnosis and Treatment, 46th ed. New York, McGraw-Hill, 2007.

CASE 54

A 54-year-old man comes to the emergency department at 2 o'clock in the morning after being awakened by an intense left-sided chest pain radiating to his back.

The patient spent the evening at a college reunion where he sampled several spicy dishes and consumed a moderate quantity of beer. His past medical history includes an appendectomy at age 18 and a cholecystectomy at age 34.

PHYSICAL EXAMINATION

VS: T 36.4°C, P 80/min, R 18/min, BP 130/90 mm Hg
PE: The abdomen is not tender, and the patient denies vomiting or nausea. He is anxious but is not pale or diaphoretic.

LABORATORY STUDIES

Plasma analysis results: Within normal limits
ECG: Normal sinus rhythm
Cardiac enzymes: Troponin and CK-MB levels normal
Endoscopy: Normal

DIAGNOSIS

Gastroesophageal reflux disease (GERD)

PATHOPHYSIOLOGY OF KEY SYMPTOMS

The major symptom of GERD is chest pain, often called heartburn. The pain is a result of inflammation of the esophagus caused by the reflux of acidic contents from the stomach. GERD does not normally occur because the lower esophageal sphincter maintains enough tone to prevent the acidic gastric contents from entering the esophagus.

The esophagus is normally isolated from the stomach by both anatomic and physiologic mechanisms. Anatomically, these are the crural diaphragm and location of the gastroesophageal junction below the diaphragmatic hiatus. Physiologically, the isolation is achieved by the contraction of the smooth muscle of the lower esophageal sphincter.

The band of smooth muscle that comprises the lower esophageal sphincter is normally contracted. During the swallowing reflex, the wave of peristalsis

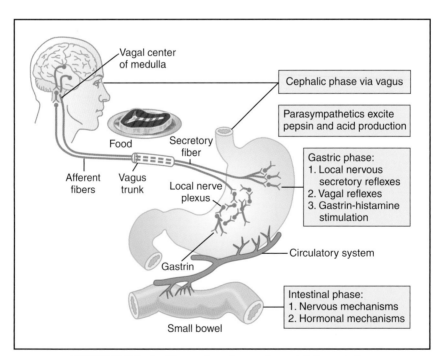

FIGURE 54–1 Phases of gastric secretion and their regulation.

descending along the esophagus causes the relaxation of the lower esophageal sphincter. Relaxation is mediated by the enteric nervous system, using nitric oxide and vasoactive intestinal peptide as neurotransmitters.

Food ingestion increases acid production by the parietal cells of the gastric mucosa. There are three separate mechanisms stimulating acid secretion: the cephalic phase mediated by the central nervous system and the vagus nerve, a gastric phase caused by the presence of food within the stomach, and an intestinal phase caused by the entry of moderately acidic chyme into the duodenum (Fig. 54-1). Acid secretion is enhanced by acetylcholine, gastrin, and histamine; and acid secretion is inhibited by somatostatin. The high rate of acid secretion results in gastric contents being much more acidic than the ingested food that originally passed through the esophagus.

Regurgitation of acidic chyme into the esophagus acutely causes pain and inflammation but chronically can lead to a change in the histology of the esophageal mucosa called Barrett's esophagus. Individuals with Barrett's esophagus are at particular risk for developing esophageal adenocarcinoma.

OUTCOME

Treatment centers on the relief of symptoms. The symptoms are caused by the reflux of acidic gastric contents through the lower esophageal sphincter and into the esophagus. Treatment strategies include diminishing the volume of the reflux, reducing the acid content of the reflux, or reestablishing the patency of the lower esophageal sphincter. The volume of the reflux can be diminished by eating smaller foods and avoiding lying down for 3 hours after meals. Gastric acid production can be acutely buffered by ingestion of antacids or diminished at the cellular level by H_2 receptor antagonists or proton pump inhibitors. Surgical treatment by laparoscopic fundoplication, in which the fundus of the stomach is sutured to a higher portion of the esophagus, is an option.

FURTHER READING

Text Sources
Carroll RG: Elsevier's Integrated Physiology. Philadelphia, Elsevier, 2007.
Copstead LC, Banasik J: Pathophysiology, 3rd ed. Philadelphia, Saunders, 2005.
Guyton AC, Hall JE: Textbook of Medical Physiology, 11th ed. Philadelphia, Saunders, 2006.

Kasper DL, Braunwald E, Fauci AS, et al: Harrison's Principles of Internal Medicine, 16th ed. New York, McGraw-Hill, 2005.
McPhee SJ, Papadakis MA, Tierney LM Jr: Current Medical Diagnosis and Treatment, 46th ed. New York, McGraw-Hill, 2007.

A 65-year-old woman comes to the clinic complaining of weakness and lethargy.
The patient indicates that for the past 6 years she has had rheumatoid arthritis and has managed the pain by daily ingestion of a nonsteroidal anti-inflammatory drug (NSAID). During the past 6 months, she noted a decrease in stamina.

PHYSICAL EXAMINATION

VS: T 36°C, P 80/min, R 18/min, BP 90/70 mm Hg, BMI 22
PE: Patient is pale and thin. Physical examination is otherwise unremarkable.

LABORATORY STUDIES

Blood analysis: Hematocrit 25%
Blood smear: Megaloblastic cells (MCV 120 fL) and hypersegmented neutrophils
Serum vitamin B_{12}: 90 pg/mL
Schilling test: Lack of absorption of vitamin B_{12}.

DIAGNOSIS

Pernicious anemia

PATHOPHYSIOLOGY OF KEY SYMPTOMS

Red blood cell synthesis depends on adequate stores of iron, amino acids, and vitamins B_6 and B_{12}. Vitamin B_{12} is a water-soluble vitamin not produced by the body; consequently, it must be a component of the diet and absorbed through the gastrointestinal system. It is a common component of foods of animal origin.

Vitamin B_{12} absorption depends on gastric production of intrinsic factor. Intrinsic factor is secreted by gastric parietal cells, which bind to vitamin B_{12} in the stomach. The B_{12} intrinsic factor complex is absorbed by sodium-coupled transport in the terminal ileum and carried to the liver by the hepatic portal system. The liver can store up to 3 years worth of vitamin B_{12}. Therefore, dietary deficiency is rare except in vegans who avoid all animal products.

Pernicious anemia results from a defect in the production of intrinsic factor. This defect can be due to an autoimmune disease or from chronic gastritis. Vitamin B_{12} is also necessary for normal nerve function, and chronic B_{12} deficiency can include neurologic symptoms such as tingling or numbness of the hands and feet and loss of balance.

The absence of vitamin B_{12} leads to the synthesis of a decreased number of red blood cells, but the individual red blood cells are larger than normal. This leads to the characterization of the disorder, which is macrocytic megaloblastic anemia.

OUTCOME

The patient is treated with an intramuscular injection of 100 μg of vitamin B_{12} and counseled on avoiding chronic NSAID use. Cyanocobalamin injection (Cobal, Cyanoject, Cyomin, Vibal) is also used.

FURTHER READING

Web Sources
http://www.nlm.nih.gov/medlineplus/ency/article/000569.htm
http://www.nhlbi.nih.gov/health/dci/Diseases/prnanmia/prnanmia_what.html
http://www.medicinenet.com/pernicious_anemia/article.htm

Text Sources
Carroll RG: Elsevier's Integrated Physiology. Philadelphia, Elsevier, 2007.
Copstead L, Banasik J: Pathophysiology, 3rd ed. Philadelphia, Saunders, 2005.

Devalia V: Diagnosing vitamin B_{12} deficiency on the basis of serum B_{12} assay, BMJ 333:654–655, 2006.
Guyton AC, Hall JE: Textbook of Medical Physiology, 11th ed. Philadelphia, Saunders, 2006.
Lagarde S, Jovenin N, Diebold MD, et al: Is there any relationship between pernicious anemia and iron deficiency? Gastroenterol Clin Biol 30:1245–1249, 2006.
McPhee SJ, Papadakis MA, Tierney LM Jr: Current Medical Diagnosis and Treatment, 46th ed. New York, McGraw-Hill, 2007.

A 38-year-old man comes to the emergency department complaining of an abrupt, severe epigastric pain.

The patient is a known alcoholic who has been seen in the emergency department for several fights and accidents related to inebriation. Today he is brought in because of an attack of pain in his epigastric region after an afternoon drinking binge. The patient describes his pain as radiating to his back, and he feels nauseated. The patient recently vomited, and he is sweating profusely.

PHYSICAL EXAMINATION

VS: T 39°C, P 98/min, R 17/min, BP 95/70 mm Hg
PE: The patient's pain worsens with walking and lying supine. His pain lessens if he sits up or leans forward. On palpation, his upper abdomen is tender, without guarding, rigidity, or rebound. His abdomen is distended. He exhibits overall weakness, pallor, and cool, clammy skin. The patient also has mild jaundice.

LABORATORY TESTS

Blood Values
    Calcium: 8 mg/dL (normal: 8.4-10.2 mg/dL)
    Glucose: 130 mg/dL (normal < 120 mg/dL)
    Blood urea nitrogen (BUN): 40 mg/dL (normal: 7-18 mg/dL)
    Bilirubin total: 4.2 mg/dL (normal: 0.1-1.0 mg/dL)
Serum Alkaline Phosphatase
    Serum amylase: 400 U/L (normal: 25-125 U/L)
    Serum lipase: 220 U/L (normal: 20-70 U/L)
    White blood cells: Leukocytosis of 10,000/uL
    Urinalysis: Proteinuria +2 (normal: 0), granular casts
Abdominal radiograph: Gallstones and a "sentinel loop" (a segment of air-filled left upper quadrant of small intestine)
CT: Enlarged pancreas
Stool test: Fatty stool sample

DIAGNOSIS

Pancreatitis

PATHOPHYSIOLOGY OF KEY SYMPTOMS

The pancreas is a complex organ with numerous endocrine and exocrine secretions. The endocrine secretions include insulin and glucagon. The exocrine secretions consist of HCO_3^- and numerous digestive enzymes, including pancreatic lipase, amylase, and zymogens of peptidases and nucleases.

Pancreatic proteases are secreted by the pancreatic acinar cells in an inactive or zymogen form. Exocrine pancreatic secretions travel through the pancreatic duct and are secreted into the duodenum. Once in the lumen of the duodenum, pancreatic trypsinogen is converted to trypsin by the duodenal enterokinase. Trypsin acts on the zymogens to convert them into active enzymes chymotrypsin and carboxypeptidase. This process ensures that the pancreatic secretions are not subjected to digestion and protein breakdown until they are in the lumen of the duodenum.

Acute pancreatitis results from the activation of the pancreatic digestive enzymes while in the pancreatic duct or the pancreatic tissues. The digestion of the pancreatic tissues results in an acute severe epigastric pain. The pain intensity increases when walking or lying flat and diminishes when sitting upright or leaning forward. Eating can also increase pain. The pain causes vomiting and strong sympathetic activation, including sweating and anxiety.

Based on the patient's history (alcoholism), his diagnosis may alternatively be chronic pancreatitis. Chronic pancreatitis is mainly caused by alcoholism or alcohol abuse. Damage caused by alcohol abuse may not appear for many years. The patient then may have a sudden onset of pancreatitis.

Serum amylase and lipase levels are elevated, reflecting damage to the pancreatic acinar cells. Destruction of pancreatic cells also results in an increase in leukocytes and an inflammation resulting in an elevation of body temperature.

Vascular volume depletion results in a drop in arterial blood pressure. The hypotension can result in acute tubular necrosis. Consequently, blood urea nitrogen levels are elevated and the urine can show proteins and granular cysts.

OUTCOME

A surgical nerve block can be performed to relieve pain. Analgesics such as meperidine should not be combined with alcohol, a risk for this patient. No fluid or foods should be given orally until the patient is free of pain and has bowel sounds. Begin with clear liquids and gradually advance the diet to solid foods. Give fluids intravenously to maintain intravascular volume and also give calcium gluconate intravenously (for hypocalcemia). Prescribe bed rest for at least a week. Depending on severity, surgery may be a possibility. Research is ongoing in the use of antiproteases to treat episodic chronic pancreatitis.

FURTHER READING

Text Sources

Carroll RG: Elsevier's Integrated Physiology. Philadelphia, Elsevier, 2007.

Copstead L, Banasik J: Pathophysiology, 3rd ed. Philadelphia, Saunders, 2005.

Guyton AC, Hall JE: Textbook of Medical Physiology, 11th ed. Philadelphia, Saunders, 2006.

Guzman EA, Rudnicki M: Intricacies of host response in acute pancreatitis. J Am Coll Surg 202:509-519, 2006.

Halangk W, Lerch MM: Early events in acute pancreatitis. Clin Lab Med 25:1-15, 2005.

Malangoni MA, Martin AS: Outcome of severe acute pancreatitis. Am J Surg 189:273-277, 2005.

McPhee SJ, Papadakis MA, Tierney LM Jr: Current Medical Diagnosis and Treatment, 46th ed. New York, McGraw-Hill, 2007.

Motoo Y: Antiproteases in the treatment of chronic pancreatitis. J Pancreas (Online) 8(4 Suppl):533-537, 2007.

Samuel I, Chaudhary A, Fisher RA, et al: Exacerbation of acute pancreatitis by combined cholinergic stimulation and duct obstruction. Am J Surg 190:721-724, 2005.

A 26-year-old woman presents with fatigue and loose "sawdust-like" bowel movements as often as three times per day. She also notes an occasional rash over her joints that is extremely itchy.

The patient was delivered of a full-term infant 9 months ago. Her symptoms began approximately 1 month post partum. The patient also has a family history of autoimmune disease.

PHYSICAL EXAMINATION

VS: T 37°C, P 80/min, R 16/min, BP 90/60 mm Hg, BMI 17

PE: The patient's weight is 5 lb less than her pre-pregnancy weight. A papulovesicular rash is seen on extensor surfaces of her shoulders, elbows, buttocks, and knees. Wheat allergy is suspected.

LABORATORY STUDIES

Colonoscopy: Nonspecific colonic edema; biopsies were negative.

CeliaGENE test: Positive for HLA-DQ2, negative for HLA-DQ8

Serologic antibody test: Negative for anti-gliadin antibody, positive for anti-endomysial antibody

Upper endoscopy: Shortening of the villi and crypt hyperplasia evident on biopsy

DIAGNOSIS

Celiac disease

PATHOPHYSIOLOGY OF KEY SYMPTOMS

The gastrointestinal tract is an epithelium-lined tube that passes through the body from the mouth to the anus. It consists of the mouth (and salivary glands), pharynx, esophagus, stomach, small intestine, large intestine, rectum, and anus (Fig. 57-1). Along this tract, digestion and absorption of nutrients takes place. Various exocrine glands and cells secrete about 7 L of fluid into the gastrointestinal tract per day. Ingested food first passes through the esophagus into the stomach where it is mixed with acid and enzymes to create chyme. The chyme passes into the small intestine, where most digestion and nearly all absorption takes place. The epithelial mucosal layer of the small intestine is covered in villi to increase the surface area

available for absorption (Fig. 57-2). From the small intestine, only approximately 1.5 L/day of watery chyme passes into the large intestine, where water and electrolytes are absorbed, leaving semisolid feces to be propelled into the rectum and then to exit the body via the anus.

In malabsorption syndromes, defects in digestion, absorption, or transport cause inadequate assimilation of dietary substances (macronutrients and/or micronutrients) and excessive fecal excretion. This produces nutritional deficiencies and gastrointestinal symptoms. Celiac disease (celiac sprue, gluten sensitivity, wheat allergy) is a disorder of impaired absorption of most nutrients.

Glutens are the storage proteins present in wheat, barley, rye, and oats. It is hypothesized that glutens stimulate an inappropriate T cell–mediated autoimmune response in the submucosa of the small

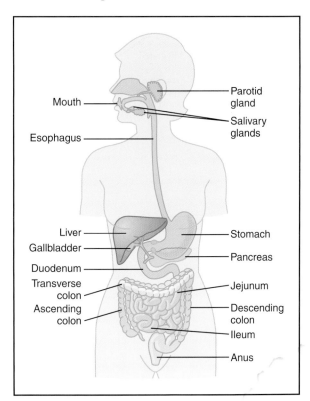

FIGURE 57–1 Alimentary tract.

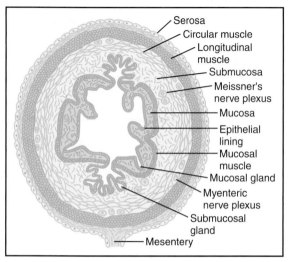

FIGURE 57–2 Typical cross section of the gut.

intestine. One target of this response is transglutamase, an enzyme that converts gliagin (a component of gluten) to a form that more strongly stimulates the T cells. This reaction causes damage to the villi of the small intestine. The exact mechanism of damage is unknown; however, it is clear that removal of gluten from the diet results in resolution of symptoms and intestinal healing.

When the villi of the small intestine are damaged, absorption is impaired, causing more than the usual 1.5 L of chyme to pass into the large intestine. In addition, the chyme is high in fats and undissolved bile salts, which stimulate and irritate the colon, causing diarrhea; it is high in unabsorbed carbohydrates, which are fermented by colonic bacteria, producing gas and fatty acids (bloating and steatorrhea).

Approximately 10% of patients with celiac disease will have dermatitis herpetiformis, which is an intensely pruritic rash over the extensor surfaces of shoulders, elbows, buttocks, knees, and scalp. The rash is brought on by ingestion of a high-gluten diet.

OUTCOME

The patient follows a gluten-free diet. Symptoms improve after 2 weeks of a strict gluten-free diet, and the patient is able to maintain a healthy BMI.

FURTHER READING

Text Sources
Carroll RG: Elsevier's Integrated Physiology. Philadelphia, Elsevier, 2007.
Copstead LC, Banasik J: Pathophysiology, 3rd ed. Philadelphia, Saunders, 2005.
Guyton AC, Hall JE: Textbook of Medical Physiology, 11th ed. Philadelphia, Saunders, 2006.

Kasper DL, Braunwald E, Fauci AS, et al: Harrison's Principles of Internal Medicine, 16th ed. New York, McGraw-Hill, 2005.
McPhee SJ, Papadakis MA, Tierney LM Jr: Current Medical Diagnosis and Treatment, 46th ed. New York, McGraw-Hill, 2007.

A 38-year-old man comes to the clinic complaining of abdominal cramping and diarrhea.

The patient has a 20-year history of alcohol abuse. He is complaining over the past 6 months of passing pale and malodorous stools that are difficult to flush.

PHYSICAL EXAMINATION

VS: T 37°C, P 72/min, R 15/min, BP 120/80 mm Hg
PE: The patient is malnourished, and his liver appears cirrhotic. His sclera are jaundiced.

LABORATORY STUDIES

Plasma analysis: Plasma K^+: 3.3 mEq/L (normal: 3.5-5.0 mEq/L)
Serum calcium: 1.9 mEq/L (normal: 2.1-2.8 mEq/L)
pH: 7.30 (normal: 7.35-7.45)
HCO_3^-: 18 mEq/L (normal: 22-28 mEq/L)
Serum triglycerides: 30 mg/dL (normal: 35-160 mg/dL)
Cholesterol: 130 mg/dL (normal < 200 mg/dL)
Fecal analysis: Positive for fat

DIAGNOSIS

Impaired fat absorption

PATHOPHYSIOLOGY OF KEY SYMPTOMS

Malabsorption is characterized as the inability to absorb ingested nutrients. The defect can be due to inadequate digestion, inadequate transport into the intestinal epithelia, or impaired movement from the intestinal epithelia into the body.

Lipid digestion is complex. Lipids are composed primarily of triglycerides and cholesterol. Ingested lipids interact with bile salts and lecithin in the lumen of the small intestine and become emulsified. Pancreatic lipase, assisted by colipase, digests the triglycerides into free fatty acids and monoglycerides (Fig. 58-1).

Cholesterol is transported across the apical surface of the intestinal epithelial cells. In addition, a fatty acid transport protein facilitates the movement of fatty acids and monoglycerides into the epithelial cell. Once within the cell, the absorbed fats combine with cholesterol and proteins in the Golgi apparatus to form chylomicrons. The chylomicrons exit the basolateral surface of the epithelial cell by exocytosis and are transported into the lacteals, through the lymphatic vessels, and enter the vena cava via the thoracic duct. Lipids are unique among dietary components in that absorbed lipids do not first pass through the liver before entering the vena cava.

Hepatic cirrhosis results in the impairment of bile acid production and secretion. The accumulation of bile pigments in the plasma results in jaundice, evidenced by a yellow discoloration of the sclera of the eye. Impaired biliary secretion results in an inability to sufficiently digest dietary fats. Dietary fats that are not digested remain in the lumen of the small intestine and then pass into the large intestine.

Poorly absorbed nutrients pass into the large intestine, where they serve as substrate for the colonic microflora. Bacterial metabolism generates intestinal gas and metabolites, which add to the osmotic load in the large intestine. The intestinal gas passes from the body as flatulence. The osmotic load impairs water absorption in the large intestine, resulting in diarrhea. Both the intestinal gas and the diarrhea result in abdominal cramps.

Lipid-soluble vitamins A, D, E, and K are absorbed mostly in micelles. Chronically impaired fat absorption also impairs absorption of these vitamins and results in a vitamin deficiency. Vitamin A deficiency can result in night blindness. Vitamin D deficiency can impair the intestinal obstruction of calcium, leading to a weakening of the bones. Bleeding disorders are characterized by vitamin K deficiency, because vitamin K is necessary for the synthesis of most of the proteins involved in the clotting cascade.

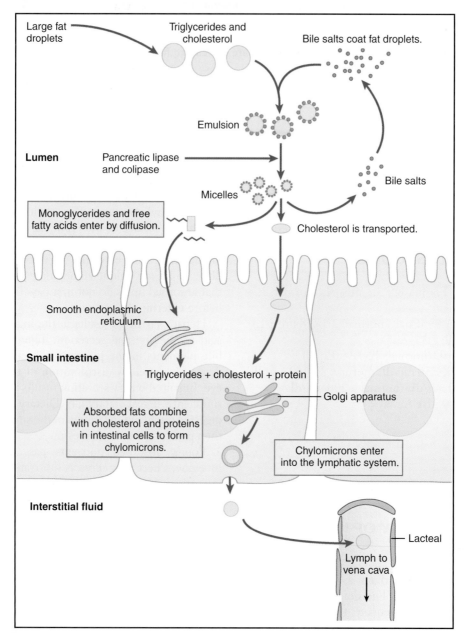

FIGURE 58–1 Products of lipid digestion are repackaged into chylomicrons in the intestinal epithelium. The combination of hepatic bile salts, pancreatic lipase, and pancreatic colipase digests fats into monoglycerides, free fatty acids, and cholesterol. These digested components enter the intestinal epithelial cells and are transported to the smooth endoplasmic reticulum. The absorbed fats combine with cholesterol and protein to form chylomicrons, which are secreted by exocytosis. The chylomicrons enter the lymphatic lacteals and are transported to the vena cava.

FURTHER READING

Text Sources

Carroll RG: Elsevier's Integrated Physiology. Philadelphia, Elsevier, 2007.

Copstead LC, Banasik J: Pathophysiology, 3rd ed. Philadelphia, Saunders, 2005.

Guyton AC, Hall JE: Textbook of Medical Physiology, 11th ed. Philadelphia, Saunders, 2006.

Kasper DL, Braunwald E, Fauci AS, et al: Harrison's Principles of Internal Medicine, 16th ed. New York, McGraw-Hill, 2005.

McPhee SJ, Papadakis MA, Tierney LM Jr: Current Medical Diagnosis and Treatment, 46th ed. New York, McGraw-Hill, 2007.

A 46-year-old man comes to the clinic complaining of abdominal cramping and severe diarrhea that has persisted for 36 hours.

The patient has just returned from a camping trip in the mountains. Both of his companions are also experiencing severe diarrhea. The diarrhea initially had loose feces but now is composed of mostly watery stools. The patient indicates he has not eaten in the past 24 hours, but he has consumed 2 L of a sports drink (Gatorade). The patient does not report nausea or a history of fever.

PHYSICAL EXAMINATION

VS: T 37°C, P 105/min, R 15/min, BP 90/70 mm Hg, BMI 29
PE: No significant findings

LABORATORY STUDIES

Plasma electrolytes:

- Sodium: 141 mEq/L (normal: 136-145 mEq/L)
- Potassium: 3.4 mEq/L (normal: 3.5-5.0 mEq/L)
- Chloride: 105 mEq/L (normal: 95-105 mEq/L)

Fecal analysis: Negative for the presence of leukocytes or blood but positive for the presence of enterotoxigenic *E. coli*.

DIAGNOSIS

Secretory diarrhea

PATHOPHYSIOLOGY OF KEY SYMPTOMS

The absorption of both dietary fluid intake and gastrointestinal secretions plays a major role in body fluid balance. In general, individuals consume 2 L of fluid each day and an additional 7 L of fluid is secreted into the lumen of the gastrointestinal tract. Of this total 9 L fluid load, only about 100 mL of fluid is lost each day in the feces.

The majority (7.5 L) of the fluid reabsorption occurs in the small intestine, and all but 100 mL of the remaining 1.5 L is absorbed in the large intestine. Chyme entering the large intestine through the ileocecal valve is predominantly fluid. There is a progressive absorption of water along the length of the small intestine, with the chyme progressing to solid feces during the 48-hour transit time through the large intestine (Fig. 59-1).

In general, diarrhea is caused by an osmotic imbalance, hypermotility, inflammation, or excessive secretion.

Osmotic diarrhea is due to the presence of poorly absorbed solutes in the intestinal lumen, such as the diarrhea accompanying milk ingestion in lactase-deficient individuals. Hypermotility diarrhea occurs when fluid passes through the intestines too quickly for normal absorption. Inflammatory diarrhea, such as that characterized by ulcerative colitis, is due to damage of the intestinal epithelial cells. Secretory diarrhea, such as is occurring in this individual, is a result of more water entering the intestinal lumen than can be absorbed.

Enterotoxic *E. coli* infection is contracted by oral ingestion of contaminated food or water. Enterotoxic *E. coli* is structurally similar to naturally occurring *E. coli*, but this strain produces enterotoxins that enhance chloride secretion by the intestinal crypt cells. At the cellular level, the toxin works through adenylyl cyclase to increase cyclic adenosine monophosphate, which opens the chloride channels (CFTR) on the apical surface of the epithelial cells. Secretion of chloride results in an electrogenic secretion of sodium. The high NaCl secretion results in osmotic movement of water into the lumen. The diarrhea results when the volume of water secreted by the intestinal crypt cells exceeds the volume of water that the small and large intestines are capable of absorbing.

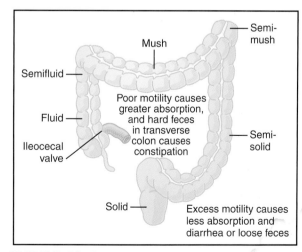

FIGURE 59–1 Absorptive and storage functions of the large intestine.

In the adult, diarrhea fluid usually has an osmolality approximately the same as plasma osmolality. The diarrhea fluid, however, contains a significant amount of potassium due to the colonic secretion of potassium. The clinical symptoms caused by persistent diarrhea, then, are an isosmotic extracellular fluid contraction and extracellular potassium depletion.

The patient's cardiovascular symptoms are hypotension and tachycardia. Isotonic fluid loss results in a drop in blood volume and, thus, a drop in arterial blood pressure. The drop in arterial blood pressure initiates the baroreflex-mediated increase in sympathetic activity and decrease in parasympathetic activity, resulting in an elevated heart rate. If sufficiently severe, the hypovolemia can result in diminished cutaneous blood flow and the patient can become pale and diaphoretic.

Hypokalemia increases the risks of cardiac arrhythmias and possibly muscle weakness. This patient does not seem to be exhibiting any symptoms related to hypokalemia, but the fluid replacement should contain potassium in addition to sodium and water. Sports drinks generally have potassium in addition to glucose and sodium.

Oral rehydration solution is particularly effective in diminishing the harmful effects of secretory diarrhea, particularly due to cholera. Glucose is absorbed in the small intestine through sodium-coupled transport. As glucose and sodium are absorbed, chloride is absorbed to maintain electroneutrality, and water is absorbed by an osmotic gradient. This enhanced absorption helps to diminish negative fluid balance, which is characteristic of the secretory diarrhea. CFTR inhibitors, which block the CFTR channel and consequently ion movement, are being investigated as a potential therapy for secretory diarrhea.

In general, most forms of diarrhea are self-limiting and gradually diminish over 24 to 72 hours. Maintaining adequate fluid intake, particularly in the form of oral rehydration solution, prevents cardiovascular collapse until fluid and electrolyte balance is restored.

OUTCOME

The patient was given 2 L of isotonic saline and was counseled to continue to consume the sports drinks. The symptoms gradually resolved over the next 24 hours.

FURTHER READING

Text Sources

Al-Awqati Q: Alternative treatment for secretory diarrhea revealed in a new class of CFTR inhibitors. J Clin Invest 110:1599-1601, 2002.

Carroll RG: Elsevier's Integrated Physiology. Philadelphia, Elsevier, 2007.

Copstead LC, Banasik J: Pathophysiology, 3rd ed. Philadelphia, Saunders, 2005.

Guyton AC, Hall JE: Textbook of Medical Physiology, 11th ed. Philadelphia, Saunders, 2006.

Kasper DL, Braunwald E, Fauci AS, et al: Harrison's Principles of Internal Medicine, 16th ed. New York, McGraw-Hill, 2005.

McPhee SJ, Papadakis MA, Tierney LM Jr: Current Medical Diagnosis and Treatment, 46th ed. New York, McGraw-Hill, 2007.

A 56-year-old man comes to his family physician complaining of fecal incontinence.
The patient had surgery 6 months earlier to treat rectal hemorrhoids. The surgery was successful, but over the past 2 months the patient indicates difficulty in determining when he needs to have a bowel movement.

PHYSICAL EXAMINATION

VS: T 37°C, P 76/min, R 15/min, BP 130/90 mm Hg, BMI 27
PE: No apparent abnormalities. Digital examination of the rectum does not show any signs of rectal prolapse.

LABORATORY STUDIES

Anal manometry: Decreased tone in the internal anal sphincter but normal tone in the external anal sphincter
Proctosigmoidoscopy: Muscle damage to the internal anal sphincter
Anal electromyography: Nerve damage

DIAGNOSIS

Fecal incontinence

PATHOPHYSIOLOGY OF KEY SYMPTOMS

Feces are normally prevented from exiting the body due to contraction of the internal anal sphincter and the external anal sphincter. The internal anal sphincter is a band of circular smooth muscle located at the distal portion of the rectum. As with all gastrointestinal sphincters, the internal anal sphincter is normally contracted. The external anal sphincter is a ring of voluntary skeletal muscle that both surrounds the internal anal sphincter and extends to the anus. The external anal sphincter is innervated by the alpha-motor neurons of the pudendal nerve and is under voluntary control. The external anal sphincter is also usually contracted.

The rectum is usually empty. When feces enter the rectum from the sigmoid colon, the rectum is distended and afferent sensory nerves initiate an increase in peristalsis that forces the feces toward the anus. The approaching wave of peristalsis relaxes the internal anal sphincter and causes the external anal sphincter

to contract. Rectal distention initiates an urge to defecate, and if the external anal sphincter is allowed to relax, defecation will commence. The defecation reflex can be augmented by contraction of the abdominal muscles to force fecal contents from the sigmoid colon into the rectum.

The defecation reflex requires intact enteric nerves, afferent sensory signals transmitted to the spinal cord, efferent parasympathetic nerves from the spinal cord, and a functional pudendal nerve (Fig. 60-1). These nerves can be disrupted by surgery, such as the surgery to repair hemorrhoids.

OUTCOME

Muscular contraction of the external anal sphincter is voluntary, and individuals can be trained to increase the tone in that sphincter. In addition, patients can alter their diet by increasing fiber, resulting in a less watery stool. In extreme cases, the damaged area of the rectal sphincter can be surgically removed and the functional ends attached to restore the circular band of muscle.

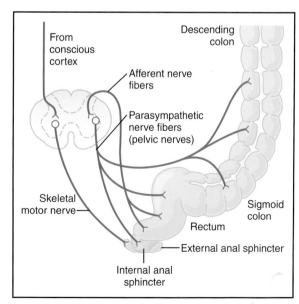

FIGURE 60–1 Afferent and efferent pathways of the parasympathetic mechanism for enhancing the defecation reflex.

FURTHER READING

Web Source

Feldman: Sleisenger & Fordtran's Gastrointestinal and Liver Disease, 8th ed. Philadelphia, Saunders, 2006. Available at http://www.mdconsult.com/das/booklist/body/87310867-2?booklist_order=title&format=AT

Text Sources

Carroll RG: Elsevier's Integrated Physiology. Philadelphia, Elsevier, 2007.

Copstead LC, Banasik J: Pathophysiology, 3rd ed. Philadelphia, Saunders, 2005.

Guyton AC, Hall JE: Textbook of Medical Physiology, 11th ed. Philadelphia, Saunders, 2006.

Kasper DL, Braunwald E, Fauci AS, et al: Harrison's Principles of Internal Medicine, 16th ed. New York, McGraw-Hill, 2005.

McPhee SJ, Papadakis MA, Tierney LM Jr: Current Medical Diagnosis and Treatment, 46th ed. New York, McGraw-Hill, 2007.

SECTION VIII

Metabolism

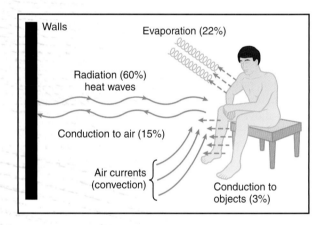

At the cellular level, metabolic processes describe the mitochondrial conversion of fuel into the high-energy phosphates needed to support cellular activity. At the organism level, metabolic processes describe substrate utilization but the physiologic focus on metabolism is tied more closely to substrate availability. Substrate availability is determined by intake, exchange with storage pools, metabolic consumption, and non-metabolic loss (Fig. VIII-1). The integrative nature of metabolism means that the regulation of metabolic activity is tied intimately with the endocrine, gastrointestinal, and renal systems and, indeed, interacts with all other physiologic systems.

Ingestion ultimately determines the availability of the primary metabolic substrates, glucose, and free fatty acids. Food intake is modulated by complex interaction of the hunger and the satiety centers in the hypothalamus (see Case 67). Layered on top of this regulation is the physical availability of substrates for ingestion.

Excess ingested food enters a variety of storage pools, including adipose, hepatic glycogen, muscle glycogen, proteins, and bone. Insulin decreases plasma glucose by increasing cellular uptake, as well as stimulating movement of glucose into storage pools and, if amino acid levels are high, stimulating protein growth (see Case 62). As plasma metabolic substrate levels fall, the storage pools are sequentially accessed

to help provide sufficient substrates or mitochondrial metabolism (see Case 66).

Mitochondria can use both glucose and free fatty acids as metabolic fuels. If both substrates are available, most tissues use glucose. In the absence of glucose, metabolic activity shifts to utilization of free fatty acids. Particularly for skeletal muscle and adipose, insulin is required for cellular uptake of glucose. In the absence of insulin, cellular glucose levels fall and mitochondria shift to metabolism of free fatty acids, generating ketones as a metabolic byproduct (see Case 61).

Whole-body metabolism consists of both basal metabolic rate and metabolism tied to activity including skeletal muscle activity. Basal metabolic rate is regulated by thyroid hormone (see Cases 63 and 64), and, consequently, alterations in thyroid hormone production alter whole-body metabolism. Cellular energetics is also tied to body core temperature. Increases in body core temperature increase metabolic activity in all tissues (see Case 68), and profound drops in body core temperature decrease the ability of all tissues to sustain metabolic activity (see Case 69).

In addition to glucose and fatty acids, calcium availability is controlled by the balance of ingestion, movement into and out of storage, and excretion. Parathyroid hormone is the primary regulator of cellular calcium levels (see Case 65), and impaired parathyroid hormone regulation alters plasma calcium levels.

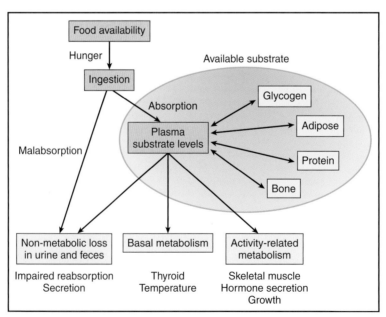

FIGURE VIII–1 The plasma concentration of the primary metabolic substrates (glucose and fatty acids) represents the balance between gastrointestinal absorption, exchange with storage pools, and loss through metabolic or non-metabolic routes.

A 6-year-old boy is brought to the pediatrician by his mother, who indicates the child is not well.

The patient is a generally healthy child who is up to date on all of his immunizations. Over the past few weeks, his mother has noticed that her son has been losing weight even though there is an increase in his appetite (polyphagia) and thirst (polydipsia). The patient says that he doesn't feel well, is tired (general malaise), can't keep up with the other kids, and has "to pee a lot" (polyuria).

PHYSICAL EXAMINATION

VS: T 36.8°C, P 80/min, R 22/min, BP 104/76 mm Hg, weight 46 lb (21 kg; 30th percentile), height 48 in (122 cm; 50th percentile)

PE: Patient has slightly decreased skin turgor. Until recently patient had been at the 50th percentile for weight and height.

LABORATORY STUDIES

Urinalysis:

- Color: light yellow (normal: colorless to dark yellow)
- Specific gravity: 1.050 (normal: 1.006 to 1.030)
- pH: 4.5 (normal: 4.6-8.0, average 6.0)
- Glucose: positive (+1) (normal: negative)
- Red blood cells: negative (normal: negative)
- Protein: negative (normal: negative)
- Ketones: positive (normal: negative)
- Leukocytes: negative (normal: negative)

Blood tests (fasting):

- Glucose: 250 mg/dL (normal: 64-128 mg/dL)
- C-peptide: 0.1 ng/ml (normal: 0.4-2.2 ng/mL)

DIAGNOSIS

Diabetes mellitus type 1

PATHOPHYSIOLOGY OF KEY SYMPTOMS

The patient's major symptoms are tied to a disruption in metabolism. The loss of weight combined with an increase in appetite reflects an increase in metabolic consumption or decrease in metabolic substrate availability. The feelings of tiredness and inactivity indicate that metabolic substrate availability is the more likely explanation. The presence of glucose and ketones in a dilute, acidic urine, the elevated plasma glucose, and the low levels of C-peptide are consistent with type 1 diabetes mellitus.

Insulin is derived from a larger pre-prohormone produced by the beta cells of the pancreas. An increase in plasma glucose is the most powerful stimulus for insulin release. In addition, ingestion of a carbohydrate meal stimulates insulin release through parasympathetic nerve activity and through the increase in gastrointestinal hormones cholecystokinin (CCK) and gastrointestinal inhibitory peptide (GIP).

Insulin decreases blood glucose by stimulating glucose uptake, utilization, and storage. Insulin enhances glucose uptake by skeletal muscle and adipose tissue by increasing the number of functional GLUT-4 transport proteins on the cell membrane (Fig. 61-1). Combined elevations in insulin and growth hormone stimulate amino acid uptake and protein synthesis in a variety of tissues. The hepatic and brain glucose transport proteins (GLUT-2 and GLUT-3, respectively) are not directly impacted by insulin. Insulin, however, increases hepatic glucose uptake and glycogen formation by increasing the activity of hexokinase and the cellular metabolic conversion of glucose. The combined actions of insulin result in a marked decrease in plasma glucose concentration.

Diabetes mellitus type 1 results from an impaired ability to secrete insulin. The exact cause is not yet known, but there appears to be an autoimmune destruction specifically of the pancreatic beta cells. Endogenous insulin production can be monitored by both plasma insulin levels and by the presence of the C-peptide fragment of the prohormone.

The lack or complete absence of insulin impairs glucose uptake, particularly by skeletal muscle. Mitochondria shift to free fatty acids as a metabolic fuel, generating ketones from the beta-oxidation of fatty acids. Consequently, diabetics exhibit a metabolic acidosis and produce an excessive amount of the ketones acetate, acetoacetate, and β-hydroxybutyrate. Diabetic ketoacidosis is a severe complication of untreated diabetes mellitus and is characterized by nausea, vomiting, and a fruity (ketone) odor on the breath.

Most of the brain tissue uses the GLUT-3 transport protein, which has a very high affinity for glucose and

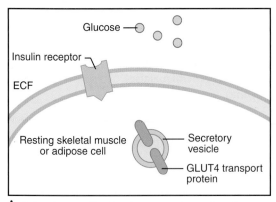

A. In the absence of insulin, glucose cannot enter the cell.

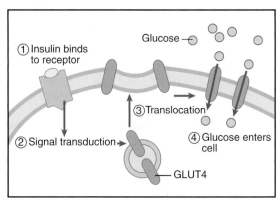

B. Insulin signals the cell to insert GLUT-4 transporters into the membrane, allowing glucose to enter the cell.

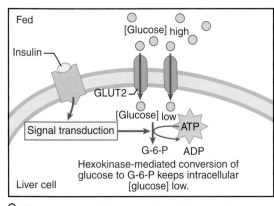

C. Hepatocyte. In the fed state, the liver cell takes up glucose and forms glycogen and fatty acids.

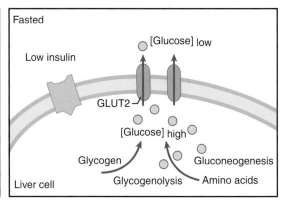

D. Hepatocyte. In the fasted state, the liver cell makes glucose from glycogen or amino acids and transports it to the blood.

FIGURE 61–1   Insulin entry by the GLUT4 transporter requires the action of insulin. In skeletal muscle and adipose tissue, glucose enters or requires insulin binding to a cell membrane receptor (**A**) and translocation of the vesicular GLUT4 transporters into the cell membrane (**B**). In contrast, glucose entry into hepatocytes (**C, D**) or neurons uses different GLUT transporters, which do not require insulin for activity.

is insulin insensitive. The brain satiety center, however, has an insulin-dependent glucose transporter. Consequently, the lack of insulin is interpreted as a decrease in blood glucose levels, leading to the hunger and polyphagia characteristic of diabetes mellitus.

Excessive production and impaired utilization lead to a marked increase in plasma glucose concentration. The elevated glucose levels alter fluid regulation. The kidney may filter more glucose than can effectively be reabsorbed, and glucose may be lost in the urine (for additional details, see Case 21). The glucose acts as an osmotic particle in the urine, leading to an osmotic diuresis. In addition, glucose acts as an osmotic particle within the plasma, stimulating the hypothalamic thirst centers. Type 1 diabetes mellitus is characterized by both a polyuria and a polydipsia.

The metabolic acidosis stimulates ventilation (respiration rate is elevated) and results in the excretion of a highly acidic urine. The urine also tests positive for ketones, indicating a shift to fatty acids as a metabolic substrate.

Insulin replacement is the principal management for patients with type 1 diabetes mellitus. Insulin can be administered by injection or by an insulin pump. Insulin dosages have to be titrated against the blood glucose concentration, and diabetic patients closely monitor carbohydrate intake to help them to achieve this balance.

FURTHER READING

Web Sources

http://www.emedicine.com/ped/topic581.htm
http://emsresource.net/vitals.shtml
http://www.nlm.nih.gov/medlineplus/ency/article/000305.htm

Text Sources

Carroll RG: Elsevier's Integrated Physiology. Philadelphia, Elsevier, 2007.

Copstead LC, Banasik J: Pathophysiology, 3rd ed. Philadelphia, Saunders, 2005.

Guyton AC, Hall JE: Textbook of Medical Physiology, 11th ed. Philadelphia, Saunders, 2006.

McPhee SJ, Papadakis MA, Tierney LM Jr: Current Medical Diagnosis and Treatment, 46th ed. New York, McGraw-Hill, 2007.

C A S E
62

A 54-year-old unresponsive man is brought to the emergency department.
The patient is a business executive and was late for an important meeting.
He was found unconscious on his office floor by his assistant. The assistant confirmed that the patient was breathing and then dialed 911. The ambulance crew arrived and provided supportive care, including initiating an intravenous line with lactated Ringers during transport to the local emergency department.

PHYSICAL EXAMINATION

VS: T 36.9°C, P 110/min, R 28/min, BP 90/70 mm Hg, BMI 31

PE: No apparent trauma. The patient is responsive to deep painful stimuli only. There is no medical alert bracelet or necklace.

LABORATORY STUDIES

Glucose (Accu-Chek): 36 mg/dL (normal: 64-128 mg/dL)

DIAGNOSIS

Hypoglycemia

PATHOPHYSIOLOGY OF KEY SYMPTOMS

Loss of consciousness can be related to a number of factors, including delivery of oxygen and glucose to the brain. This patient was found in an environment with adequate oxygen; and if vascular structures are intact, blood pressure should be sufficient to ensure central nervous system blood flow. The low blood glucose level is consistent with the finding of hypoglycemic shock.

Regulation of plasma glucose levels is complex, depending on glucose consumption and storage in a variety of tissues (Fig. 62-1). Pancreatic insulin decreases plasma glucose levels by both promoting storage and tissue utilization.

Hepatic glycogen is a glucose storage molecule whose synthesis is stimulated by insulin. Insulin increases the activity of the enzyme hexokinase, converting intracellular glucose to glucose-6-phosphate, and, ultimately, to glycogen. This process depletes cellular glucose levels, facilitating the entry of plasma glucose into the hepatocytes by diffusion. Glycogen can be mobilized back into glucose when plasma glucose levels fall.

Insulin indirectly enhances fat deposition in adipose tissue. Excess glucose entering the hepatocytes is converted into triglycerides and free fatty acids. Free fatty acids and triglycerides are released from the liver and, along with glucose, are absorbed by the adipocytes and stored as fats. Although glucose cannot be directly recovered from fat, free fatty acids can replace glucose as a metabolic substrate for mitochondria and preserve the remaining glucose for those tissues that use predominantly glucose for metabolic fuel, such as the brain.

Insulin, in combination with growth hormone, stimulates amino acid uptake by tissues and protein synthesis. Although amino acids cannot be directly generated from glucose, glucose can be generated from amino acids by hepatic and renal gluconeogenesis.

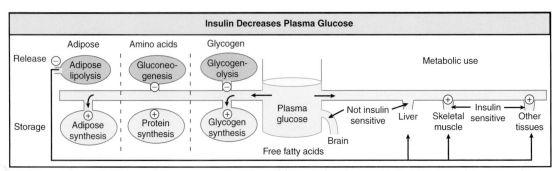

FIGURE 62–1 Plasma glucose levels represent the balance between gastrointestinal glucose absorption, movement into and out of storage pools, and metabolism by mitochondria. Insulin stimulates adipose protein and glycogen synthesis, and the uptake of glucose into skeletal muscle for metabolic use.

Consequently, body protein represents a glucose storage pool that can be used in extreme need.

Cellular uptake of glucose is facilitated by a family of sodium-coupled glucose transport proteins and GLUT proteins. Insulin stimulates glucose uptake by skeletal muscle and a variety of other tissues that utilize the GLUT-4 transport protein. Neuronal tissue uses a different isoform, GLUT-3, which is not insulin sensitive but which has a very high affinity for glucose. Glucose transport into neuronal tissue persists until plasma glucose levels drop below 50 mg/dL. A decrease in glucose below this level impairs neuronal metabolism and can cause confusion or a coma (insulin shock).

Treatment centers on rapidly restoring plasma glucose levels or infusion of glucagon, a hormone that increases plasma glucose levels. The patient was administered one ampule of D50 (50% dextrose in water). He rapidly regained consciousness and indicated that he is an insulin-dependent diabetic. In his rush to make preparations for his big meeting, he failed to eat breakfast after taking his normal morning dose of insulin.

FURTHER READING

Web Sources

http://www.emedicine.com/med/topic1123.htm
http://www.nlm.nih.gov/medlineplus/ency/article/000386.htm

Text Sources

Carroll RG: Elsevier's Integrated Physiology. Philadelphia, Elsevier, 2007.

Copstead LC, Banasik J: Pathophysiology, 3rd ed. Philadelphia, Saunders, 2005.

Guyton AC, Hall JE: Textbook of Medical Physiology, 11th ed. Philadelphia, Saunders, 2006.

McPhee SJ, Papadakis MA, Tierney LM Jr: Current Medical Diagnosis and Treatment, 46th ed. New York, McGraw-Hill, 2007.

A 30-year-old woman visits her primary care doctor with concerns about a growth on her neck.

The patient also complains about anxiety and irritability. She has noticed a 6-pound loss of weight over the past 2 months despite an increase in her appetite. She also feels uncomfortable when in a warm room.

PHYSICAL EXAMINATION

VS: T 38°C, P 110/min, R 18/min, BP 140/90 mm Hg, BMI 26
PE: Thyroid gland is enlarged symmetrically. Skin is warm and moist to the touch. Exophthalmos is evident by her protruding eyes. Onycholysis is present in her nails.

LABORATORY STUDIES

Blood analysis (thyroid panel):

- Serum TSH: 0.1 mIU/mL (normal: 0.4-6.0 mIU/mL)
- Thyroxine: 40 µg/dL (normal: 4.5-11.2 µg/dL)
- Triiodothyronine: 280 ng/dL (normal: 95-190 ng/dL)
- TSH receptor antibody: positive (normal: negative)

DIAGNOSIS

Graves' disease

PATHOPHYSIOLOGY OF KEY SYMPTOMS

The patient's major complaints—hyperactivity, weight loss, and warm intolerance—are all characteristic of an elevated metabolic rate. The enlargement of the thyroid gland and the exophthalmos are consistent with an elevation of thyroid hormone mediating the disturbances. Plasma analysis showing an elevated T_3 and T_4 confirm her hyperthyroid status.

Thyroid hormone is an iodinated derivative of the amino acid tyrosine. Thyroid hormone synthesis is controlled by peptides released from the hypothalamus and the anterior pituitary. The hypothalamus releases thyrotropin-releasing hormone (TRH), which acts on the anterior pituitary to release thyroid stimulating hormone (TSH). TSH binds to receptors on the follicle cells of the thyroid gland to stimulate iodide uptake and thyroid hormone synthesis. Mature thyroid hormone has either three iodides (T_3) or four iodides (T_4) attached to the tyrosine. The majority of thyroid hormone released by the thyroid gland is T_4, but T_3 has a stronger biologic activity. The combination of T_3 and T_4 together is referred to as thyroid hormone (Fig. 63-1).

Although thyroid hormone is synthesized from an amino acid, thyroid hormone is transported and acts in a manner analogous to the steroid hormones. In the plasma, only 1% of the thyroid hormone is free and the remainder is bound to thyroxine-binding globulin or other plasma proteins. Thyroid hormone crosses the cell membrane and binds to a nuclear receptor in the target tissues. In addition, T_4 is converted to T_3 by $5'$ deiodinases in many tissues. The biologic effects of thyroid hormone are tied to transcription and translation of proteins.

Thyroid hormone increases metabolic rate by increasing the size and density of mitochondria. In addition, thyroid hormone plays a permissive role in the growth and development of many tissues,

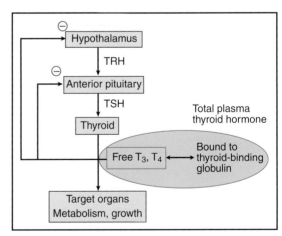

FIGURE 63–1 Free T_3 and T_4 provide feedback control for pituitary thyroid-stimulating hormone (TSH) release. Most circulating thyroid hormone is bound to thyroid-binding globulin. Free thyroid hormone levels produce both the biologic effects and the negative feedback signal regulating TSH release. TRH, thyroid-releasing hormone.

particularly the nervous system. Thyroid hormone can potentiate the action of additional hormones such as the catecholamines.

Thyrotoxicosis occurs when patients have serum T_4 and T_3 levels that are excessive for that individual (hyperthyroidism). Graves' disease is the most common cause of thyrotoxicosis. In Graves' disease, antibodies develop against the TSH receptor on the thyroid gland. The antibodies mimic the action of TSH and activate the receptors, resulting in stimulation of the thyroid gland and thyroid hormone synthesis. Stimulation of the TSH receptors causes an enlargement of the thyroid gland (goiter), and the elevated thyroid hormone levels cause the remainder of the patient's symptoms, such as the protruding eyeballs or exophthalmos.

The high T_3 and T_4 levels normally act by negative feedback to suppress the hypothalamic production of TRH and the anterior pituitary production of TSH. Antibody production, however, is not controlled by this negative feedback mechanism. Consequently, the high secretions of thyroxine cannot turn off the excessive stimulation of the thyroid.

Treatment options for individuals with Graves' disease include suppressing the immune system, clearing the antibodies from the plasma, suppressing the thyroid gland, thyroid gland removal, or blocking the actions of thyroid hormone.

FURTHER READING

Text Sources

Carroll RG: Elsevier's Integrated Physiology. Philadelphia, Elsevier, 2007.

Copstead LC, Banasik J: Pathophysiology, 3rd ed. Philadelphia, Saunders, 2005.

Guyton AC, Hall JE: Textbook of Medical Physiology, 11th ed. Philadelphia, Saunders, 2006.

McPhee SJ, Papadakis MA, Tierney LM Jr: Current Medical Diagnosis and Treatment, 46th ed. New York, McGraw-Hill, 2007.

A 48-year-old woman visits her family practitioner complaining of fatigue, weakness, and weight gain.

The patient also states that she experiences frequent muscle cramping and always feels cold. When questioned, she indicates that she has experienced an increase in constipation and headaches during the past 2 months.

PHYSICAL EXAMINATION

VS: T 36°C, P 50, R 16, BP 100/64 mm Hg, BMI 32
PE: The patient is an overweight postmenopausal female. Her skin is pale, dry, and thin, and her hair is brittle.

LABORATORY STUDIES

Red blood cell count: 3.9 million cells/μL (normal: 4.2 to 5.4 million cells/μL)
Blood analysis (thyroid panel):

- Serum TSH: 6.4 mIU/mL (normal: 0.4-6.0 mIU/mL)
- Thyroxine (T_4): 3.9 μg/dL (normal: 4.5-11.2 μg/dL)
- Triiodothyronine (T_3): 80 ng/dL (normal: 95-190 ng/dL)
- TSH receptor antibody: Negative (normal: negative)
- Thyroid antibodies: Positive (normal: negative)

DIAGNOSIS

Hypothyroidism (Hashimoto's thyroiditis)

PATHOPHYSIOLOGY OF KEY SYMPTOMS

The patient's presenting symptoms of fatigue, weight gain, and cold intolerance all indicate an abnormally low metabolic rate. The thin skin and brittle hair also indicate impaired protein synthesis. Thyroid hormone is a major hormone controlling basal metabolism. The thyroid panel confirms hypothyroidism.

Thyroid hormone is an amino acid derivative synthesized in the thyroid gland (Fig. 64-1). The thyroid gland consists of numerous follicles containing colloid surrounded by follicular cells. Follicular cells absorb iodide by sodium-coupled transport and accumulate the iodide within the colloid. The follicular cells also synthesize the large protein thyroglobulin and the enzymes necessary to attach the iodide to the tyrosine. Tyrosine residues bind to the thyroglobulin and are iodinated sequentially within the colloid. Each tyrosine can bind up to two iodides and, after iodination, two tyrosine residues join to form the mature thyroid hormones T_3 and T_4. The thyroglobulin bound to thyroid hormone is absorbed back into the follicular cell. The T_3 and T_4 are separated from the thyroglobulin and secreted into the blood.

Hypothyroidism can result from a number of causes, including the lack of dietary iodide. The iodide present in seawater is adequate to support normal thyroid function. In regions removed from the ocean, hypothyroidism and goiter are common findings. The addition of iodide to salt ensures that the lack of dietary iodide does not limit thyroid hormone production.

In Hashimoto's disease, an autoimmune response is directed against the thyroid tissue. Initially, follicle destruction releases T_3 and T_4 from the colloid, creating a transient hyperthyroid state (hashitoxicosis). The destruction of the follicles, however, means that that region of the thyroid gland will no longer be able to produce hormone. Ultimately, thyroid hormone levels fall and the patient exhibits signs of hypothyroidism. The diagnosis of Hashimoto's disease is confirmed by the presence of the anti-thyroid antibodies.

Secretion of hypothalamic thyrotropin-releasing hormone (TRH) and pituitary thyroid-stimulating hormone (TSH) is controlled by negative feedback from circulating thyroid hormone levels. Hypothyroidism causes an increase in TRH and TSH production. The elevated TSH can cause hypertrophy of the thyroid gland in the goiter, but the thyroid tissue does not produce hormone.

Treatment of hypothyroidism involves replacement therapy using the synthetic thyroid hormone levothyroxine. The appropriate dose is initially estimated, and TSH levels are monitored to ensure a physiologically appropriate dose.

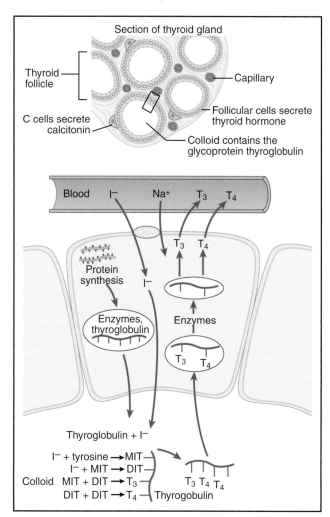

FIGURE 64–1 Thyroid hormone is synthesized within the colloid of thyroid follicles. The thyroid follicular cells actively transport iodide (I⁻) into the follicle, where it combines with the tyrosine residues attached to the protein thyroglobulin to make T_3 and T_4. The T_3 and T_4 are separated from the protein and secreted into the blood. MIT, monoiodinated tyrosine; DIT, diiodinated tyrosine.

FURTHER READING

Web Source
http://www.mayoclinic.com/health/hashimotos-disease/DS00567

Text Sources
Carroll RG: Elsevier's Integrated Physiology. Philadelphia, Elsevier, 2007.

Copstead LC, Banasik J: Pathophysiology, 3rd ed. Philadelphia, Saunders, 2005.

Goldman L, Ausiello D: Cecil Medicine, 23rd ed. Philadelphia, Saunders, 2007.

Guyton AC, Hall JE: Textbook of Medical Physiology, 11th ed. Philadelphia, Saunders, 2006.

McPhee SJ, Papadakis MA, Tierney LM Jr: Current Medical Diagnosis and Treatment, 46th ed. New York, McGraw-Hill, 2007.

C A S E

65

A 58-year-old woman is referred to an internist due to high calcium levels found during treatment for a fracture of her femur.

The patient's femur was fractured at the midshaft by a compression. The injury should not have been severe enough to break the bone. During treatment, the patient was noted to have high calcium levels and was referred for further study.

PHYSICAL EXAMINATION

VS: T 37°C, P 80/min, R 15/min, BP 116/76 mm Hg, BMI 26

PE: The patient appears healthy and exercised regularly before the injury. The left femur is immobilized, and the injury appears to be healing well.

LABORATORY STUDIES

Plasma analysis:

- Serum calcium: 14.2 mg/dL (normal: 8.4-10.2 mg/dL)
- Serum phosphorus (inorganic): 2.1 mg/dL (normal: 3.0-4.5 mg/dL)
- PTH levels: 2200 pg/mL (normal: 230-630 pg/mL)

DIAGNOSIS

Hyperparathyroidism

PATHOPHYSIOLOGY OF KEY SYMPTOMS

The patient's major symptoms are tied to bone integrity and calcium balance. Bone weakness can be localized, for example, owing to poor circulation or a growing tumor. Alternatively, the bone weakness can be generalized phenomena affecting all the bones in the body. Compromised bone integrity can be due to the loss of the organic bone matrix or the loss of calcium hydroxyapatite crystals.

Within the body, calcium balance is maintained by regulating dietary intake and absorption against renal excretion. Ninety-nine percent of body calcium is stored in bone complexed to phosphate as hydroxyapatite crystals. The remaining 1% is distributed within the cells (particularly the endoplasmic sarcoplasmic reticulum) and in the extracellular fluid. Normal plasma calcium concentration is 10 mg/dL, 50% of which

circulates as ionized (free) calcium, 40% complexed to plasma proteins, and 10% complexed to phosphate, citrate, and other nonprotein anions. Ionized calcium levels represent the balance between dietary absorption, exchange with storage pools, and renal excretion (Fig. 65-1).

Parathyroid hormone (PTH) increases plasma ionized calcium levels through a variety of mechanisms. It increases the renal conversion of vitamin D into its active form, 1,25-dihydroxycholecalciferol (also called vitamin D_3). Vitamin D_3 enhances the absorption of ingested calcium across the intestine and into the body. PTH activates osteoclasts and stimulates calcium reabsorption from bone stores. PTH has two major renal actions. It directly stimulates the distal tubule and collecting duct reabsorption of calcium, decreasing the renal excretion of calcium, and it also stimulates the renal excretion of phosphate, removing anions in the plasma that would otherwise bind calcium. Phosphate excretion increases the percentage of calcium that is in the ionized form.

Ionized plasma calcium provides a dominant negative feedback control of PTH release. Hypercalcemia

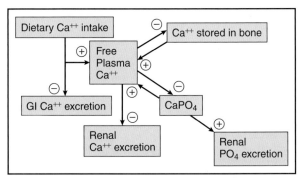

FIGURE 65–1 Parathyroid hormone increases free plasma Ca^{++}. Free plasma Ca^{++} represents the balance between dietary Ca^{++} uptake, exchange with the bone Ca^{++} storage pool, binding to PO_4, and renal Ca^{++} loss. Parathyroid hormone increases dietary Ca^{++} uptake by increasing vitamin D synthesis, increases osteoclast activity to release Ca^{++} stored in the bone, increases renal PO_4 excretion, and decreases renal Ca^{++} excretion. All these actions increase free plasma Ca^{++} levels.

inhibits PTH secretion, and hypocalcemia stimulates PTH release. The combined elevation of plasma calcium levels and PTH in this patient indicates that the negative feedback control of PTH is not functional. Disruption of negative feedback is characteristic of many endocrine tumors, including the parathyroid adenoma.

Hyperparathyroidism disrupts calcium regulation. Excessive stimulation of bone reabsorption causes depletion of hydroxyapatite crystals, weakening the bone. The persistent elevation in plasma calcium facilitates the formation of calcium-containing kidney stones. In severe cases, anorexia, nausea, and vomiting may occur, as can depression. The constellation of potential hyperparathyroid symptoms is summarized as "bones, stones, abdominal groans, and psychic moans."

Osteoporosis is a significant concern for postmenopausal women and can contribute to bone weakness. The patient's symptoms, however, are not indicative of osteoporosis. In osteoporosis, plasma calcium levels are normal in spite of the excessive bone demineralization. In addition, osteoporosis leads to a weakness at the neck of the femur instead of at the midshaft, as occurred in this patient.

Surgical parathyroidectomy is the best option to treat hyperparathyroidism. Removal of the parathyroid glands, however, can cause hypoparathyroidism, characterized by hypocalcemic paresthesias and tetany.

FURTHER READING

Text Sources

Carroll RG: Elsevier's Integrated Physiology. Philadelphia, Elsevier, 2007.

Copstead LC, Banasik J: Pathophysiology, 3rd ed. Philadelphia, Saunders, 2005.

Guyton AC, Hall JE: Textbook of Medical Physiology, 11th ed. Philadelphia, Saunders, 2006.

McPhee SJ, Papadakis MA, Tierney LM Jr: Current Medical Diagnosis and Treatment, 46th ed. New York, McGraw-Hill, 2007.

A 16-year-old girl is brought to a physician by her parents because of the patient's dramatic weight loss.

The patient dances 4 days a week at a private studio. During the past 2 months, she has not been interested in eating and now is weak and unable to complete the dance regimens. Her last menstrual period was 4 months ago.

PHYSICAL EXAMINATION

VS: T 35.5°C, P 55/min, R 15/min, BP 90/66 mm Hg, BMI 15

PE: The patient is thin with minimal subcutaneous fat stores. Leg muscles are well toned, but arm and upper body muscles are weak. Complexion is pale, and capillary refill after compression of a finger nailbed is slow. The patient denies that there is any problem.

LABORATORY STUDIES

Pregnancy test: Negative
Hemacrit: 32% (normal: 36-46%)

DIAGNOSIS

Starvation (anorexia nervosa)

PATHOPHYSIOLOGY OF KEY SYMPTOMS

This patient's symptoms are due to a negative caloric balance maintained for a long duration. Caloric restriction causes the loss of energy substrates, with depletion first of carbohydrates and then adipose and finally catabolism of muscle (Fig. 66-1). Blood pressure and body temperature fall, and the hypotension, combined with anemia, causes a pale complexion and slow capillary refill.

Glucose and fatty acids are the two metabolic substrates used by mitochondria. Fasting causes decreased glucose utilization and increased breakdown of glucose stores (Fig. 66-2). These changes are mediated by the starvation-induced increases in cortisol and growth hormone and decrease in insulin. The decrease in insulin reduces the uptake of glucose by skeletal muscle and other tissues.

Hepatic glycogen is the most labile of the glucose storage pools and is mobilized by glucagon and catecholamines early in fasting. In the absence of insulin, hexokinase activity is low and hepatic glycogen is broken down to form glucose. The glucose diffuses out of the hepatocytes using the GLUT-2 transporter. Hepatic glycogen is stored in a hydrated form, so that each gram of glycogen is tied to 2 g of water. Glycogenolysis causes both the loss of tissue glycogen stores and the loss of the water that normally is bound to them. Metabolism of glycogen stores also occurs during carbohydrate restriction, and the early weight loss associated with low carbohydrate diets is due to depletion of glycogen and water. Re-introduction of carbohydrates into the system, however, stimulates the recent assess of glycogen, along with the water weight gain.

Adipose tissue represents an energy storage pool that is mobilized by growth hormone and glucocorticoids during fasting lasting more than 1 day. Although adipose cannot be directly converted to glucose, adipolysis releases the free fatty acids and triglycerides to support mitochondrial metabolism. Mitochondrial metabolism of fatty acids causes the formation of ketone bodies.

Body protein and amino acid stores are the least labile form of energy storage. Cortisol is the major stress hormone of the body and, during prolonged starvation, glucocorticoids stimulate the catabolism

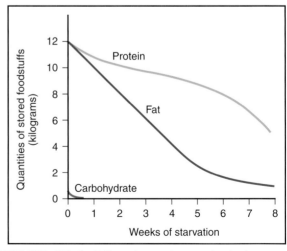

FIGURE 66–1 Effect of starvation on the food stores of the body.

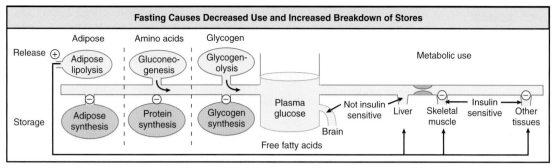

FIGURE 66–2   Plasma glucose levels represent the balance between gastrointestinal glucose absorption, movement into and out of storage pools, and metabolism by mitochondria. Fasting causes lipolysis and glycoglycogenolysis, and gluconeogenesis.

of proteins. Insulin, glucagon, catecholamines, and growth hormone levels are all suppressed. The amino acids are used for subsequent gluconeogenesis by the liver and kidney. This process ensures that at least a minimal level of plasma glucose remains to support brain metabolism.

Prolonged starvation leads to reduced metabolism, characterized by weakness, hypothermia, and the depletion of body protein stores. The cardiovascular system in particular has diminished activity, characterized by hypotension and bradycardia.

Anorexia nervosa is an eating disorder accompanied by body image distortion and a fear of gaining weight. Prolonged starvation leads to atrophy of the intestinal lumen. Consequently, foods must be gradually introduced to allow growth of the intestinal mucosa. If not, the diet will not be absorbed and will pass into the colon where it will be metabolized by colonic microflora, leading to cramping and diarrhea. Nutritional support should be followed by counseling to address the underlying cause for the eating disorder.

FURTHER READING

Text Sources
Carroll RG: Elsevier's Integrated Physiology. Philadelphia, Elsevier, 2007.
Copstead LC, Banasik J: Pathophysiology, 3rd ed. Philadelphia, Saunders, 2005.

Guyton AC, Hall JE: Textbook of Medical Physiology, 11th ed. Philadelphia, Saunders, 2006.
McPhee SJ, Papadakis MA, Tierney LM Jr: Current Medical Diagnosis and Treatment, 46th ed. New York, McGraw-Hill, 2007.

C A S E

67

A 23-year-old woman comes to her family physician complaining about weight gain.
The patient has gained 20 pounds since graduating from college 2 years ago and is now finding routine activities, such as climbing stairs, difficult. She was active in intramural sports while in college but has not found an organized physical activity since graduating. She works for a publishing firm and spends most of her time sitting at a desk. Her job requires a lot of overtime hours, and she admits to having a poor diet while working.

PHYSICAL EXAMINATION

VS: T 37.2°C, P 82/min, R 15/min, BP 130/85 mm Hg, BMI 31
PE: Patient is otherwise healthy.

LABORATORY STUDIES

Cholesterol: 242 mg/dL (recommended: < 200 mg/dL)
Triglycerides: 178 mg/dL (normal: 35-160 mg/dL)
Fasting blood glucose: 105 mg/dL (normal: 70-110 mg/dL)
LDL: 148 (recommended: < 130 mg/dL)
HDL: 46 (normal female: 50-60 mg/dL)

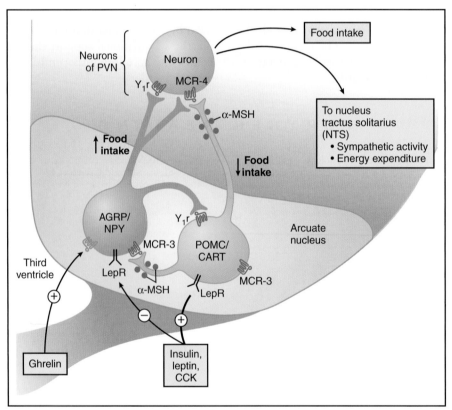

FIGURE 67–1 Control of energy balance by two types of neurons of the arcuate nuclei: (1) pro-opiomelanocortin (POMC) neurons that release alpha-melanocyte–stimulating hormone (α-MSH) and cocaine- and amphetamine-regulated transcript (CART), decreasing food intake and increasing energy expenditure; and (2) neurons that produce agouti-related protein (AGRP) and neuropeptide Y (NPY), increasing food intake and reducing energy expenditure. α-MSH released by POMC neurons stimulates melanocortin receptors (MCR-3 and MCR-4) in the paraventricular nuclei (PVN), which then activate neuronal pathways that project to the nucleus tractus solitarius (NTS) and increase sympathetic activity and energy expenditure. AGRP acts as an antagonist of MCR-4. Insulin, leptin, and cholecystokinin (CCK) are hormones that inhibit AGRP-NPY neurons and stimulate adjacent POMC-CART neurons, thereby reducing food intake. Ghrelin, a hormone secreted from the stomach, activates AGRP-NPY neurons and stimulates food intake. LepR, leptin receptor; Y_1R_1, neuropeptide Y_1 receptor. *(Redrawn from Barsh GS, Schwartz MW: Nat Rev Genet 3:589, 2002).*

TABLE 67–1   Neurotransmitters and Hormones that Influence Feeding and Satiety Centers in the Hypothalamus

Decrease Feeding (Anorexigenic)	Increase Feeding (Orexigenic)
Alpha-melanocyte-stimulating hormone (α-MSH)	Neuropeptide Y (NPY)
Leptin	Agouti-related protein (AGRP)
Serotonin	Melanin-concentrating hormone (MCH)
Norepinephrine	Orexins A and B
Corticotropin-releasing hormone	Endorphins
Insulin	Galanin (GAL)
Cholecystokinin (CCK)	Amino acids (glutamate and γ-aminobutyric acid)
Glucagon-like peptide (GLP)	Cortisol
Cocaine- and amphetamine-regulated transcript (CART)	Ghrelin
Peptide YY (PYY)	

DIAGNOSIS

Obesity

PATHOPHYSIOLOGY OF KEY SYMPTOMS

The patient's symptoms are tied to an imbalance between caloric intake and metabolic expenditure. An increase in body weight reduces physical stamina, and a reduced physical stamina often diminishes the quantity of calories expended by exercise. Changes in lifestyle often disrupt both eating patterns and activity patterns and can lead to changes in body weight. Eating patterns are regulated by complex interaction of physiologic factors such as hunger, environmental factors, and cultural factors.

At the level of physiology, food intake is regulated predominantly by the hunger and satiety centers of the hypothalamus. The hunger center is tonically active and contributes to appetite. After a sufficient quantity and quality of food is ingested, the hypothalamic satiety center is activated, which inhibits the hunger center. There are two major theories regarding activation of the satiety center, one suggesting that glucose utilization is the appropriate activator and a second suggesting that the body fat stores provide a signal that regulates the satiety center.

Within the hypothalamus, the pro-opiomelanocortin (POMC) neurons secrete alpha-melanocyte–stimulating hormone and the cocaine- and amphetamine-related transcript (CART), both of which decrease food intake and increase energy expenditure. Insulin, leptin, and cholecystokinin (CCK) activate the POMC neurons (Fig. 67-1). Increased food intake is mediated by the neurons that produce neuropeptide Y (NPY) and the agouti-related protein (AGRP). Ghrelin activates the AGRP/NPY neurons, stimulating hunger. There are overriding neurotransmitters and hormones that influence the feeding and satiety centers (Table 67-1).

In contrast to caloric intake, metabolic expenditure is only loosely regulated. Basal metabolic rate is influenced by thyroid hormone, and the catecholamines can increase metabolic rate. Most of the metabolic expenditure is due to activity, which is regulated by behavioral, rather than physiologic, mechanisms.

A 2006 study by the National Institutes of Health estimated that 26% of U.S. adults are obese and that 16% of children and adolescents younger than age 19 years are obese. These percentages have increased dramatically during the past 20 years. Obesity is a significant medical problem, because obese individuals are at increased risk for type 2 diabetes mellitus, heart disease, stroke, arthritis, and cancer.

Effect of weight loss requires the balance of calories consumed/calories expended be altered in favor of expended calories. The calories consumed can be reduced by shifting intake to foods lower in calories, particularly the calories tied to fat. Caloric expenditure is maintained most effectively by lifestyle changes incorporating both increased activity and regular physical exercise.

FURTHER READING

Web Sources

http://www.cdc.gov/nchs/products/pubs/pubd/hestats/overweight/
overwght_adult_03.htm
http://www.cdc.gov/nccdphp/dnpa/obesity

Text Sources

Carroll RG: Elsevier's Integrated Physiology. Philadelphia, Elsevier, 2007.

Copstead LC, Banasik J: Pathophysiology, 3rd ed. Philadelphia, Saunders, 2005.

Guyton AC, Hall JE: Textbook of Medical Physiology, 11th ed. Philadelphia, Saunders, 2006.

McPhee SJ, Papadakis MA, Tierney LM Jr: Current Medical Diagnosis and Treatment, 46th ed. New York, McGraw-Hill, 2007.

Ogden CL, Carroll MD, Flegal KM: High Body Mass Index for Age among US Children and Adolescents, 2003-2006. JAMA 2008;299 (20): 2401-2405.

An 18-year-old girl comes to the university clinic complaining of fever, chills, headache, and aching joints.

Prior to today, the patient has been generally healthy and is up to date on all immunizations.

PHYSICAL EXAMINATION

VS: T 39°C, P 96/min, R 26/min, BP 105/85 mm Hg
PE: The patient has a sore throat and a nonproductive cough. Her skin is dry, and she appears mildly dehydrated.

LABORATORY STUDIES

Influenza antigen test from throat swab: Positive for influenza type A

DIAGNOSIS

Influenza

PATHOPHYSIOLOGY OF KEY SYMPTOMS

The patient's major symptoms are tied to an infectious process. Increased activity of the immune system generates pyrogens that alter the hypothalamic temperature set point and cause an elevation in body core temperature. The changes in the vital signs are secondary to the fever.

Body core temperature results from the balance of heat gain and heat loss. Body core temperature is sensed in the anterior hypothalamus and regulated around a set point. If body core temperature falls below the set point, heat gain mechanisms are activated and heat lost mechanisms are inhibited. If body core temperature rises above the set point, heat lost mechanisms are activated and heat gain mechanisms are inhibited.

There are numerous pyrogenic substances that increase set point, including interleukin-1, interleukin-6, selected interferons, prostaglandins, and bacterial endotoxins. Many of these substances mediate the febrile response to infection. Prostaglandins, in particular, can play a central role in the resetting of the hypothalamic set point.

Influenza causes a transient increase in set point and, therefore, body core temperature. During the initial stages of the infection, temperature set point is elevated to 39°C. Body core temperature at 37°C is lower than the set point, and generating a "too cold" error signal, so heat gain mechanisms are activated. These include diminished cutaneous blood flow, shivering, and behavioral mechanisms such as putting on additional clothes or covering under blankets. Elevation of core temperature to 39°C brings the hypothalamic set point in body core temperature back into balance (Fig. 68-1).

After the infection is cleared from the body, pyrogen production ceases. Hypothalamic set point returns to 37°C, but body core temperature is still at 39°C. This imbalance generates a "too hot" error signal, activating heat lost mechanisms, such as increased cutaneous blood flow, sweating, and the removal of clothing. Lowering of core temperature to 37°C brings the body core temperature and hypothalamic set point back into balance.

The elevated body core temperature increases most body reactions. Increased temperature causes an increase in heart rate. Increase in temperature also increases mitochondrial metabolic rate and therefore increases oxygen consumption and depletes body glucose and fatty acids stores. The increase metabolism stimulates an increase in ventilation. The increase in

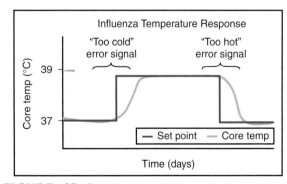

FIGURE 68–1 Influenza results in a transient increase in body core temperature. The increase in body core temperature is initiated after an elevation in the hypothalamic set point. Return of body temperature toward normal occurs only after the set point has returned to 37°C.

body core temperature also increases renal blood flow. The combination of enhanced metabolism and activation of the elimination systems allows the immune system to be more effective.

Prostaglandins play a central role in the resetting of the hypothalamic set point. Agents such as aspirin and other nonsteroidal anti-inflammatory drugs (NSAIDs) block prostaglandin synthesis and consequently return the hypothalamic set point to 37°C. This causes a transient decrease in body core temperature but diminishes the immune system's effectiveness. After the NSAID is metabolized, and the infection persists, the set point will again return to 39°C and the heat gain mechanisms will be activated.

FURTHER READING

Text Sources

Carroll RG: Elsevier's Integrated Physiology. Philadelphia, Elsevier, 2007.

Copstead LC, Banasik J: Pathophysiology, 3rd ed. Philadelphia, Saunders, 2005.

Guyton AC, Hall JE: Textbook of Medical Physiology, 11th ed. Philadelphia, Saunders, 2006.

McPhee SJ, Papadakis MA, Tierney LM Jr: Current Medical Diagnosis and Treatment, 46th ed. New York, McGraw-Hill, 2007.

A 20-year-old man is brought to the emergency department after camping in the winter with some friends. He became cold and wet during a rainstorm during the night and, in the morning, his friends had difficulty waking him.

PHYSICAL EXAMINATION

VS: T 32°C (rectal), P 50/min, R 8/min, BP 90/70 mm Hg, BMI 26
PE: The patient is conscious but confused. His skin is pale, and the lips, fingers, and toes are cyanotic and cold. Corneal reflexes are diminished. The patient is shivering uncontrollably and has difficulty speaking.

LABORATORY STUDIES

ECG: Sinus bradycardia

DIAGNOSIS

Hypothermia

PATHOPHYSIOLOGY OF KEY SYMPTOMS

The patient's symptoms are tied to severe hypothermia. The pronounced drop in core temperature slows all metabolic activity and causes activation of the heat-conservation and heat-generation mechanisms.

Body core temperature reflects the balance of heat generation and heat transfer with the environment.

Heat generation is predominantly from metabolism and from muscle movement. Heat exchange with the environment occurs by conduction, convection, radiation, and evaporation (Fig. 69-1). Conduction is the direct transfer of heat by contact. Conductive exchange of heat with the air is minimized by the insulating ability of the skin and by reducing cutaneous blood flow, particularly to the extremities. Clothing with insulating capabilities also diminishes the conductive loss of heat to the air. Convection enhances heat exchange by exchange of air in contact with the body surface. Radiation allows transfer of heat by infrared energy. Evaporation facilitates the cooling of skin by sweating or when the skin surface becomes wet.

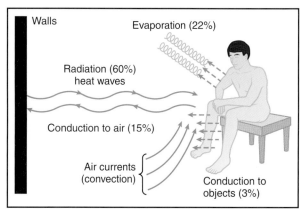

FIGURE 69–1   Mechanisms of heat loss from the body.

TABLE 69–1 Heat Loss and Heat Gain Mechanisms	
Enhance Heat Loss/Diminish Heat Gain When Ambient Temperature Is Lower Than Body Temperature	**Diminish Heat Loss/Enhance Heat Gain When Ambient Temperature Is Lower Than Body Temperature**
Increase cutaneous blood flow	Decrease cutaneous blood flow
Increase sweating (even when ambient temperature is higher than body temperature)	Piloerect
	Huddle or take ball posture
Remove clothing	Move to warmer environment
Move to cooler environment	Increase activity and movement
Decrease metabolic rate	Shivering
Take sprawled posture	Metabolize brown adipose (infants)
	Increase metabolic rate

Core body temperature is maintained around 37°C by the hypothalamus. Output from the hypothalamus controls both the physiologic and behavioral adjustments that alter heat exchange with the environment. The physiologic mechanisms of heat gain and heat loss are listed in Table 69-1.

Cutaneous blood flow represents a major route for balancing heat exchange with the environment. Skin has normal capillaries serving in a nutritive function of the skin, and the extremities (fingers and hands, toes and feet, and head) have extensive venous plexuses that allow a large volume of blood to flow through the surface of the skin. The increase in cutaneous blood flow brings warm blood from the body core to the surface of the skin where the heat can be lost in the environment. Decreases in cutaneous blood flow assist heat conservation.

Following a moderate drop in core temperature, cutaneous vasoconstriction can be supplemented by increasing heat generation from shivering. Skeletal muscle contraction generates heat as a byproduct, and shivering is an uncoordinated skeletal muscle contraction. The severity of shivering increases proportional to the hypothermia.

Assessing the status of an individual with hypothermia presents specific challenges. Cold blood has significantly diminished buffering capacity, so laboratory analysis conducted at 37°C will underestimate the pH and overestimate the P_{CO_2} and the P_{O_2}.

Treatment for hypothermia consists of first limiting additional heat loss from the body and then gradually warming the body. If possible, warming should begin initially with the core before warming the shell. Warming extremities before warming the core results in the return of cool blood toward the heart, where it can cause fatal arrhythmias.

FURTHER READING

Web Source

http://www.mayoclinic.com/health/hypothermia/DS00333

Text Sources

Carroll RG: Elsevier's Integrated Physiology. Philadelphia, Elsevier, 2007.

Copstead LC, Banasik J: Pathophysiology, 3rd ed. Philadelphia, Saunders, 2005.

Guyton AC, Hall JE: Textbook of Medical Physiology, 11th ed. Philadelphia, Saunders, 2006.

McPhee SJ, Papadakis MA, Tierney LM Jr: Current Medical Diagnosis and Treatment, 46th ed. New York, McGraw-Hill, 2007.

SECTION IX

Endocrinology

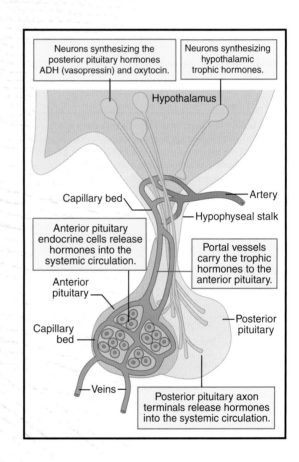

Neurons synthesizing the posterior pituitary hormones ADH (vasopressin) and oxytocin.

Neurons synthesizing hypothalamic trophic hormones.

Hypothalamus

Capillary bed

Artery

Hypophyseal stalk

Anterior pituitary endocrine cells release hormones into the systemic circulation.

Portal vessels carry the trophic hormones to the anterior pituitary.

Anterior pituitary

Posterior pituitary

Capillary bed

Veins

Posterior pituitary axon terminals release hormones into the systemic circulation.

The endocrine system and the nervous system integrate and coordinate metabolism, fluid balance, and reproduction. The endocrine system relies on hormones as chemical messengers that circulate in the bloodstream before binding to a receptor on the target tissue. Hormone molecular structure falls into one of three classes: peptide/protein, steroid, or amino acid derivative.

More important is the target tissue receptor location. The water-soluble hormones (peptides, proteins, and catecholamines) bind to receptors on the extracellular surface of the cell membrane. The hormones are the

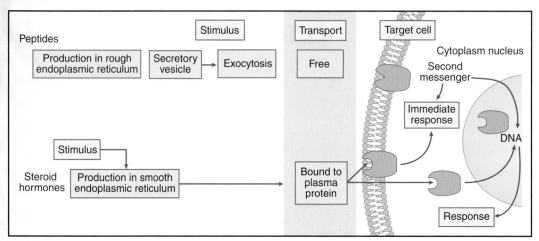

FIGURE IX–1 Peptide and steroid endocrine agents exhibit different patterns of action. Peptide hormones are synthesized in advance and released by exocytosis following an appropriate stimulus. Once released, they travel within the plasma until binding with a receptor on the cell surface of the target tissue and quickly activating intracellular second messenger systems. In contrast, steroid hormones are synthesized on demand following an appropriate stimulus. After release, steroid hormones travel bound to plasma protein, enter the cell by diffusion, and bind an intracellular receptor, ultimately affecting DNA transcription and translation.

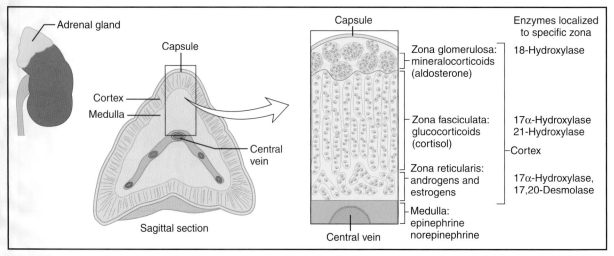

FIGURE IX–2 The adrenal gland has an inner medulla and an outer cortex consisting of three main zones. The adrenal medulla consists of chromaffin tissue that synthesizes epinephrine and, to a lesser extent, norepinephrine and dopamine. The location of specific enzymes in the zones of the adrenal cortex allows regional synthesis of a variety of steroid hormones. The zona glomerulosa has the enzyme 18-hydroxylase and can synthesize the mineralocorticoid aldosterone. The zona fasciculata has the enzyme 17α-hydroxylase and can synthesize the glucocorticoid cortisol. The zona reticularis has the additional enzyme 17,20-desmolase and can synthesize androgens and estrogens.

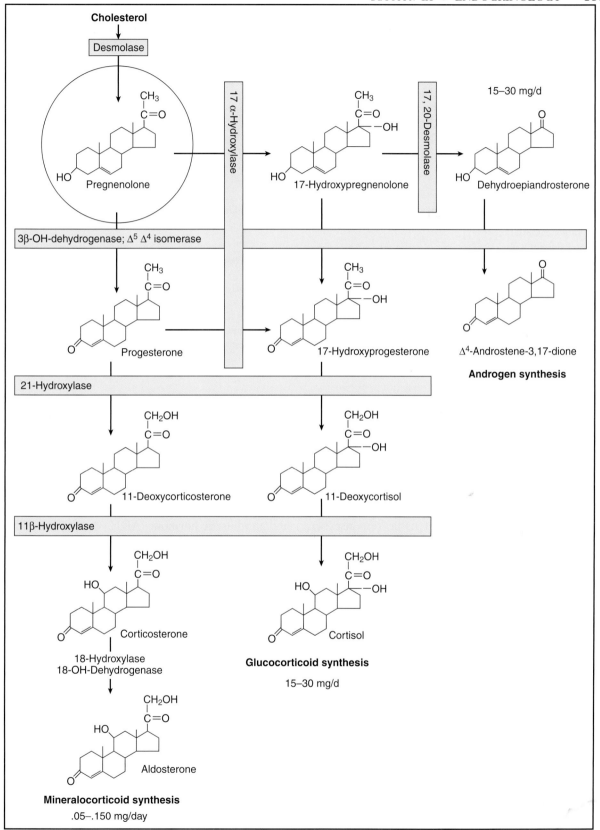

FIGURE IX–3   The pathways of adrenal steroid biosynthesis show the sites of enzymatic action. A congenital deficiency in any of the adrenal enzymes will diminish the synthesis of some hormones and inappropriately increase the synthesis of other hormones. For example, a 21-hydroxylase deficiency inhibits both glucocorticoid and mineralocorticoid production but results in increased adrenal and androgen production.

TABLE IX–1   Hypothalamic and Anterior Pituitary Hormones

Hypothalamic Hormone	Pituitary Hormone	Intermediate Target	Final Target
Corticotropin-releasing hormone (CHR)	Adrenocorticotropic hormone (ACTH)	Adrenal cortex cortisol	Liver, adipose tissue stress response
Thyroid hormone–releasing hormone (THRH)	Thyroid-stimulating hormone (TSH)	Thyroid hormones T_3 and T_4	Most tissues (metabolism, growth)
Prolactin inhibitory hormone (PIH), dopamine	Prolactin	None	Breast milk production
Prolactin-releasing hormone (PRH)			
Growth hormone–releasing hormone (GHRH)	Growth hormone (GH)	Liver, insulin-like growth factors (IGFs)	Most tissues (growth, metabolism)
Growth hormone–inhibiting hormone (GHIH) (somatostatin)			
Gonadotropin-releasing hormone (GnRH)	Follicle-stimulating hormone (FSH)	Female ovary (estrogen)	Many tissues Secondary sexual characteristics
		Male testis (estrogen)	Sertoli cells Sperm maturation
	Luteinizing hormone (LH)	Female corpus luteum (progesterone)	Many tissues Reproduction
		Male testis (testosterone)	Many tissues Secondary sexual characteristics

first messengers, and binding to a receptor generates an intracellular response mediated by second messenger systems. The second messenger systems can generate an immediate response or can interact with nuclear transcription elements to generate a long-term response. In contrast, the receptors for lipid-soluble hormones (steroids and thyroid hormone) are within or close to the nucleus. Target tissue responses to steroid hormones generally involve transcription and translation of proteins, a process that takes hours before a biologic effect is apparent. Some lipid-soluble hormones can bind to cell membrane receptors and generate an immediate response. The biologic significance of this new route for steroid hormone action is actively being investigated (Fig. IX-1).

An adrenal gland sits on the superior pole of each kidney and is roughly triangular. Histologically, the adrenal gland can be divided into an outer cortex and an inner medulla. Beginning from the outside of the adrenal gland, the adrenal cortex consists of the outer glomerulus zone that secretes the mineralocorticoid aldosterone (see Case 72), the fasciculata zone that secretes the glucocorticoid cortisol (see Cases 70 and 71), and the reticularis zone that secretes glucocorticoids and some sex steroids (Figs. IX-2 and IX-3). All adrenal cortical hormones are derived from cholesterol. The hormones secreted by the different zones of the adrenal gland are determined by the limited expression of

appropriate synthetic enzymes. The adrenal medulla is a catecholamine-secreting region that augments the action of the sympathetic nervous system (see Case 73).

The pituitary gland is a complex structure that releases eight different hormones. The posterior pituitary is the neuronal structure, secreting oxytocin and antidiuretic hormone (ADH, vasopressin). These peptides are synthesized by cell bodies located in nuclei within the hypothalamus. The anterior pituitary gland is predominantly an endocrine structure that releases six peptide hormones: adrenocorticotropic hormone (ACTH), thyroid-stimulating hormone (TSH), follicle-stimulating hormone (FSH), luteinizing hormone (LH), growth hormone (GH), and prolactin.

Hypothalamic control of anterior pituitary hormone release is by stimulation (hypothalamic releasing hormones), inhibition (hypothalamic inhibitory hormones), or some combination of the two (Table IX-1). ACTH, TSH, FSH, and LH are controlled predominantly by hypothalamic releasing factors. GH is under dual control by both the releasing hormone and an inhibiting hormone (see Case 74). Prolactin is unique in that its major control is by an inhibiting hormone (see Case 75). The co-localization of these endocrine tissues in a single small gland results in pathologic processes that often overlap many endocrine systems (see Case 76).

A 38-year-old man is transported to the emergency department after having fainted at home.

The patient is a recent immigrant to the United States from equatorial Africa. During the past year he has become progressively weak and lethargic. He had tuberculosis 2 years ago, which was managed medically. The patient has had vomiting and diarrhea for the past 24 hours, and his family reports a weight loss of about 15 pounds during the past 3 months.

PHYSICAL EXAMINATION

VS: T 39.5°C, P 120/min, R 28/min, BP 80/65 mm Hg
PE: Patient is disoriented and is having difficulty remaining conscious. He is sweating and appears malnourished. Excessive pigmentation is present on the lips and gums and in the palmar creases of the hands.

LABORATORY STUDIES

Plasma studies:

- Sodium: 135 mEq/L (normal: 136-145 mEq/L)
- Potassium: 5.2 mEq/L (normal: 3.5-5.0 mEq/L)
- Chloride: 100 mEq/L (normal: 95-105 mEq/L)
- Blood urea nitrogen: 25 mg/dL (normal: 7-18 mg/dL)

Tetracosactide test: Resting plasma cortisol 50 nmol/L (normal at 4:00 PM: 82-413 nmol/L); 60 minutes after injection: Increased to 100 nmol/L (normal response: increase > 330 nmol/L)

DIAGNOSIS

Acute adrenal insufficiency (Addisonian crisis)

PATHOPHYSIOLOGY OF KEY SYMPTOMS

The patient's symptoms affect a variety of systems. Hypotension indicates a defect of the cardiovascular and/or renal systems. The abnormal electrolytes suggest defects in the renal or mineralocorticoid systems. Progressive weight loss, vomiting, and diarrhea indicate abnormal metabolic regulation. The adrenal cortex is an endocrine gland that impacts all of these systems.

Adrenocortical insufficiency, first described by the physician Addison, is characterized by destruction of adrenal tissue or by defective adrenal steroid synthesis. The clinical symptoms result from the lack of aldosterone, a lack of cortisol, or an overproduction of pituitary adrenocorticotropic hormone (ACTH). Adrenocortical insufficiency may be mild, but an additional stress such as an infection may cause a sudden worsening of the condition, called an Addisonian crisis.

Cortisol production is essential to allow the body to adjust to stress. Plasma cortisol levels show a wide diurnal variation, being highest in the morning and lowest at night.

Cortisol increases the plasma glucose level by stimulating hepatic gluconeogenesis and by diminishing tissue glucose uptake. Cortisol suppresses the immune system activity and causes deposition of fat and glycogen, particularly in the trunk area. The absence of cortisol impairs metabolic regulation. Low plasma cortisol leads to hypoglycemia, weakness, fatigue, and weight loss. The complete absence of cortisol is fatal.

Cortisol exhibits a marked diurnal variation in plasma levels, with the highest level at 8 AM being more than four times as high as the lowest level at night (Fig. 70-1). Consequently, a patient's plasma cortisol level must be matched against an appropriate range for that time of day.

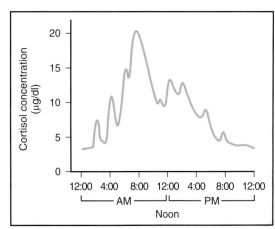

FIGURE 70–1 Typical pattern of cortisol concentration during the day. Note the oscillations in secretion as well as a daily secretory surge an hour or so after awaking in the morning.

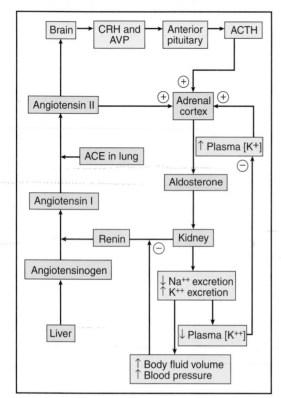

FIGURE 70–2 Aldosterone release is stimulated by increases in plasma potassium, angiotensin II, and ACTH. The normal release of aldosterone is tied to plasma potassium and angiotensin II, with a minor role for ACTH. This multiple control reflects the actions of aldosterone to increase renal potassium excretion and to decrease renal sodium excretion. AVP, vasopressin; CRH, corticotropin-releasing hormone.

Aldosterone is a mineralocorticoid tied most directly to potassium regulation, but with an important role on sodium and, consequently, extracellular fluid volume (Fig. 70-2). Aldosterone decreases plasma potassium by stimulating cellular uptake of potassium and by increasing renal potassium excretion. Aldosterone also stimulates renal sodium retention, which increases circulating fluid volume. A deficiency in aldosterone accounts for the hypotension, hyponatremia, and hyperkalemia present in this patient. The hypotension is due in part to sodium depletion and the consequent decrease in circulating fluid volume. Hypotension, resulting in diminished cerebral blood flow, is likely causing the disorientation and syncope in this patient.

ACTH normally stimulates adrenal production of cortisol, and cortisol is the primary negative feedback regulator on hypothalamic corticotropin-releasing hormone (CRH) and pituitary ACTH release. Melanocyte-stimulating hormone (MSH) is part of the same parent protein as ACTH. Consequently, stimulation of ACTH synthesis and release also causes an increase in MSH levels. MSH stimulates the melanocytes and causes the darkening of the skin. In patients with existing skin pigment, evidence of increased MSH activity is still evident in excessive pigmentation at the gum lines and in the palmar creases of the hands.

Infusion of an ACTH analogue such as tetracosactide can be used to test adrenal cortical function. The lack of a response to tetracosactide indicates that the effect is in the adrenal gland itself. In contrast, a significant increase in cortisol after tetracosactide infusion indicates that the adrenal cortex is intact and functional and that the defect lies in the pituitary or hypothalamus.

Primary adrenocortical insufficiency is often caused by an autoimmune destruction of the adrenal cortex. Tuberculosis infection can directly destroy the adrenal cortex, and thus it contributes to a large number of cases of adrenocortical insufficiency in regions of the world where it is still common.

FURTHER READING

Text Sources
Carroll RG: Elsevier's Integrated Physiology. Philadelphia, Elsevier, 2007.
Copstead L, Banasik J: Pathophysiology, 3rd ed. Philadelphia, Saunders, 2005.
Guyton AC, Hall JE: Textbook of Medical Physiology, 11th ed. Philadelphia, Saunders, 2006.

Kronenberg HM, Melmed S, Polonsky KS, Larsen PR: Williams Textbook of Endocrinology, 11th ed. Philadelphia, Elsevier Saunders, 2007.
McPhee SJ, Papadakis MA, Tierney LM Jr: Current Medical Diagnosis and Treatment, 46th ed. New York, McGraw-Hill, 2007.

A 35-year-old woman comes to her physician's office with the complaint of recent rapid weight gain and excessive sweating.

What initiated her visit was a recent panic attack that frightened her. Her face looks swollen compared with the rest of her body. She complains of recent weakness, backaches, and headaches, and her periods have lately been irregular. Over the past month, she has noticed frequent bruising with slow healing. She is not on any birth control or using any medication except for acetaminophen for the headaches.

PHYSICAL EXAMINATION

VS: T: 37°C, P 68/min, R 14/min, BP 130/86 mm Hg, BMI 33
PE: The patient's face is round and her trunk is swollen, but her arms and legs are thin. She sounds depressed. She has supraclavicular fat pads.

LABORATORY STUDIES

Pregnancy test (HCG): Negative
Glucose tolerance: Abnormal, consistent with insulin resistance
Plasma cortisol levels: 4 PM: 25 μg/dL (normal: 3-15 μg/dL). Dexamethasone is given orally at 11 PM. At around 8 AM the next morning, cortisol levels are 35 μg/dL (normal: < 5 μg/dL).
24-Hour urine collection for free cortisol: Abnormally high
Plasma ACTH: 7 pg/mL (normal: > 20 pg/mL)
MRI of the pituitary: Normal
CT of abdomen and chest: Adrenal tumor

DIAGNOSIS

Cushing's syndrome (primary hypercortisolism from adrenal tumor)

PATHOPHYSIOLOGY OF KEY SYMPTOMS

The majority of the patient's symptoms reflect the disruption of the endocrine control of growth and glucose metabolism. This includes the weight gain and then an increase in fat deposits in central areas of the body, weakness, and the loss of muscle mass in the extremities.

Cortisol is the primary glucocorticoid secreted by the adrenal cortex. Secretion is controlled by the hypothalamic corticotropin-releasing hormone (CRH), which stimulates the release of adrenocorticotropic hormone (ACTH) from the anterior pituitary. ACTH stimulates cortisol synthesis and release. Plasma cortisol levels provide a negative feedback inhibition of the release of both ACTH and CRH (Fig. 71-1). Cortisol acts on a variety of target tissues to broadly suppress immune function and to alter glucose and amino acid metabolism. These actions allow the body to adapt to stressful situations, and cortisol is appropriately described as the body's major stress hormone.

Cortisol increases plasma glucose levels but preserves body glycogen stores (Fig. 71-2). It stimulates hepatic gluconeogenesis, the production of glucose from the amino acids. It also stimulates protein breakdown in many regions of the body, resulting in a decrease in

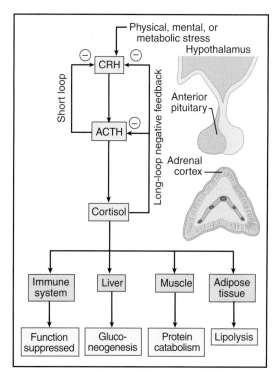

FIGURE 71–1 Cortisol is released in response to physical, mental, and metabolic stress. Cortisol increases the plasma glucose level through a variety of mechanisms (shown in Figure 71-2) and suppresses the action of the immune system. Circulating cortisol levels provide the normal feedback signal inhibiting CRH and ACTH.

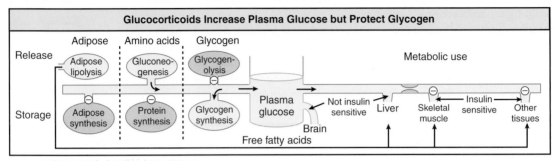

FIGURE 71–2 Plasma glucose levels represent the balance between gastrointestinal glucose absorption, movement into and out of storage pools, and metabolism by mitochondria. Glucocorticoids increase plasma glucose levels by stimulating gluconeogenesis and inhibiting glucose uptake by skeletal muscle.

muscle mass and a decrease in the protein structure of the skin. The decrease in muscle mass leads to the atrophy of the arms and legs, and a decrease in skin proteins allows the skin to be more easily damaged (striae) by physical stretch. Cortisol also stimulates the hepatic uptake of amino acids and enhances their conversion into glucose. The high hepatic glucose levels stimulate hepatic glycogen synthesis. Hepatic glycogen deposition contributes to the enlargement of the trunk and abdomen.

Glucocorticoids inhibit cellular glucose utilization, another action that helps to preserve high plasma glucose levels. Insulin is released in response to the high glucose levels, and target tissues such as skeletal muscle and adipose have a diminished responsiveness to insulin in the presence of high glucocorticoid levels. The combination of enhanced glucose production and diminished glucose utilization leads to an elevation in plasma glucose, much as occurs in type 2 diabetes mellitus. These metabolic changes are also characteristic of the transition from glucose to fatty acids as a metabolic substrate, such as occurs during starvation.

Cortisol action on adipose is more complex. Cortisol depletes adipose stores in the extremities, such as the arms and legs. In contrast, cortisol increases adipose synthesis in the trunk and especially in the fat pads of the neck and shoulders (supraclavicular fat pads). Hypercortisolemia leads to the central deposition of fat and the appearance of a "buffalo hump" on the shoulders and a round face.

The dexamethasone suppression test assesses the pituitary and adrenal cortex function. Normally, addition of an exogenous steroid (dexamethasone) should markedly reduce ACTH release and therefore adrenal cortisol release. An abnormal dexamethasone suppression test confirms the abnormal cortisol production.

High plasma cortisol levels can result from either overproduction by an adrenal tumor (primary hypercortisolism, characterized by low ACTH) or excessive ACTH production from either a pituitary or lung tumor (secondary hypercortisolism). ACTH levels can be assessed by radioimmunoassay to distinguish between primary and secondary hypercortisolism, and imaging can confirm the location of the tumor.

Adrenal androgens and mineralocorticoids share many common synthetic steps with cortisol. Consequently, adrenal tumors can also produce excessive amounts of androgens and mineralocorticoids, allowing the patient to exhibit symptoms of virilization and mineralocorticoid excess.

FURTHER READING

Web Source
http://www.mayoclinic.com/health/cushings-syndrome/DS00470

Text Sources
Carroll RG: Elsevier's Integrated Physiology. Philadelphia, Elsevier, 2007.

Copstead L, Banasik J: Pathophysiology, 3rd ed. Philadelphia, Saunders, 2005.

Guyton AC, Hall JE: Textbook of Medical Physiology, 11th ed. Philadelphia, Saunders, 2006.

Kronenberg HM, Melmed S, Polonsky KS, et al: Williams Textbook of Endocrinology, 11th ed. Philadelphia, Saunders, 2007.

McPhee SJ, Papadakis MA, Tierney LM Jr: Current Medical Diagnosis and Treatment, 46th ed. New York, McGraw-Hill, 2007.

A 45-year-old woman comes in for her regular check-up and complains about a constant thirst and having to get up frequently in the night to urinate.

The patient has a history of high blood pressure. It is possible that she may be noncompliant with her medications because her blood pressure has remained high regardless of the medications she was prescribed or the dosage taken.

PHYSICAL EXAMINATION

VS: T 37°C, P 85/min, R 17/min, BP 145/110 mm Hg, BMI 32
PE: Well-nourished female in no apparent distress

LABORATORY STUDIES

Plasma Analysis:

- Glucose: 95 mg/dL (normal: 70-110 mg/dL)
- Ca^{++}: 9.2 mg/dL (normal: 8.4 to 10.2 mg/dL)
- Na^+: 146 mEq/L (normal: 136 to 145 mEq/L)
- Cl^-: 100 mEq/L (normal: 95-105 mEq/L)
- K^+: 3.2 mEq/L (normal: 3.5 to 5.0 mEq/L)
- Plasma aldosterone (recumbent): 25 ng/dL (normal: 2-16 ng/dL)
- Plasma renin activity: 0.8 ng/mL/hr (normal: 1.9 to 3.7 ng/mL/hr)

CT: Tumor on the left adrenal gland

DIAGNOSIS

Conn's syndrome (hyperaldosteronism)

PATHOPHYSIOLOGY OF KEY SYMPTOMS

The patient's presenting symptoms of nocturia and polydipsia, along with the persistent hypertension, are indicative of a fluid and electrolyte imbalance. The elevated plasma sodium and low plasma potassium are consistent with an elevated aldosterone level as the underlying cause. The normal plasma glucose levels exclude diabetes mellitus as a potential cause for the polydipsia and polyuria.

Aldosterone is the primary mineralocorticoid secreted by the adrenal cortex. It stimulates reabsorption of sodium and secretion of potassium in the renal distal tubules. The reabsorption of sodium contributes to the development of hypertension, and the excessive excretion of potassium can lead to muscular weakness and possibly tetany.

Aldosterone secretion is under multiple controls and is increased by elevation in plasma potassium, by an elevation in angiotensin II, and by an elevation in adrenocorticotropic hormone (ACTH) (see Fig. 70-2, p. 190). Plasma potassium is the most potent of the stimuli governing aldosterone release, and aldosterone is the major hormone regulating body potassium balance. The finding of hypokalemia alone does not immediately suggest hyperaldosteronism, because most diuretics used to treat hypertension are potassium wasting and will deplete body potassium stores.

The endocrine and electrolyte profile in this patient suggests primary hyperaldosteronism. Plasma potassium levels are low and therefore are not stimulating adrenal aldosterone synthesis. Plasma renin activity is also low, indicating that angiotensin II is not stimulating aldosterone synthesis. ACTH plays only a minor role in aldosterone release, and ACTH elevation would be characterized by symptoms related to glucocorticoid excess.

Aldosterone directly stimulates renal H^+ secretion in the late tubular segments. Consequently, hyperaldosteronism causes a metabolic alkalosis, characterized by an elevation in pH and high plasma bicarbonate levels. Metabolic acid-base disturbances develop slowly, and, consequently, a respiratory compensation by increasing the plasma CO_2 levels would be expected.

Treatment for Conn's syndrome due to unilateral adrenal adenoma is by adrenalectomy. Hyperaldosteronism due to other causes may be medically managed by spironolactone or by dexamethasone.

FURTHER READING

Web Sources

http://www.labtestsonline.org/understanding/conditions/conn
.html
http://www.urologyhealth.org/adult/index.cfm?cat=04&topic=113
http://www.cushings-help.com/conns_syndrome.htm
http://www.nlm.nih.gov/medlineplus/encyclopedia.html

Text Sources

Carroll RG: Elsevier's Integrated Physiology. Philadelphia, Elsevier, 2007.

Copstead L, Banasik J: Pathophysiology, 3rd ed. Philadelphia, Saunders, 2005.
Guyton AC, Hall JE: Textbook of Medical Physiology, 11th ed. Philadelphia, Saunders, 2006.
Kronenberg HM, Melmed S, Polonsky KS, et al: Williams Textbook of Endocrinology, 11th ed. Philadelphia, Saunders, 2007.
McPhee SJ, Papadakis MA, Tierney LM Jr: Current Medical Diagnosis and Treatment, 46th ed. New York, McGraw-Hill, 2007.

A 56-year-old woman presents to the emergency department with chest pain, sweating, extreme anxiety, abdominal pain, pale skin, and a racing heart.

The patient has experienced these symptoms intermittently over the past month, and they usually subside after 15 to 20 minutes. This time the symptoms are more severe. She states that her hobby is gardening and noticed that these episodes occur when she is lifting a heavy bag of soil or when she runs inside to catch the phone. These episodes happen several times a week.

PHYSICAL EXAMINATION

VS: T 98.7°F, P 128/min, R 17/min, BP 146/95 mm Hg, BMI 25
PE: Patient is pale and diaphoretic

LABORATORY STUDIES

Blood test:

- Epinephrine: 80 mg/dL (normal: 20 mg/dL)
- Norepinephrine: 400 mg/dL (normal: 60 ng/dL)

24-Hour urine specimen:

- Metanephrine: 1235 μg/24 hr (normal: 24-96 μg/24 hr)
- Total urine catecholamines: 1420 μg/24 hr (normal: 14-110 μg/24 hr)

Abdominal CT: Tumors on adrenal glands

DIAGNOSIS

Pheochromocytoma

PATHOPHYSIOLOGY OF KEY SYMPTOMS

The patient's symptoms are consistent with marked activation of the sympathetic nervous system. The duration and intermittent nature of the episodes, however, are more consistent with an endocrine action rather than an autonomic nervous system action.

The sympathetic nervous system consists of the sympathetic nerves and the adrenal medulla. Norepinephrine is a neurotransmitter at the postganglionic sympathetic nerve terminals. The adrenal medulla receives preganglionic sympathetic nerves from the spinal cord (Fig. 73-1), but, rather than function as a postganglionic nerve, the adrenal medulla secretes the catecholamines epinephrine and norepinephrine into the bloodstream, where they act as hormones.

The sympathetic nervous system mediates the "fight or flight" response. Sympathetic nerve activity increases arterial blood pressure through a variety of mechanisms. Sympathetic nerves increase heart rate (β_1-adrenergic receptor) and myocardial contractility (β_1-adrenergic receptor), as well as constrict arteriolar and venous vascular smooth muscle (α_1-adrenergic receptor). Constriction of the arterioles reduces blood flow to the skin, particularly the extremities, causing the skin to be pale and cold. The increased heart rate and arterial pressure dramatically increases the workload on the heart, possibly contributing to the patient's chest pain. Sweating is increased during sympathetic activity through the actions of the sympathetic cholinergic nerves that innervate the sweat glands.

The catecholamines and epinephrine, in particular, have strong metabolic actions, stimulating glycogenolysis and gluconeogenesis. In addition, epinephrine stimulates lipolysis in adipose tissue (β_3-adrenergic receptor).

Catecholamines have a relatively short half-life in the body. The intermittent release of catecholamines by a pheochromocytoma and the short biologic half-life combined to make detection of elevated plasma catecholamine levels difficult. Consequently, 24-hour urine collection is used and the urine analyzed for catecholamine metabolites to assist the diagnosis. Of the multiple catecholamine metabolites, metanephrine levels are the most sensitive and specific test for pheochromocytomas. Urinary catecholamine concentrations may be normalized to creatinine levels to compensate for variations in 24-hour urine volume.

The increasing frequency and severity of the episodes is likely due to growth of the tumor. The episodes of catecholamine release can be initiated by compression of the tumor, possibly caused by abdominal muscle contraction or by external palpation. Although the adrenal medulla normally secretes predominantly epinephrine, pheochromocytomas predominantly secrete norepinephrine.

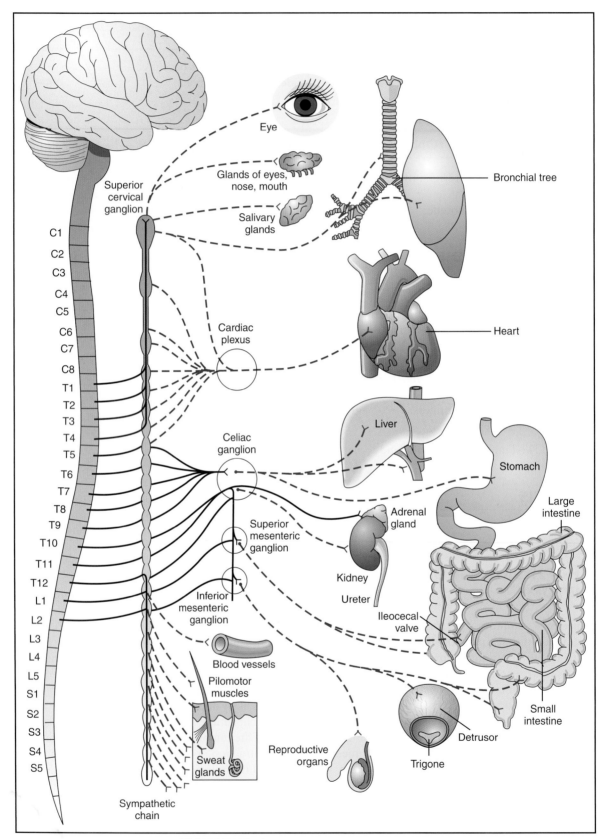

FIGURE 73–1   Distribution of sympathetic nerves.

FURTHER READING

Web Source

www.mayoclinic.com/pheno

Text Sources

Carroll RG: Elsevier's Integrated Physiology. Philadelphia, Elsevier, 2007.

Copstead L, Banasik J: Pathophysiology, 3rd ed. Philadelphia, Saunders, 2005.

Guyton AC, Hall JE: Textbook of Medical Physiology, 11th ed. Philadelphia, Saunders, 2006.

Kronenberg HM, Melmed S, Polonsky KS, et al: Williams Textbook of Endocrinology, 11th ed. Philadelphia, Saunders, 2007.

McPhee SJ, Papadakis MA, Tierney LM Jr: Current Medical Diagnosis and Treatment, 46th ed. New York, McGraw-Hill, 2007.

A 33-year-old woman comes to her primary care physician complaining of amenorrhea, headaches, profuse sweating, and joint pains associated with changes in the sizes of her hands and feet.

The patient reports massive growth of her hands and feet as well as protrusion of her lower jaw. She believes the shape of her face has changed, becoming sharper. She also complains of sudden weakness, even when just "carrying the clothes hamper upstairs." She first noticed these changes about 6 months ago when she was home for the holidays and saw some high school and early college pictures of herself. Her mother brought to her attention how her features seemed much larger. After that she says she became more aware of her bodily changes. She came in because she says she knows something is wrong and that there is a definite distinction from how she looks now from how she used to look. Her husband and she are also trying to conceive and have been unsuccessful due to amenorrhea for the past 8 months.

PHYSICAL EXAMINATION

VS: T 99.1°F, P 65/min, R 14/min, BP 130/80 mm Hg, weight 132 lb, BMI 24

PE: Marked enlargement of facial features, as well as tongue, feet, and hands; soft doughy handshake; thyroid gland enlargement, and possible visceral enlargement; loss of visual field (typically associated with disease)

LABORATORY STUDIES

Pregnancy test (hCG): Negative
Growth Hormone: 40 ng/mL (normal: 0-5 ng/mL)
Fasting IGF-I: 31 ng/mL (normal: < 20 ng/mL)
Prolactin: 100 ng/mL (normal: < 20 ng/mL)
Glucose: 1.5 ng/mL
Glucose suppression test: after 75-g glucose, GH was 8 µg/L (normal: < 1 µg/L)
BUN and liver enzymes: Normal
MRI: Pituitary tumor

DIAGNOSIS

Acromegaly

PATHOPHYSIOLOGY OF KEY SYMPTOMS

The patient's initial complaint centers around growth of the cartilage and soft tissue of the body. Growth is a complex process requiring many hormones in a permissive role, but growth hormone (GH) and the insulin-like growth factors (IGFs) are the dominant controllers of growth.

GH is a peptide released from the anterior pituitary (Fig. 74-1). The hypothalamus secretes two peptides that control GH release: growth hormone–releasing hormone (GHRH) and somatostatin, which is also called growth hormone–inhibiting hormone (GHIH). GH acts directly on multiple tissues to increase blood glucose and also stimulates the hepatic release of IGFs, which mediate growth in numerous tissues.

GH increases plasma glucose concentration by stimulating lipolysis and adipose tissue and glycogen breakdown in the liver and muscle (Fig. 74-2). It inhibits the insulin-dependent uptake of glucose in skeletal muscle and other insulin-sensitive tissues. Impaired glucose uptake by skeletal muscle shifts the metabolic fuel to free fatty acids, augmenting the breakdown of fat stores. GH inhibits gluconeogenesis, which preserves the amino acid pool to support protein synthesis. Patients with GH overproduction can develop type 2 diabetes mellitus.

GH levels vary throughout the day, and, consequently, a single plasma sample for GH is of limited diagnostic use. Glucose ingestion normally inhibits GH release, so glucose challenge testing can be used to identify the abnormal regulation of GH. For this patient, the high GH level in spite of the glucose challenge confirms the diagnosis of acromegaly, because it indicates that GH production and release is not under normal control. Plasma IGF-I levels are more stable, and an elevation in IGF-I provides a useful indication of overproduction of GH.

GH overproduction is generally caused by a pituitary adenoma. The growth of pituitary tumors can result in visual field defects (bilateral temporal hemianopia) because of the location of the pituitary immediately posterior to the optic chiasm. Compression of surrounding brain tissue can also cause headaches. In addition, the pituitary adenoma can impair the normal release of other pituitary hormones.

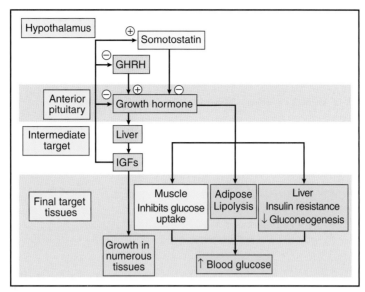

FIGURE 74–1 Pituitary growth hormone (GH) release is under dual control, stimulated by growth hormone–releasing hormone (GHRH) and inhibited by somatostatin. The hypothalamus regulates GH release. Once released, GH acts directly on tissues to increase blood glucose levels. GH also causes the release of insulin-like growth factors (IGFs) from the liver, and IGFs stimulate growth in numerous tissues.

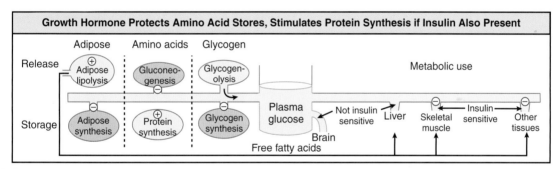

FIGURE 74–2 Plasma glucose levels represent the balance between gastrointestinal glucose absorption, movement into and out of storage pools, and metabolism by mitochondria. Growth hormone stimulates adipolysis and glycogenolysis, and shifts skeletal muscle metabolism to use of free fatty acids.

The amenorrhea is likely a consequence of the impaired follicle-stimulating hormone and luteinizing hormone release.

The physical consequence of GH overproduction depends on the life stage of the patient. GH overproduction before puberty leads to gigantism, because the growth processes occur before closure of the epiphyseal plates in the long bones. GH production after puberty only affects the cartilage and soft tissue, a disease process termed "acromegaly."

Treatment is centered on removal or destruction of the pituitary adenoma or pharmacologic blockade of the GH release. Removal can be accomplished by surgical methods, and destruction of the gland can be done by irradiation. Because many hormones are produced by the anterior pituitary, either surgical or radiation therapies may result in defective production of the other pituitary hormones.

FURTHER READING

Text Sources

Carroll RG: Elsevier's Integrated Physiology. Philadelphia, Elsevier, 2007.

Copstead L, Banasik J: Pathophysiology, 3rd ed. Philadelphia, Saunders, 2005.

Guyton AC, Hall JE: Textbook of Medical Physiology, 11th ed. Philadelphia, Saunders, 2006.

Kronenberg HM, Melmed S, Polonsky KS, et al: Williams Textbook of Endocrinology, 11th ed. Philadelphia, Saunders, 2007.

McPhee SJ, Papadakis MA, Tierney LM Jr: Current Medical Diagnosis and Treatment, 46th ed. New York, McGraw-Hill, 2007.

A 42-year-old man comes to his physician because of a decrease in sexual desire and erectile dysfunction.

The patient noticed visual problems and headaches during the past month. The decrease in sexual desire began about 2 months ago and was accompanied by erectile dysfunction.

PHYSICAL EXAMINATION

VS: T 37°C, P 76/min, R 15/min, BP 128/86 mm Hg, BMI 28
PE: There is a small amount of growth of the breasts (gynecomastia). Stimulation of the nipples produces a small amount of milk (galactorrhea). Testicular size is small (hypogonadism). The remainder of the examination was unremarkable.

LABORATORY STUDIES

Testosterone: 300 ng/dL (normal: 500-900 ng/dL)
Thyroxine: 8 µg/dL (normal: 5-12 µg/dL)
Prolactin: 300 ng/mL (normal: < 20 ng/mL)
Pituitary MRI: Macroprolactinoma (8 cm in diameter)

DIAGNOSIS

Hyperprolactinemia

PATHOPHYSIOLOGY OF KEY SYMPTOMS

The patient's major symptoms are centered around reproduction. Erectile dysfunction can have many causes: vascular, neural, endocrine, and psychologic. The decrease in libido, accompanied by hypogonadism, suggests a drop in testosterone levels. Galactorrhea is an unusual finding in males and indicates an elevated prolactin level. Headaches and visual disturbances are consistent with a problem in the pituitary, the site of prolactin production.

Prolactin is an important hormone of pregnancy, stimulating the growth of the breast epithelial cells and the production of milk. Prolactin levels increase during the last trimester of pregnancy, in preparation for nursing (Fig. 75-1). After delivery, prolactin levels fall to baseline over the next 8 to 12 weeks. There is a surge in prolactin production for about 1 hour during and after nursing that persists as long as the mother continues to nurse. The prolactin surges allow milk production to continue until the infant is weaned.

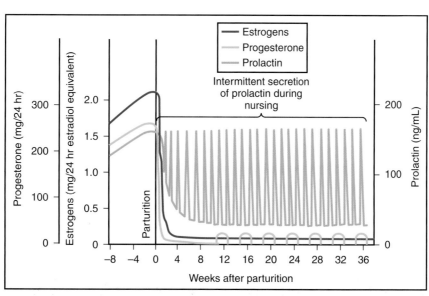

FIGURE 75–1 Changes in rates of secretion of estrogens, progesterone, and prolactin for 8 weeks before parturition and 36 weeks thereafter. Note especially the decrease of prolactin secretion back to basal levels within a few weeks after parturition but also the intermittent periods of marked prolactin secretion (for about 1 hour at a time) during and after periods of nursing.

The prolactin stimulation of breast epithelial cell growth and lactation is diminished in males but can still occur. The male breasts have a rudimentary duct structure necessary to support lactation. The low levels of circulating estrogen and progesterone in males prevent the growth and maturation of the breast tissues that are characteristic of females.

The physiologic role for prolactin in males, if any, is not yet understood.

Elevated prolactin suppresses gonadotropin releasing hormone (GnRH) and, consequently, follicle-stimulating hormone and luteinizing hormone. In males, the low levels of luteinizing hormone cause a reduction in testosterone production by the testicular Leydig cells and a decrease in testicular size. In females, the prolactin suppression of GnRH contributes to the suppression of ovulation that is seen in nursing mothers.

In addition to the effects of elevated prolactin, this patient's symptoms are also related to a tumor mass effect. As a pituitary tumor increases in size, it begins to compress the optic chiasm, creating a characteristic visual field defect (bilateral temporal hemianopia). Both the increase in tumor size and the visual disturbance can contribute to the headaches.

As pituitary tumors continue to grow, they begin to compress the remainder of the pituitary gland. The patient should be evaluated for hypopituitarism secondary to the adenoma.

The initial goal of treatment is to reduce prolactin secretion and tumor size. Prolactin release is normally under inhibitory control by hypothalamic prolactin inhibitory hormone, which is chemically identical to dopamine. Dopamine (D_2) receptor agonists, such as bromocriptine mesylate or cabergoline, may inhibit prolactin secretion and reduce tumor size. Radiation therapy or surgery can be used if dopamine agonists cannot attenuate tumor growth.

FURTHER READING

Web Source

http://www.emedicine.com/med/topic1098.htm

Text Sources

Carroll RG: Elsevier's Integrated Physiology. Philadelphia, Elsevier, 2007.

Copstead L, Banasik J: Pathophysiology, 3rd ed. Philadelphia, Saunders, 2005.

Guyton AC, Hall JE: Textbook of Medical Physiology, 11th ed. Philadelphia, Saunders, 2006.

Kronenberg HM, Melmed S, Polonsky KS, et al: Williams Textbook of Endocrinology, 11th ed. Philadelphia, Saunders, 2007.

McPhee SJ, Papadakis MA, Tierney LM Jr: Current Medical Diagnosis and Treatment, 46th ed. New York, McGraw-Hill, 2007.

A 28-year-old woman complains to her obstetrician of amenorrhea and milk discharge from her nipples.

The patient was involved in a motorcycle accident 3 months ago. Injuries were mostly superficial, but the impact was sufficient to break her helmet. The patient indicated she just has not "felt right since the accident." She is constantly tired, has gained 5 pounds, and drinks and urinates more than before the accident.

PHYSICAL EXAMINATION

VS: T 36.5°C, P 84/min, R 15/min, BP 95/60 mm Hg, BMI 29

PE: A small amount of white fluid can be expressed from the nipples. The patient appears otherwise healthy. Gynecologic examination does not reveal any evidence of pregnancy.

LABORATORY STUDIES

Pregnancy test: Negative
FSH levels: 2 mIU/mL (normal: 4-30 mIU/mL)
LH levels: 2 mIU/mL (normal: 5-30 mIU/mL)
Cortisol level: 2 µg/dL (normal: 3-15 µg/dL)
Thyroxine (T$_4$): 3 µg/dL (normal: 5-12 ug/dL)
Triiodothyronine (T$_3$): 60 ng/dL (normal: 115-190 ng/dL)
Prolactin levels: 70 ng/mL (normal: < 20 ng/mL)

DIAGNOSIS

Panhypopituitarism

PATHOPHYSIOLOGY OF KEY SYMPTOMS

The patient exhibits a variety of symptoms involving the reproductive system, cardiovascular system, fluid balance, and metabolism. In most cases, the symptoms reflect a diminished end organ response from the targets of pituitary gland hormones. In one instance, the symptom of galactorrhea reflects the overproduction of pituitary prolactin. This grouping of symptoms is characteristic of damage to the pituitary stalk, separating the pituitary from the hypothalamic control.

The pituitary gland is a mixed neuronal and endocrine structure that is connected to the hypothalamus by the hypophyseal stalk (Fig. 76-1). The posterior pituitary is neural in origin and secretes the hormones oxytocin and antidiuretic hormone (ADH,

vasopressin). The cell bodies synthesizing these hormones are in the supraoptic and paraventricular nuclei of the hypothalamus. The anterior pituitary is a glandular tissue that secretes six physiologically important hormones: adrenocorticotropic hormone (ACTH), follicle-stimulating hormone (FSH), growth hormone (GH), luteinizing hormone (LH), prolactin, and thyroid-stimulating hormone (TSH). Pituitary gland secretions control metabolism, reproduction, growth,

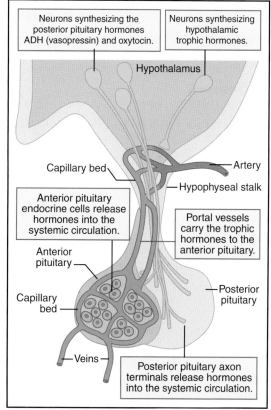

FIGURE 76-1 The hypothalamus and pituitary have complex neural and endocrine interactions. Neurons in the hypothalamus synthesize oxytocin and antidiuretic hormone. The hormones are transported within axon terminals to the posterior pituitary for release. In contrast, the anterior pituitary is an endocrine gland. Hormone release is controlled by releasing inhibitory peptides that pass from the hypothalamus to the anterior pituitary by a vascular hypothalamic-hypophyseal portal system.

and fluid balance. Consequently, the pituitary is often referred to as the master gland.

Hypothalamic control of anterior pituitary hormone release is by hypothalamic releasing hormones and hypothalamic inhibitory hormones. ACTH is controlled by corticotropin-releasing hormone. Thyroid hormone is controlled by thyroid hormone–releasing hormone. FSH and LH are both controlled by a single hypothalamic peptide, gonadotropin-releasing hormone. Growth hormone is under dual control by both growth hormone–releasing hormone and a growth hormone and inhibiting hormone (somatostatin). Prolactin is predominantly controlled by an inhibitory hypothalamic peptide, prolactin inhibitory hormone (dopamine).

Head trauma can disrupt the pituitary stalk, damaging the blood vessels that carry the hypothalamic hormones down to the pituitary. For the five hormones controlled predominantly by releasing factors, this will result in the decrease in the pituitary production and release of the hormone. For prolactin, disruption of the pituitary stalk removes the normal inhibition on prolactin production and, consequently, prolactin production is increased.

The patient currently is experiencing symptoms of prolactin excess and of deficiency in LH, FSH, and TSH. Although the patient is not experiencing symptoms related to ACTH deficiency, the symptoms may become evident if the patient is subjected to stress.

Treatment involves restoring end organ hormone levels to their preinjury values. This may necessitate treatment with a combination of thyroid hormone, estrogen, and cortisol. Endogenous prolactin production can be diminished by treatment with a dopamine analogue.

FURTHER READING

Web Source
http://www.emedicine.com/MED/topic1137.htm

Text Sources
Carroll RG: Elsevier's Integrated Physiology. Philadelphia, Elsevier, 2007.
Copstead L, Banasik J: Pathophysiology, 3rd ed. Philadelphia, Saunders, 2005.

Guyton AC, Hall JE: Textbook of Medical Physiology, 11th ed. Philadelphia, Saunders, 2006.
Kronenberg HM, Melmed S, Polonsky KS, et al: Williams Textbook of Endocrinology, 11th ed. Philadelphia, Saunders, 2007.
McPhee SJ, Papadakis MA, Tierney LM Jr: Current Medical Diagnosis and Treatment, 46th ed. New York, McGraw-Hill, 2007.

SECTION X

Reproduction

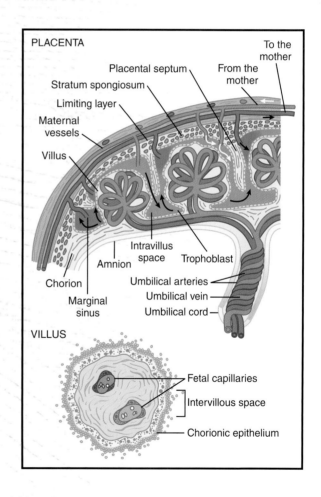

PLACENTA

Placental septum

Stratum spongiosum

Limiting layer

Maternal vessels

Villus

To the mother

From the mother

Intravillus space

Amnion

Trophoblast

Chorion

Marginal sinus

Umbilical arteries

Umbilical vein

Umbilical cord

VILLUS

Fetal capillaries

Intervillous space

Chorionic epithelium

Physiologic regulation of the human reproduction systems is centered on the production and joining of the haploid germ cells. During the fertile years, males produce sperm in the testes and females produce ova in the ovaries. The testes in the ovaries are also the sites of synthesis of the major reproductive hormones—testosterone in the male and estrogen and progesterone in the female (Fig. X-1).

The female reproductive years are marked at the onset by puberty and end with menopause (see Case 77). During these years, an ovarian monthly cycle leads to the production of hormones that regulate the uterine menstrual cycle. Puberty is initiated by a pulsatile secretion of gonadotropin-releasing hormone (GnRH) from the hypothalamus. GnRH secretion continues throughout the reproductive years, acting on the anterior pituitary to control the release of follicle-stimulating hormone (FSH) and luteinizing hormone (LH) (see Case 78).

The first half of the ovarian cycle is dominated by FSH, which stimulates the maturation of an ovarian follicle (see Case 79). The maturing follicle secretes estrogen, which acts on the uterine endometrium to stimulate growth and proliferation. At the midpoint of the cycle the high estrogen levels lead to a marked increase in LH secretion, which causes the follicle to rupture and release the egg. The second half of the ovarian cycle is dominated by LH, which stimulates the remnants of the follicle (corpus luteum) to secrete progesterone. Progesterone causes an increase in the uterine endometrial secretion and inhibits the contraction of uterine smooth muscle. If a fertilized ovum does not implant, the corpus luteum degenerates, progesterone production ceases, and a portion of the uterine endometrium is lost in the menstrual flow (see Case 80). During menstruation, a primary follicle begins to mature in the ovary and the cycle begins again.

In the absence of testosterone in utero, female secondary sexual characteristics develop. At puberty, ovarian production of estrogen and progesterone stimulate the maturation of the female secondary sexual characteristics.

The male reproductive years also begin at puberty, but males do not show the cyclic monthly changes that characterize the female reproductive years. Hypothalamic and pituitary function are similar to that described for females. After puberty, hypothalamic GnRH stimulates the pituitary release of LH and FSH (see Case 85). LH stimulates testosterone production in the testicular Leydig cells. Testosterone stimulates the development of male secondary sexual characteristics in utero (see Case 86) and, along with the testosterone metabolite dihydrotestosterone (DHT) (see Case 87), the maturation of the male secondary sexual characteristics during puberty and their maintenance throughout life. There is a gradual decline in male reproductive fertility after the age of 50, but men have remained fertile into their 60s and 70s.

Testosterone stimulates the production and the maturation of sperm from the spermatogonia. The maturation of sperm is nurtured by the testicular Sertoli cells, whose action is stimulated by pituitary FSH. Sperm, along with secretions from the prostate gland and seminal vesicles, are secreted from the urethra as semen during the ejaculation phase of intercourse. Ejaculation is preceded by an erection of the penis, mediated by vasodilation and engorgement of blood in the corpus cavernosa (see Case 88).

Sexual intercourse results in the deposition of sperm into the female vagina. Intercourse during the days immediately around ovulation can result in fertilization, the successful joining of a sperm and an egg. The fertilized egg has a normal chromosome complement and begins a process of cell division and development, leading to a blastocyst. The blastocyst can implant into the uterine endometrium (see Case 81) and further develop into a fetus and placenta.

The human gestation period is about 36 weeks, commonly divided into three trimesters each of 12 weeks. During this time, the placenta plays an essential role in the exchange of nutrients and wastes between the maternal and fetal circulations. Disruption of placental function can limit growth of the fetus and possibly be fatal (see Cases 82 and 83). Maternal diet and metabolism must adapt to support the needs of the growing fetus, often presenting a metabolic challenge for the mother (see Case 84).

FIGURE X–1 Concept map of the male and female reproductive systems. Both systems share common hypothalamic and pituitary hormones, which are named for their role in the female. **A,** The male reproductive system is specialized for the production and ejaculation of sperm. **B,** The female reproductive system is specialized both for the production and release of an ovum and also for fertilization, implantation, development, and birth.

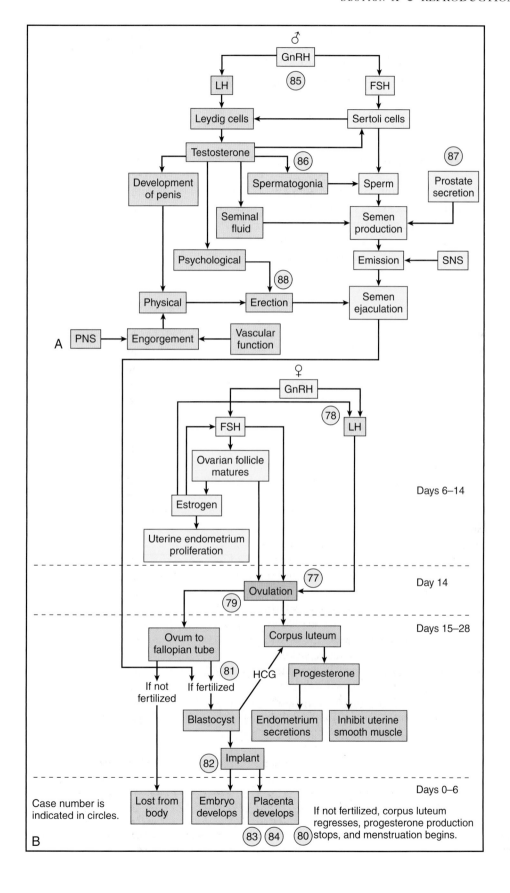

A 50-year-old woman presents to the office for her annual physical examination. The patient complains of night sweats, hot flashes, and vaginal dryness. She also reports irregular menstruation. The patient lives with her husband and is concerned about the menopause symptoms. She has a history of mild hypothyroidism, obesity, and eczema. She is currently taking levothyroxine and topical corticosteroids.

PHYSICAL EXAMINATION

VS: T 98.0°F, P 70/min, R 16/min, BP 130/90 mm Hg, weight 125 lb, BMI 33
PE: Pelvic examination is unremarkable.

LABORATORY STUDIES

CBC: Within normal limits
CHEM-7: Within normal limits
FSH: 80 U/L (normal: premenopausal 4-30 U/L)
LH: 170 U/L (normal: premenopausal 5-150 U/L)

DIAGNOSIS

Female menopause

PATHOPHYSIOLOGY OF KEY SYMPTOMS

Menopause is the time when women's reproductive cycles end and is part of the natural aging process. Menopause can be induced earlier by surgical removal of the ovaries or occur because of abnormalities of the pituitary or hypothalamus.

After age 35, ovarian mass and fertility begin to decline. Perimenopause describes the gradual depletion of primary follicles. During perimenopause, menstrual cycles decrease by approximately 3 days due to a shortened follicular phase. Hormonal levels will be irregular, but the diminished maturation of follicles will reduce inhibin secretion and lead to a rise in follicle-stimulating hormone (FSH). Ultimately, hormone levels will stabilize in menopause with a high FSH and low estradiol levels but estrone levels remain stable (Figs. 77-1 and 77-2). The fluctuating hormone levels of perimenopause may contribute to the increased incidence of endometrial hyperplasia or carcinoma, uterine polyps, and leiomyoma observed among women of perimenopausal age.

In the uterus, menstruation becomes irregular and then stops (menopause) as the ovaries stop producing estrogen in response to gonadotropin. Decreased estrogen secretion leads to less abundant endometrial growth. The cessation of menstruation occurs when the ovaries no longer respond to pituitary FSH and luteinizing hormone (LH).

The symptoms of menopause are due to the absence of estrogen. The severity of the symptoms varies considerably between individuals. The symptoms include hot flashes, atrophy of genitalia and breasts, and osteoporosis.

Hot flashes occur in 80% of women, often beginning before menstruation ceases. Hot flashes are feelings of intense heat and flushing and can lead to excessive sweating. An increase in pulsatile release of gonadotropin-releasing hormone (GnRH) from the hypothalamus is believed to trigger the hot flashes by affecting temperature regulation in the hypothalamus. The abrupt decrease in the hypothalamic temperature set point causes a sensation that the body core temperature is inappropriately high, leading to physical and behavioral actions to dissipate heat.

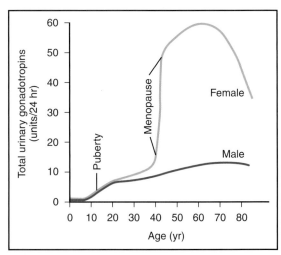

FIGURE 77–1 Total rates of secretion of gonadotropic hormones throughout the sexual lives of female and male humans, showing an especially abrupt increase in gonadotropic hormones at menopause in the female.

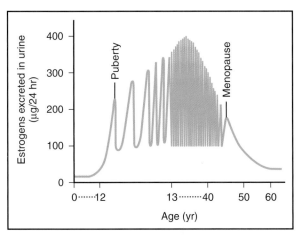

FIGURE 77-2 Estrogen secretion throughout the sexual life of the female human.

Vaginal atrophy is also the result of decreased estrogen. The vaginal mucosa thins and lubrication decreases. Vaginal cytologic examination shows predominantly parabasal cells, indicating lack of epithelial maturation due to low estrogen levels.

Osteoporosis occurs in late menopause.

OUTCOME

Estrogen replacement therapy, as a treatment to reduce the symptoms associated with menopause, is controversial. Data from the Women's Health Initiative study indicate that women should not use combination progestin-estrogen therapy for more than 3 or 4 years. This is because the increased risk of cardiovascular disease, cerebrovascular disease, and breast cancer with this regimen outweighed the benefits.

New therapies such as selective estrogen receptor modulators (SERMs) are replacing the use of estrogen replacement. These drugs mimic the beneficial effects of estrogen on bone yet do not have detrimental effects on uterine and breast tissue. A support group can be helpful.

FURTHER READING

Web Source
http://www.nhlbi.nih.gov/whi/index.html

Text Sources
Carroll RG: Elsevier's Integrated Physiology. Philadelphia, Elsevier, 2007.

Copstead L, Banasik J: Pathophysiology, 3rd ed. Philadelphia, Saunders, 2005.

Guyton AC, Hall JE: Textbook of Medical Physiology, 11th ed. Philadelphia, Saunders, 2006.

McPhee SJ, Papadakis MA, Tierney LM Jr: Current Medical Diagnosis and Treatment, 46th ed. New York, McGraw-Hill, 2007.

A 17-year-old girl visits the pediatrician because of an 8-month absence of a menses. The patient joined a cross country team at high school 3 years ago and is training for the upcoming state championships. She has ranged between the 25th and 55th percentile for both height and weight since her second birthday but has progressively lost weight during the past 2 years. All other developmental milestones were met at an appropriate age. Both parents are of normal height and stature.

PHYSICAL EXAMINATION

VS: T 37°C, P 90/min, R 22/min, BP 100/80 mm Hg, BMI 17
PE: Physical examination reveals a well-toned female athlete with minimal subcutaneous body fat.

LABORATORY STUDIES

Pregnancy test (hCG): Negative
Radiography: Normal hypothalamus and pituitary
LH: 0.4 IU/mL (normal: 0.9 to 10.6 IU/mL)
Prolactin: 12 ng/mL (normal: < 20 ng/mL)
Injection of GnRH stimulates the release of both FSH and LH.

DIAGNOSIS

Hypothalamic amenorrhea

PATHOPHYSIOLOGY OF KEY SYMPTOMS

Gonadotropin releasing hormone (GnRH) is produced and secreted by neurons in the hypothalamus and travels through the hypothalamohypophyseal portal system to the anterior pituitary to stimulate the release of follicle-stimulating hormone (FSH) and luteinizing hormone LH). The reproductive cells and glands are the targets for FSH and LH. For females, FSH stimulates ovarian follicles to mature and to release estrogen and LH stimulates the corpus luteum to secrete progesterone (Fig. 78-1).

The initial event in puberty is the onset of pulsatile GnRH secretion by the hypothalamus. The absence of pulsatile GnRH secretion is called idiopathic hypogonadotropic hypogonadism. This syndrome is often accompanied by a defect in olfaction, and the combination of the hypogonadotropic hypogonadism and anosmia is called Kallmann's syndrome.

GnRH and reproductive hormone levels vary significantly throughout the lifespan. GnRH stimulates FSH and LH secretion in utero and during the first 18 months post partum. Levels of all three hormones fall by age 2 and remain low throughout childhood. During puberty, GnRH pulsatile secretion increases and the FSH and LH stimulation of estrogen and progesterone production allows females to reach reproductive maturity (Fig. 78-2).

After puberty, hypothalamic GnRH secretion can be diminished by significant weight loss, exercise, or stress. In these cases, the patient may cease menstruating, a syndrome called hypothalamic amenorrhea. Confirmation of this diagnosis is obtained by a normal FSH and LH released after injection of exogenous

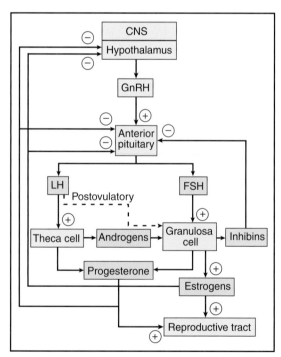

FIGURE 78–1 Complex regulation of estrogen and progesterone production. FSH stimulates estrogen secretion by ovarian granulosa cells, and LH stimulates progesterone secretion by the ovary. Complex negative feedback loops inhibit both hypothalamic and anterior pituitary hormone secretion. –, negative feedback; +, positive feedback.

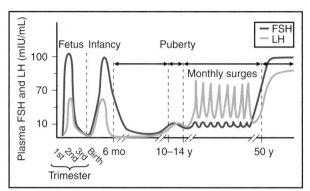

FIGURE 78–2 Plasma FSH and LH levels show peaks in utero and during infancy, monthly cycling during the reproductive years, and sustained elevation after menopause. In utero, FSH and LH secretion is stimulated by human chorionic gonadotropin. After puberty, FSH and LH secretion is stimulated by GnRH and inhibited by estrogen and progesterone. After menopause, impaired secretion of ovarian estrogen and progesterone results in elevated FSH and LH levels.

GnRH. An individual with an impaired pituitary production of FSH or LH would also show low hormone levels (FSH and estrogen) but elevated GnRH levels. Finally, a lack of ovarian response to GnRH would result in an individual with low estrogen and progesterone but high levels of GnRH, FSH, and LH.

Disruption of communication between the hypothalamus and pituitary can lead to a defect in FSH and LH production. Prolactin, in contrast, is controlled by prolactin inhibitory factor (dopamine) from the hypothalamus. Damage to the hypothalamohypophyseal stalk will cause the simultaneous increase in prolactin release and inhibition of the release of all of the other anterior pituitary hormones. The normal prolactin levels in this patient, along with normal computed tomographic findings, indicate that the communication between the hypothalamus and the pituitary is intact.

FURTHER READING

Text Sources

Carroll RG: Elsevier's Integrated Physiology. Philadelphia, Elsevier, 2007.

Copstead L, Banasik J: Pathophysiology, 3rd ed. Philadelphia, Saunders, 2005.

Guyton AC, Hall JE: Textbook of Medical Physiology, 11th ed. Philadelphia, Saunders, 2006.

McPhee SJ, Papadakis MA, Tierney LM Jr: Current Medical Diagnosis and Treatment, 46th ed. New York, McGraw-Hill, 2007.

Rexford SA: Body fat, leptin, and hypothalamic amenorrhea. N Engl J Med 351:959-962, 2004.

A 24-year-old woman presents to her gynecologist with concerns regarding her menstrual cycle.

The patient complains of very irregular menstrual periods (fewer than eight a year) that are very heavy. She also noticed dark, coarse hair growing on her face, upper arms, chest, and abdomen, which she stated is extremely embarrassing. The patient also complains of persistent acne on her face. She is married without children. She and her husband have been trying for a pregnancy for about 3 months now but have been unsuccessful.

PHYSICAL EXAMINATION

VS: T 98.8°F, P 82/min, R 14/min, BP 125/80 mm Hg, weight 145 lb, height 5'3"
PE: Patient is overweight with a BMI of 26. The majority of the excess fat is centralized around her abdominal area. There is some dark, coarse hair.

LABORATORY STUDIES

Transvaginal ultrasonography: A 2-5 fold ovarian enlargement with thickened tunica albuginea and approximately 20 follicles 1 to 5 mm in diameter without a dominant follicle; endometrium is thin. The findings are consistent with polycystic ovary disease.
Blood test: Elevated LH/FSH ratio > 2.5
Testosterone: 130 ng/dL (normal: 20-80 ng/dL)
Prolactin: 18 ng/dL (normal: < 20 ng/dL)
Glucose tolerance test: Abnormal
Thyroid Hormone (TH): 7 μg/dL (normal: 5-12 μg/dL)

DIAGNOSIS

Polycystic ovary syndrome

PATHOPHYSIOLOGY OF KEY SYMPTOMS

During the reproductive years the ovaries undergo cyclic changes that are integral to normal reproductive function. After the onset of menstruation, follicle-stimulating hormone (FSH) from the hypothalamus stimulates the maturation of the primordial follicles. Numerous follicles begin the maturation process, but one follicle becomes dominant and continues to mature into a graafian follicle, surrounded by thecal cells that produce androgens and granulosa cells that produce estrogens and progesterone. The nondominant follicles regress and degenerate. Ovulation occurs on day 14, when the mature follicle ruptures, releasing the ova. The granulosa cells in the remnants of the ruptured follicle become the corpus luteum and secrete progesterone and estrogen.

Polycystic ovary syndrome is often called Stein-Leventhal syndrome. In this syndrome a number of primordial follicles begin the maturation process but no single follicle emerges as the dominant follicle. In the absence of the development of a primary follicle, ovulation does not occur. Polycystic ovary syndrome occurs in 10% of females in the United States and is the leading cause of female infertility.

Failure of the follicle to mature also causes reduced estrogen and progesterone production. The cyclic changes of the uterine endometrium associated with the menstrual cycle are normally stimulated by estrogen and progesterone. Consequently, women with polycystic ovary syndrome will have irregular or completely absent menses.

Androgen production by the thecal cells of the primordial follicles continues throughout the ovarian cycle, leading to many the external symptoms of polycystic ovary syndrome. These symptoms are generally thought of as male secondary sexual characteristics and include increased hair growth on the face and trunk, excessive oil production by the sebaceous glands leading to acne, and possibly male pattern baldness or thinning of hair.

The exact causes of polycystic ovary syndrome are not yet known, but the syndrome tends to occur in families. Cysts can occur in women without the disease, so the presence of cysts alone does not indicate the development of the syndrome.

Obesity is both associated as a risk factor for developing the syndrome and as a symptom of the disease. Part of this association may be due to the relationship between obesity and diminished insulin sensitivity. Women with polycystic ovary syndrome frequently have decreased insulin sensitivity and increased insulin production, as is characteristic with type 2 diabetes mellitus. The decreased insulin sensitivity likely accounts for the abnormal glucose tolerance test of this patient.

Treatment options depend on the desired clinical outcome. Estrogen-based birth control pills can help restore regular menstrual cycling but not ovulation. Ovulation can be restored by treatment with clomiphene. 5α-Reductase inhibitors such as finasteride can be used to block the intracellular conversion of testosterone into dihydrotestosterone and, in doing so, reduce the development of many of the male secondary sexual characteristics. Finally, weight loss has been effective at diminishing many of the symptoms of polycystic ovary syndrome.

FURTHER READING

Web Sources

http://www.mayoclinic.com/health/polycystic-ovary-syndrome/
DS00423
http://www.mdconsult.com/about/book/88498341-2/instruct.
html?DOCID=1531

Text Sources

Carroll RG: Elsevier's Integrated Physiology. Philadelphia, Elsevier, 2007.

Copstead L, Banasik J: Pathophysiology, 3rd ed. Philadelphia, Saunders, 2005.
Guyton AC, Hall JE: Textbook of Medical Physiology, 11th ed. Philadelphia, Saunders, 2006.
McPhee SJ, Papadakis MA, Tierney LM Jr: Current Medical Diagnosis and Treatment, 46th ed. New York, McGraw-Hill, 2007.

A 28-year-old nulliparous woman visits her gynecologist complaining of pelvic pain accompanying her menses.

The patient states that the pain begins around 1 week before her menses and becomes increasingly severe until flow slackens, at which time the pubic pain subsides. The intervals of pain have been getting progressively worse over the past few months. The patient states that her menses are no longer regular or consistent and that they "feel heavier than they used to be." She also complains of some discomfort during intercourse. The patient states that all of these symptoms have started within the last 6 months and that previously she only had mild cramping with menstruation. She is sexually active and uses condoms for contraception.

PHYSICAL EXAMINATION

VS: T 98.6°F, P 70/min, R 16/min, BP 120/70 mm Hg, BMI 24
PE: Pelvic examination is unremarkable.

LABORATORY STUDIES

MRI: Lesions along the uterus
Laparoscopy and tissue biopsy: Endometrial tissue on the ovaries and uterine tubes

DIAGNOSIS

Endometriosis

PATHOPHYSIOLOGY OF KEY SYMPTOMS

The female reproductive cycle is a recurring set of changes in the uterus and ovaries that enables successful uterine implantation of a zygote. The uterine wall consists of an external parametrium, a middle

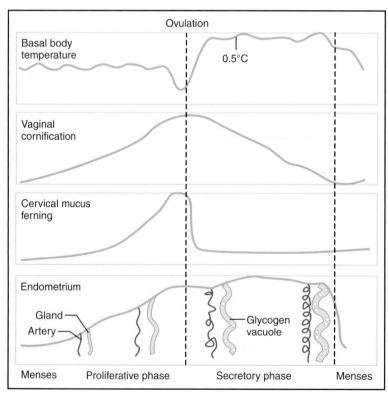

FIGURE 80–1 Uterine and vaginal changes during the menstrual cycle. After menstruation the uterine endometrium increases in size and vaginal cornification and secretions provide a nutritive environment for sperm. After ovulation the uterine endometrium enters the secretory phase, providing a suitable environment for implantation of a fertilized ovum.

myometrium, and the internal endometrial lining. During the first half of the reproductive cycle, an ovarian follicle matures and grows in response to anterior pituitary follicle-stimulating hormone (FSH) release. Estrogen produced by the maturing follicle stimulates the growth of the epithelia, glands, blood vessels, and connective tissue that comprise the endometrium. The first half of the uterine reproductive cycle is called the proliferative phase. The duration of the proliferative phase is presented typically 14 days, but it can vary greatly (Fig. 80-1).

At the midpoint of the reproductive cycle, the primary follicle ruptures, releasing an ovum in a process called ovulation. During the next week, the egg is transported along the fallopian tubes and passes through the uterus. The remnants of the primary follicle form the corpus luteum, which persists for 11 days and then spontaneously degenerates.

The corpus luteum is stimulated to secrete progesterone by pituitary luteinizing hormone (LH). Progesterone stimulates an increase in the endometrial secretions, and the deposition of glycogen in the endometrial tissue. The blood vessels continue to grow and become coiled. At this point, the uterine endometrium is ideally prepared for implantation of a fertilized blastocyst. Failure of ovum fertilization or implantation results in atrophy of the corpus luteum.

At 12 to 14 days after ovulation the corpus luteum begins to atrophy, diminishing progesterone secretion. In the absence of progesterone, the uterine endometrium retracts and degenerates. The blood vessels constrict, creating necrotic patches of endometrial tissue that separate from the endometrial wall. This necrotic tissue and secretions become menstrual flow. The menstrual flow exits the body through the cervix and vagina.

Occasionally, the tissue normally found in the uterine endometrium spreads into the peritoneal cavity and can cause a painful inflammatory response known as endometriosis. The ectopic endometrial tissue is often found around the ovaries and in the dependent portions of the peritoneum. Although not in the uterus, this ectopic endometrial tissue responds to the same hormonal signals for growth during the proliferative phase of the uterine cycle and growth and secretion during secretory phase of the uterine cycle. As progesterone levels fall at the end of the secretory phase, the ectopic endometrial tissue remains in the peritoneum but still necrotizes, setting up an inflammatory response. Inflammation contributes to the reported pain during the menstrual cycle and also results in adhesion and scarring. The occasions can contribute to sensations of pain that may not be limited to the menstrual period. Scar tissue, particularly involving the ovaries or the fallopian tubes, can disrupt the normal release and transport of the ovum and cause infertility.

Treatment may involve oral contraceptive therapy to regulate hormonal balance and pelvic pain. Over-the-counter pain relievers can be used as needed. If the pain is severe, surgical removal of the endometrial tissue may be necessary.

FURTHER READING

Web Sources

http://www.endometriosisassn.org/index.html
http://www.endo-resolved.com/index.html
http://www.mayoclinic.com/health/endometriosis/DS00289
Stoppler MC: MedicineNet from WebMD: Endometriosis, March 2007. http://www.medicinenet.com/endometriosis/article.htm

Text Sources

Carroll RG: Elsevier's Integrated Physiology. Philadelphia, Elsevier, 2007.
Copstead L, Banasik J: Pathophysiology, 3rd ed. Philadelphia, Saunders, 2005.

Guyton AC, Hall JE: Textbook of Medical Physiology, 11th ed. Philadelphia, Saunders, 2006.
McPhee SJ, Papadakis MA, Tierney LM Jr: Current Medical Diagnosis and Treatment, 46th ed. New York, McGraw-Hill, 2007.
Olive DL, Lindheim SR, Pritts EA: New medical treatments for endometriosis. Best Pract Res Clin Obstet Gynecol 18:319-328, 2004.
Osteen KG, Bruner-Tran KL, Eisenberg E: Reduced progesterone action during endometrial maturation: a potential risk factor for the development of endometriosis. Fertil Steril 83:529-537, 2005.

A 24-year-old woman comes to the emergency department complaining of severe left lower quadrant pelvic pain and abnormal vaginal bleeding.

The patient states that the pain began abruptly 1 hour ago. She describes pain as 10 on a scale of 10 and states it radiates to her lower back. She denies nausea or vomiting. She states she has a history of abnormal periods and pelvic inflammatory disease, with the last period ending 8 weeks ago.

PHYSICAL EXAMINATION

VS: T 99°F, P 92/min, R 22/min, BP 142/76 mm Hg
PE: Tenderness in left inguinal region on palpation

LABORATORY STUDIES

CBC: Hematocrit 37% (normal: 38% to 42%); leukocytosis
β-hCG: Positive (2000 mIU/mL)
Progesterone: 12 ng/mL
Transvaginal and transabdominal ultrasound: No intrauterine pregnancy. Normal intrauterine sac, swollen left fallopian tube with an apparent mass.
Culdocentesis: Nonclotting blood aspirated from cul-de-sac

DIAGNOSIS

Ectopic pregnancy

PATHOPHYSIOLOGY OF KEY SYMPTOMS

Female reproductive fertility is limited to the brief period of time (around 24 hours) after ovulation. After ovulation, the ovum enters the fimbriae of the fallopian tube and is transported to the uterus during the next 6 days. Pregnancy requires the fertilization of the egg shortly after it enters the fallopian tube. During the remaining time while passing through the fallopian tube the fertilized egg matures into a blastocyst and successfully implants onto the uterine endometrium (Fig. 81-1). One region of the blastocyst becomes the embryo, and a different region of the blastocyst digests the uterine endometrium and matures into a placenta. The placenta and the embryo have the same genetic composition and, consequently, chorionic villous sampling can be used to genotype the embryo. A blastocyst that implants in a region of the body other than the uterus is termed an "ectopic pregnancy."

The incidence of ectopic pregnancy is 1:150 live births. Of those, 98% are located in the fallopian tubes. Ova released from the surface of the ovary travel through a small space in the peritoneum before entering the fimbriae of the fallopian tube. Ova fertilized before they enter the fallopian tube can implant in the peritoneum, abdominal viscera, the ovary, or the cervix. Conditions that predispose a patient to ectopic pregnancy are a history of infertility, pelvic inflammatory disease, ruptured appendix, and prior tubal surgery. Currently, in the United States, undiagnosed ectopic pregnancy is the most common cause of maternal death during the first trimester.

At 12 to 14 days after ovulation the ovarian corpus luteum degenerates and ceases progesterone production. The decline in progesterone production causes spasm of the blood vessels of the uterine endometrium, creating necrotic patches. In the absence of progesterone, the uterine myometrium begins rhythmic contractions. The combination of vascular contraction and enhanced uterine muscle activity lead to a sloughing of part of the uterine endometrium as menses.

Successful implantation requires a continuous production of progesterone. The blastocyst secretes the hormone human chorionic gonadotropin (hCG), which stimulates the corpus luteum to continue to produce progesterone during the first trimester of pregnancy. The continued high level of progesterone prevents menstruation and also diminishes the contraction of the uterine smooth muscle.

Production of hCG can be used to assess the viability of the fetus. Normally, as the blastocyst implants and the fetus grows, hCG levels should double every 48 hours. If hCG production is diminished, this indicates a problem with the developing fetus. Implantation in a region that is not the uterine endometrium attenuates both nutrient availability and vascular supply and impedes placental and/or fetal development. Inadequate hCG production is one of the characteristics of an ectopic pregnancy.

Implantation in the fallopian tube presents a structural barrier to the growth of the fetus. As the fetus grows, the wall of the fallopian tube is stretched and may spontaneously rupture. Because of the small diameter

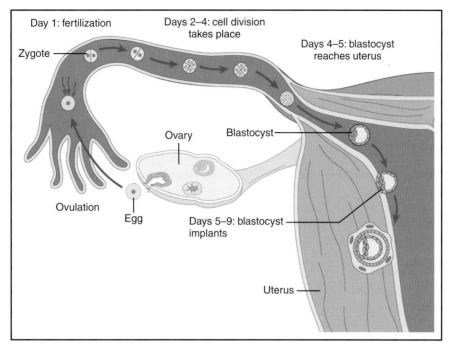

FIGURE 81–1   Fertilization in the fallopian tube and implantation in the uterus occur during normal pregnancy. Conception occurs when sperm and ovum unite in the fallopian tube. The fertilized ovum begins a series of mitotic cell divisions and reaches the blastocyst stage before implanting in the uterus.

of the tube, isthmic pregnancies tend to rupture earliest, at 6 to 8 weeks' gestation. Ampullary pregnancies rupture later, generally at 8 to 12 weeks. Interstitial pregnancies are the last to rupture, usually at 12 to 16 weeks. Interstitial rupture creates a critical situation because it is very close to uterine and ovarian vessels and can cause massive hemorrhage.

Ultrasonography and laparoscopy can be used to confirm the site of implantation. Transvaginal ultrasonography can determine if the pregnancy is in the uterus. The combination of a positive hCG test and a transvaginal sonogram that does not visualize an intrauterine pregnancy indicates an ectopic pregnancy.

OUTCOME

Because of the positive culdocentesis, a laparotomy or laparoscopy should be done immediately.

FURTHER READING

Web Sources
http://www.americanpregnancy.org
http://www.medicinenet.com/ectopic_pregnancy/article.htm

Text Sources
Carroll RG: Elsevier's Integrated Physiology. Philadelphia, Elsevier, 2007.

Copstead L, Banasik J: Pathophysiology, 3rd ed. Philadelphia, Saunders, 2005.
Guyton AC, Hall JE: Textbook of Medical Physiology, 11th ed. Philadelphia, Saunders, 2006.
McPhee SJ, Papadakis MA, Tierney LM Jr: Current Medical Diagnosis and Treatment, 46th ed. New York, McGraw-Hill, 2007.

C A S E

82

A 40-year-old pregnant woman visits her obstetrician after noting vaginal bleeding. The bleeding is a small volume and began during the previous night. Fetal age is estimated at 32 weeks' gestation. Chorionic villi sampling did not reveal any genetic abnormalities. There have been two prior pregnancies, one ending in a 10-week miscarriage and the other a normal labor and vaginal delivery 3 years previously. The patient developed gestational diabetes at week 34, four weeks before delivery.

PHYSICAL EXAMINATION

VS: T 99.0°F, P 84/min, R 24/min, BP 130/90 mm Hg, weight 145

PE: Patient looks normal for a 32-week pregnancy. There is localized uterine pain.

LABORATORY STUDIES

Fetal:

- Ultrasound: Fetus is normal for gestational age.
- Fetal heart rate: Normal

Maternal:

- Glucose tolerance test: Borderline elevated
- Estriol levels: Normal for gestational age

DIAGNOSIS

Placental abruption

PATHOPHYSIOLOGY OF KEY SYMPTOMS

The third trimester is a time of rapid fetal growth and maturation. The maternal fetal interface is created by the fetal placenta and the maternal uterus to facilitate the delivery of nutrients and removal of wastes from the fetus. The close approximation of fetal placental capillaries and the maternal uterine capillaries provides a very large surface area to facilitate diffusional will exchange (Fig. 82-1). In addition, fetal characteristics enhance the movement of oxygen and glucose. Fetal hemoglobin has a higher affinity for oxygen then does maternal hemoglobin, enhancing the delivery of oxygen to the fetus. Fetal hematocrit is higher than maternal hematocrit, enhancing the oxygen-carrying capacity of the fetal blood. Glucose delivery to the fetus is enhanced by the high maternal plasma glucose levels. Throughout gestation, the growing fetus places additional demands on nutrient and waste exchange at the placenta.

Fetal viability is assessed by observing a correlation between fetal heart rate and fetal movement. Both tachycardia and bradycardia can be signs of fetal distress, as is a decreased variability in the fetal heart rate. Cardiotocography is used to simultaneously measure fetal heart rate and the strength of uterine contractions during labor. Fetal heart rate should decrease during the uterine contractions but return to normal shortly after the uterine contraction ceases.

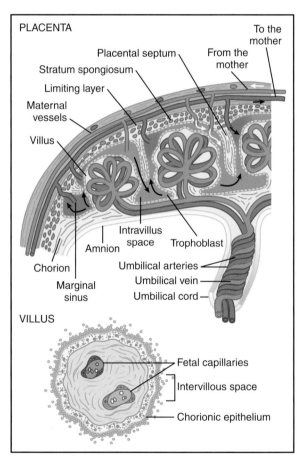

FIGURE 82–1 **Top,** Organization of the mature placenta. **Bottom,** Relation of the fetal blood in the villus capillaries to the mother's blood in the intervillous spaces. (*Modified from Gray H, Goss CM: Anatomy of the Human Body, 25th ed. Philadelphia, Lea & Febiger, 1948; and from Arey LB: Developmental Anatomy: A Textbook and Laboratory Manual of Embryology, 7th ed. Philadelphia, Saunders, 1974.*)

A drop in maternal serum estriol indicates a decline in fetal viability. Estriol synthesis requires adequate function of both the placenta and the fetal adrenal gland. Steroid precursors produced in the fetal liver are converted into dehydroepiandrosterone sulfate in the fetal adrenal gland and then converted to estriol in the placenta. After synthesis, estriol circulates in the maternal plasma in both a free and a glucuronide conjugated form. Unconjugated serum estriol is a useful index of fetal health because it assesses function of both the fetal adrenal gland and the placenta.

Damage to the placenta poses significant health risks for both the mother and the fetus. Placental abruption is the separation of a region of the placenta (of fetal origin) from the maternal uterine myometrium. The health risks are tied to both the quantity of the placenta that is damaged as well as hemorrhage. Loss of placental tissue decreases the surface area available for exchange of nutrients and wastes between the fetal and maternal circulations. Hemorrhage can create an immediate health risk to the mother and potentially generate a delayed immune sensitization.

Rhesus factor (Rh) is a red blood cell surface antigen that was first identified in primates. An individual who is Rh negative lacks the antigen. During labor and delivery, mothers who are Rh negative are treated with RhoGAM to diminish the chance of antibodies developing because of exposure to fetal (potentially Rh positive) blood. Although development of antibodies does not represent a risk for the current pregnancy, the antibodies can generate an immune response against future Rh-positive fetuses. Placental abruption allows mixing of the fetal and maternal blood while the fetus is still in utero.

Likely treatment includes admission to the hospital, bed rest, and observation. Serial ultrasonography and fetal heart rate monitoring are used to assess fetus health, and estradiol levels are used to assess the fetal and placental viability. Fetal surfactant production begins at 28 weeks' gestational age, and sufficient surfactant availability is a major factor in the decision to induce an early labor. Corticosteroid treatment can be used to accelerate the maturation of the type II alveolar epithelial cells that produce surfactant.

FURTHER READING

Text Sources
Carroll RG: Elsevier's Integrated Physiology. Philadelphia, Elsevier, 2007.
Copstead L, Banasik J: Pathophysiology, 3rd ed. Philadelphia, Saunders, 2005.

Guyton AC, Hall JE: Textbook of Medical Physiology, 11th ed. Philadelphia, Saunders, 2006.
McPhee SJ, Papadakis MA, Tierney LM Jr: Current Medical Diagnosis and Treatment, 46th ed. New York, McGraw-Hill, 2007.

A pregnant 34-year-old woman arrives in the emergency department by ambulance after suffering a seizure while waiting in the optometrist's office.

The patient is at 29 weeks' gestation, and this is her third pregnancy. She has a history of hypertension and diabetes but managed these conditions well during her previous pregnancies. However, with this pregnancy, she experienced excessive swelling in comparison to the past two and reports a decrease in urine production. The patient had an acute decrease in visual acuity 2 days ago and had a seizure while in the waiting room at the optometrist's office. She arrived at the emergency department 45 minutes later.

PHYSICAL EXAMINATION

VS: T 98°F, P 100/min, R 20/min, BP 160/110 mm Hg
PE: The patient is anxious and recovering from the unexpected seizure. Ophthalmoscope shows retinal hemorrhage. The patient has edema of the hands and feet. The remainder of the physical examination is appropriate for a 29-week gestation.

LABORATORY STUDIES

Ultrasonography: Fetal growth restriction
Blood tests:

- Platelets: 80,000/mL (normal: 150,000-350,000/mL)
- Aspartate aminotransferase: 80 IU/L (normal: 7-27 IU/L)
- Lactate dehydrogenase: 650 IU/L (normal: 50-150 IU/L)
- Alanine aminotransferase: 40 IU/L (normal: 1-21 IU/L)
- Uric acid: 12 mg/dL (normal 2-7 mg/dL)
- Fasting blood glucose level: 105 mg/dL (normal: 70-110 mg/dL)

24-hour urine collection:

- 300 mL (normal: > 500 mL/24 hr)
- 8 g protein (normal: < 1 g/24 hr)

DIAGNOSIS

Eclampsia

PATHOPHYSIOLOGY OF KEY SYMPTOMS

Fetal growth during the final trimester places a significant demand on exchange of nutrients and waste products between the placenta and the uterus. Placental function, if impaired, can restrict the growth of the fetus and result in damage to a variety of maternal organs, creating a syndrome of preeclampsia. Five percent of patients with preeclampsia progress to eclampsia, with the distinction being the occurrence of seizures.

Preeclampsia and eclampsia result from damage to the vascular component of the placenta. Although the exact cause is not known, an immunologic disruption may be a significant contributing factor. Symptoms of preeclampsia result from impairment of the kidney, cardiovascular system, liver, hematopoietic state, central nervous system, and placenta. Damage to the wide variety of organs resulted in elevation in the number of serum enzymes.

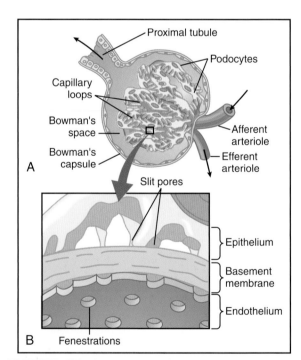

FIGURE 83–1 A, Basic ultrastructure of the glomerular capillaries. **B,** Cross section of the glomerular capillary membrane and its major components: capillary endothelium, basement membrane, and epithelium (podocytes).

During pregnancy, renal function increases by as much as 50%. If renal function fails to increase sufficiently, there is a relative impairment of renal function, as indicated by the oliguria, by the presence of proteins in the urine, and by the elevated uric acid levels. The oliguria in the presence of normal fluid intake results in an increase in body fluid volume. Proteinuria results from damage to the glomerular capillaries and basement membrane, possibly from the immunologic system (Fig. 83-1).

A significant hypertension is a consequence of enhanced fluid retention and blood volume expansion. The increase in preload causes an increase in cardiac output. Normally during pregnancy, the drop in peripheral vascular resistance from vasodilation of the uterine blood vessels offsets the increase in cardiac output and blood pressure remains normal.

The central nervous system symptoms are related to hypertension, vascular damage, and abnormal clotting. All three of these cardiovascular disorders initially can lead to headaches and visual disturbances and, in eclampsia, seizures. Vascular damage to the retina may be visible on ophthalmoscope examination and may contribute to diminished visual acuity.

Hepatic injury in eclampsia is likely due to increased hemolysis, enhanced coagulation, or hepatic vascular damage. The liver enlarges and can become tender to palpation during eclampsia. Hepatic injury can be monitored by elevated liver enzymes.

Impaired placental function is at the root of most of the symptoms of preeclampsia. For the fetus, impaired placental function can restrict nutrient availability and diminish growth. Consequently, fetal growth restriction is a characteristic of preeclampsia.

Preeclampsia is difficult to manage and is best treated by having labor and delivery as soon as the fetus is viable. Expulsion of the placenta at delivery results in a fairly rapid recovery of maternal organ function. Epidemiologic studies, however, indicate that women with preeclampsia are at risk for future development of hypertension and/or renal disease. The incidence of preeclampsia in women at risk may be reduced by treatment with aspirin and by ensuring adequate calcium intake.

FURTHER READING

Web Source
http://www.emedicine.com/emerg/topic796.htm

Text Sources
Carroll RG: Elsevier's Integrated Physiology. Philadelphia, Elsevier, 2007.

Copstead L, Banasik J: Pathophysiology, 3rd ed. Philadelphia, Saunders, 2005.
Guyton AC, Hall JE: Textbook of Medical Physiology, 11th ed. Philadelphia, Saunders, 2006.
McPhee SJ, Papadakis MA, Tierney LM Jr: Current Medical Diagnosis and Treatment, 46th ed. New York, McGraw-Hill, 2007.

C A S E
84

A 32-year-old woman has an appointment with her gynecologist for a normal prenatal checkup.

The patient is pregnant with gestational age estimated at 32 weeks. This is her first pregnancy. Her mother is overweight and has recently been diagnosed with type 2 diabetes.

PHYSICAL EXAMINATION

VS: T 38.5°C, P 85/min, R 22/min, BP 130/90 mm Hg, BMI 33

PE: The patient presents as a typical 32-week pregnant woman.

LABORATORY STUDIES

Glucose tolerance test: Abnormal

DIAGNOSIS

Gestational diabetes

PATHOPHYSIOLOGY OF KEY SYMPTOMS

Pregnancy dramatically alters maternal steroids and peptide hormone production. For the steroids, this includes marked increases in the production of the estrogens, progesterone, aldosterone, and deoxycorticosterone. For the peptides, this includes insulin, plasma renin, angiotensinogen, and human chorionic gonadotropin. Placental secretions include thyrotropin, adrenocorticotropic hormone (ACTH), and somatostatin. The endocrine "overproduction" is necessary to support the growth and development of the fetus and to allow maternal changes necessary to provide a nurturing environment for the fetus.

Insulin is produced by the pancreas in response to an elevation in blood glucose. Insulin acts to decrease plasma glucose by stimulating cellular glucose uptake in a variety of tissues, especially the liver and skeletal muscle (Fig. 84-1). One consequence of the changing endocrine environment is that the maternal tissues lose their sensitivity to insulin. As tissues become less responsive to glucose, fasting plasma glucose levels rise, plasma insulin levels rise, and the body is unable to efficiently store ingested glucose. Gestational diabetes results from a loss of tissue insulin sensitivity during the third trimester of pregnancy and resembles type 2 diabetes mellitus. Gestational diabetes develops in around 4% of pregnancies in the United States.

Gestational diabetes is confirmed by an abnormal response to a glucose tolerance test. Normally, ingestion of a glucose load will cause a moderate increase in plasma glucose, stimulating pancreatic insulin secretion. Insulin causes the cellular uptake of glucose, attenuating the rise in plasma glucose. In addition, the insulin helps clear the glucose from the body over the next 3 hours. An abnormal glucose tolerance test is one in which the fasting glucose is greater than 95 mg/dL or, following ingestion, the plasma glucose level rises higher than 180 mg/dL at 1 hour after ingestion or remains elevated (>155 mg/dL at 2 hours or >140 mg/dL at 3 hours).

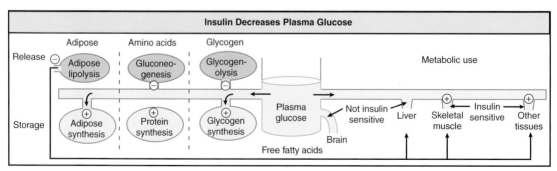

FIGURE 84–1 Plasma glucose levels represent the balance between gastrointestinal glucose absorption, movement into and out of storage pools, and metabolism by mitochondria. Insulin stimulates adipose synthesis and glycogen synthesis, and enhances glucose uptake in skeletal muscle.

Gestational diabetes presents risks for both the infant and the mother. Insulin is a growth factor as well as a glucose regulatory hormone. The combination of high insulin and high glucose stimulates fetal growth and can result in an abnormally large infant with extra fat. In addition, the fetus becomes acclimated to the high insulin levels and the separation from the maternal glucose stores at birth can cause a significant hypoglycemia.

Mothers who develop gestational diabetes also have an increased risk for gestational hypertension. In addition, patients who develop gestational diabetes are at risk for developing type 2 diabetes mellitus later in life.

FURTHER READING

Web Sources

http://diabetes.niddk.nih.gov/dm/pubs/gestational/
http://www.diabetes.org/gestational-diabetes.jsp
http://www.mayoclinic.com/health/gestational-diabetes/DS00316

Text Sources

Carroll RG: Elsevier's Integrated Physiology. Philadelphia, Elsevier, 2007.

Copstead L, Banasik J: Pathophysiology, 3rd ed. Philadelphia, Saunders, 2005.
Guyton AC, Hall JE: Textbook of Medical Physiology, 11th ed. Philadelphia, Saunders, 2006.
McPhee SJ, Papadakis MA, Tierney LM Jr: Current Medical Diagnosis and Treatment, 46th ed. New York, McGraw-Hill, 2007.

A 17-year-old boy with an absence of signs of puberty visits the pediatrician.
The patient has had a range between the 25th and 55th percentile for both height and weight since his second birthday. All other developmental milestones were met at an appropriate age. Both parents are of normal height and stature.

PHYSICAL EXAMINATION

VS: T 37°C, P 90/min, R 22/min, BP 100/80 mm Hg, height 5 ft 10 in, weight 130 lb, BMI 18.5

PE: Physical examination reveals a normal prepubertal male in spite of his age, with no signs of secondary sexual characteristic development. The patient appears underdeveloped, with little muscle mass. His voice is high pitched. He has sparse pubic and axillary hair, underdeveloped testes (volume < 4 ml), and a small phallus. Evaluation of cranial nerve I shows normal smelling ability.

LABORATORY STUDIES

MRI: Normal hypothalamus and pituitary
LH: 0.6 IU/mL (normal: 0.9 to 10.6 IU/mL)
Testosterone: 80 ng/dL (normal: 300-1000 ng/dL)
Injection of 100 μg GnRH stimulates a lower than normal release of both FSH and LH.

DIAGNOSIS

Secondary hypogonadotropic hypogonadism

PATHOPHYSIOLOGY OF KEY SYMPTOMS

Gonadotropin-releasing hormone (GnRH) is produced and secreted by neurons in the hypothalamus and travels through the hypothalamohypophyseal portal system to the anterior pituitary to stimulate the release of follicle-stimulating hormone (FSH) and luteinizing hormone (LH) (Fig. 85-1). The reproductive cells and glands are the targets for FSH and LH. For females, FSH stimulates ovarian follicles to mature and to release estrogen. For males, FSH stimulates testicular Sertoli cells to produce paracrine molecules necessary for the mitosis of spermatogonia into mature sperm. For females, LH stimulates the corpus luteum to secrete progesterone.

For males, LH stimulates testicular Leydig cells to secrete testosterone.

The hypothalamic pituitary gonadal axis is active late in gestation and remains active during the first

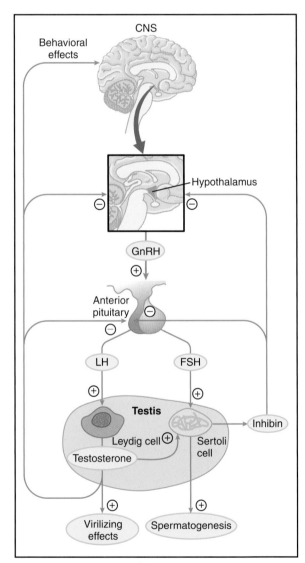

FIGURE 85–1 Feedback regulation of the hypothalamic-pituitary-testicular axis in males. Stimulatory effects are shown by ⊕ and negative feedback inhibitory effects are shown by ⊖. GnRH, Gonadotropin-releasing hormone; LH, luteinizing hormone; FSH, follicle-stimulating hormone.

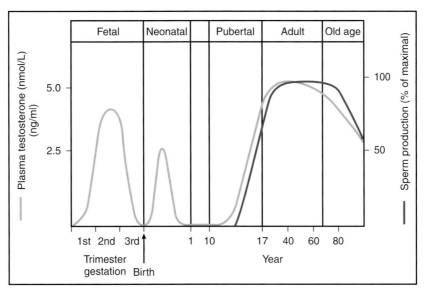

FIGURE 85–2   The different stages of male sexual function as reflected by average plasma testosterone concentrations *(red line)* and sperm production *(blue line)* at different ages. *(Modified from Griffin JF, Wilson JD: The testis. In Bondy PK, Rosenberg LE [eds]: Metabolic Control and Disease, 8th ed. Philadelphia, Saunders, 1980.)*

few months post partum. By 6 months post partum, hypothalamic secretion of GnRH is markedly attenuated and remains low until puberty. The initial event in puberty is the onset of pulsatile GnRH secretion by the hypothalamus. GnRH stimulates the pituitary to release FSH and LH. FSH and LH stimulate the growth and development of the testes, including the secretion of testosterone (Fig. 85-2).

Testosterone acts on a variety of tissues to stimulate the development of secondary sexual characteristics. These include growth of the external genitalia, enlargement of the larynx, development of pubic hair, skeletal muscle growth, a growth spurt followed by closure of the epiphyseal plates, and increased growth of the epidermis and sebaceous glands.

In the absence of GnRH there is no stimulation for the maturation of the testes or the secretion of testosterone and thus no production of the testosterone metabolite dihydrotestosterone (DHT). In the absence of testosterone and DHT, secondary male sexual characteristics will not develop.

Congenital idiopathic hypogonadotropic hypogonadism affects an estimated 1 in 10,000 people and is more common in males then females. In Kallmann syndrome, magnetic resonance imaging would reveal a lesion. In addition, an impaired ability to smell (anosmia) accompanies the idiopathic hypogonadic hypogonadism in Kallmann syndrome.

Treatment involves maintenance of normal testosterone production. This can be achieved by treatment with long-acting testosterone ester given intramuscularly every 2 weeks until virilization is achieved or by pulsatile injection of GnRH to stimulate pituitary FSH and LH secretion. The pulsatile injection is necessary because the steady infusion of GnRH causes downregulation of the receptors in the pituitary and a consequent diminished responsiveness to the releasing hormone. Dietary support is necessary to allow the normal growth of muscle mass and bone characteristic of puberty.

FURTHER   READING

Text Sources
Carroll RG: Elsevier's Integrated Physiology. Philadelphia, Elsevier, Philadelphia, 2007.
Copstead L, Banasik J: Pathophysiology, 3rd ed. Philadelphia, Saunders, 2005.

Guyton AC, Hall JE: Textbook of Medical Physiology, 11th ed. Philadelphia, Saunders, 2006.
McPhee SJ, Papadakis MA, Tierney LM Jr: Current Medical Diagnosis and Treatment, 46th ed. New York, McGraw-Hill, 2007.

A 1-year-old boy is referred to a surgeon because of bilateral absence of testes within the scrotum.

The absence of the testes was noted at birth and has persisted through the first year of life. All other developmental aspects are normal.

PHYSICAL EXAMINATION

VS: T 37°C, P 90/min, R 22/min, BP 88/40 mm Hg
PE: Scrotal sack is empty to palpation.

LABORATORY STUDIES

Ultrasonography: Testes are located within the inguinal canal.

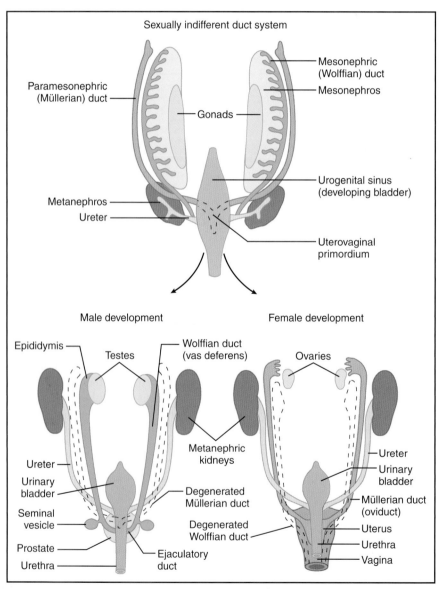

FIGURE 86–1 Both male and female genitalia are present early in fetal development. The development of the testes in the male genitalia is driven by the testis-determining factor on the short arm of the Y chromosome. Differentiation of the fetal gonad to the testis allows production of testosterone and the anti-müllerian hormone, leading to development of the male phenotype.

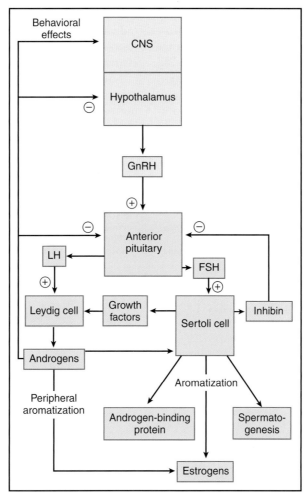

FIGURE 86–2   The anterior pituitary stimulates endocrine secretions of the testis. LH from the anterior pituitary stimulates androgen production by the testicular Leydig cells, with androgens providing a negative feedback inhibition at the level of both hypothalamus and anterior pituitary. FSH stimulates Sertoli cell secretions, including the hormone inhibin, which provides a negative feedback signal diminishing FSH released by the anterior pituitary. –, Negative feedback; + positive feedback.

DIAGNOSIS

Cryptorchidism

PATHOPHYSIOLOGY OF KEY SYMPTOMS

Early during fetal development, both male and female genitalia are present (Fig. 86-1). The development of the testes and the male external genitalia is stimulated by the testis-determining factor on the short arm of the Y chromosome. The developing testes secrete testosterone and anti-müllerian hormone. Testosterone stimulates the growth of the male external genitalia,

and the anti-müllerian hormone causes a regression of the female reproductive structures.

During the third trimester of male development in utero, the testes normally descend through the inguinal canal into the scrotum. By the first year of age, about 1% of male infants exhibit cryptorchidism, in which the testes are located in an extrascrotal position.

Temperatures within the scrotum are 1° to 2°C cooler than abdominal temperature. This lower temperature facilitates the development and maturation of spermatogonia. Males with cryptorchidism retain the testes in the body core, where they are exposed to normal abdominal temperature. Consequently, men who were born with undescended testes have diminished sperm counts.

Leydig cell and Sertoli cell function are not impaired at testicular temperatures of 37°C. In utero, pituitary luteinizing hormone stimulates Leydig cells to produce androgens such as testosterone (Fig. 86-2). Androgens stimulate the growth of the male secondary sexual characteristics. In addition, pituitary follicle-stimulating hormone and androgens both stimulate the growth and maturation of the Sertoli cells. Because the higher testicular temperature does not inhibit the production of testicular hormones, individuals with cryptorchidism continue to produce testosterone and can develop male secondary sexual characteristics.

Surgical correction of cryptorchidism usually occurs during the first year of life and may help restore normal spermatogenesis. If not, the tubules can become fibrotic, leading to a permanent impairment of spermatogenesis and subsequent infertility.

FURTHER READING

Text Sources

Carroll RG: Elsevier's Integrated Physiology. Philadelphia, Elsevier, 2007.

Copstead L, Banasik J: Pathophysiology, 3rd ed. Philadelphia, Saunders, 2005.

Guyton AC, Hall JE: Textbook of Medical Physiology, 11th ed. Philadelphia, Saunders, 2006.

McPhee SJ, Papadakis MA, Tierney LM Jr: Current Medical Diagnosis and Treatment, 46th ed. New York, McGraw-Hill, 2007.

A 65-year-old man comes to the clinic complaining of difficulty in urinating.

The patient states that over the past month he has had to get out of bed three to five times a night to urinate. He complains that his bladder is not completely empty during voiding. The patient states that he finds himself "stopping and starting again several times while urinating." He also complains of finding it difficult to postpone urination. The patient also describes his urinary stream as "weak." He states that he had two urinary tract infections within the last 3 months.

PHYSICAL EXAMINATION

VS: T 37°C, P 72/min, R 18/min, BP 128/80 mm Hg, BMI 28

PE: Examination of lower abdomen shows a distended bladder but no pain on palpation. Digital rectal examination reveals a smooth, firm and elastic enlargement of the prostate, with no induration.

LABORATORY STUDIES

Urinalysis: Negative for hematuria and negative for urinary tract infection

Prostate specific antigen (PSA): Normal

DIAGNOSIS

Benign prostatic hyperplasia

PATHOPHYSIOLOGY OF KEY SYMPTOMS

Urine produced by the kidneys is transported through the ureter and stored in the bladder before elimination from the body. During the micturition reflex, contraction of the detrusor muscle of the bladder wall increases pressure in the bladder. This, along with the relaxation of the internal and external sphincter, allows urine to exit the body through the urethra.

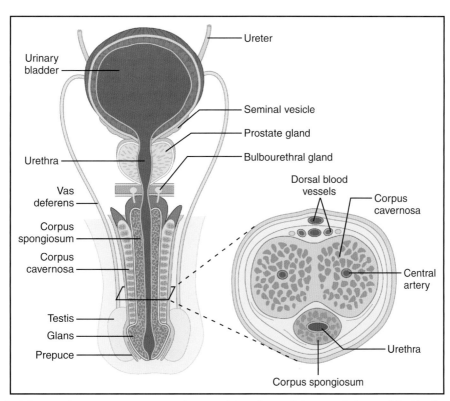

FIGURE 87–1 The paired corpora cavernosa provide most of the volume of the penis. Dilation of the blood vessels supplying the corpora cavernosa allows them to become engorged with blood, causing the penis to become erect and rigid.

In males, the urethra passes through the center of the prostate gland before entering the penis (Fig. 87-1). Enlargement of the prostate gland can cause external compression of the ureter and impair micturition. The patient's symptoms—difficulty in urination, bladder distention, weak urinary stream, and urinary frequency—result from obstruction of the ureter and impaired emptying of the bladder.

Benign prostatic hyperplasia (BPH) is a nonmalignant enlargement of the prostate gland, which continues to grow throughout life. Consequently, the incidence of BPH increases with age. Clinical symptoms of bladder outlet obstruction occur in 75% of men older than 80 years of age. BPH results in a symmetrical growth of the prostate gland, in contrast to the asymmetrical enlargement of the prostate gland characteristic of prostatic cancer. Enlargement of the prostate gland can be identified during digital rectal examination. The normal level of prostate-specific antigen is consistent with the absence of prostate cancer.

Development and maturation of the prostate gland is a secondary male sexual characteristic controlled by the testosterone metabolite dihydrotestosterone (DHT). Testosterone is converted into DHT by the cellular enzyme 5α-reductase. Intracellular conversion of testosterone into DHT in the target tissues is necessary for the development of many of the male secondary sexual characteristics.

OUTCOME

Treatment of BPH is based on suppression of androgen production, blockade of the conversion of androgens into DHT, or blockade of the cellular androgen receptor. Finasteride inhibits the isoform of 5α-reductase that is found in the prostate. Reducing the size of an enlarged prostate, however, requires weeks or months.

The prostate gland also has a significant amount of smooth muscle cells. Contraction of these smooth muscle cells is mediated by α_1-adrenergic receptors. Consequently, α_1-adrenergic receptor blockade can cause a more immediate relief of urethral obstruction.

FURTHER READING

Text Sources

Carroll RG: Elsevier's Integrated Physiology. Philadelphia, Elsevier, 2007.

Copstead L, Banasik J: Pathophysiology, 3rd ed. Philadelphia, Saunders, 2005.

Guyton AC, Hall JE: Textbook of Medical Physiology, 11th ed. Philadelphia, Saunders, 2006.

McPhee SJ, Papadakis MA, Tierney LM Jr: Current Medical Diagnosis and Treatment, 46th ed. New York, McGraw-Hill, 2007.

Wein AJ, Kavoussi LR, Novick AC, et al: Campbell-Walsh Urology Review Manual, Philadelphia, Saunders Elsevier, 2007.

A 60-year-old man visits his primary care physician complaining of an inability to have sex with his wife.

The patient reports an inability to achieve erections in at least 75% of intercourse attempts over the past 6 months and a complete absence of nocturnal erections.

He has a 3-year history of hypertension, which has been controlled by a calcium channel blocker. In addition, the patient has mild hyperlipidemia, which is controlled with dietary modification. He has a 1-year history of chest pain with moderate physical exertion and is being treated with aspirin and nitroglycerin. He is a social drinker and smokes one pack of cigarettes per day.

PHYSICAL EXAMINATION

VS: T 37°C, P 86/min, R 22/min, BP 130/90 mm Hg, BMI 33
PE: Patient is obese and leads a sedentary lifestyle. Physical examination does not reveal any other abnormalities.

LABORATORY STUDIES

Cholesterol: 250 mg/dL (normal: < 200 mg/dL)
Triglycerides: 180 mg/dL (normal: 35-160 mg/dL)

DIAGNOSIS

Erectile dysfunction

PATHOPHYSIOLOGY OF KEY SYMPTOMS

The male erection response is due to the engorgement of blood vessels in the corpus cavernosa (see Fig. 87-1). These vascular changes require the interplay of the vascular endothelial cells, sympathetic and parasympathetic nervous system, the central nervous system, and a permissive role played by the endocrine system. Disorders in any of these systems can result in erectile dysfunction, defined as "an inability to achieve and maintain an erection sufficient for satisfactory sexual performance."

The penis is normally in a flaccid state, in which sympathetic nervous system tone constricts the smooth muscle of the penile erectile tissue, limiting blood flow into the corpus cavernosa. Endothelin and prostaglandins produced in the vascular wall augment the arteriolar vasoconstriction.

Appropriate psychologic or tactile stimulation causes an increase in parasympathetic activity and a withdrawal of sympathetic tone. The neurally

mediated vasodilation causes blood to become trapped in the corpus cavernosa, leading to an erection.

The erectile response is initiated by an increase in parasympathetic nerve activity working through the NANC (nonadrenergic, noncholinergic) neurotransmitters, predominantly nitric oxide (NO) and vasoactive intestinal peptide (VIP). An increase in the activity of the NANC nerves dilates the vascular smooth muscle and causes an increase in blood flow. The increase in blood flow creates a shear stress on the vascular endothelium, stimulating NO production by the endothelial cells. It is the endothelial NO that mediates the maintenance of an erection (Fig. 88-1).

At the cellular level, nitric oxide acts on smooth muscle to increase the production of cyclic guanosine

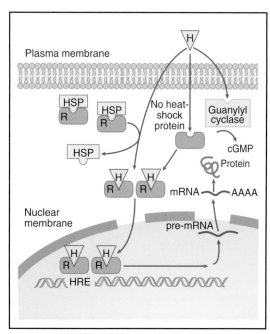

FIGURE 88–1 Lipophilic signaling molecules (H) bind to intracellular receptors (R). About half of the steroid receptors are coupled to heat-shock proteins (HSPs), which dissociate when the steroid binds the receptor. Nitric oxide binds to soluble guanylyl cyclase, generating cGMP and, from that point, follow the normal G protein–coupled second messenger pathway.

monophosphate (GMP) and activates protein kinase G (PKG). PKG acts to reduce calcium release from the sarcoplasmic reticulum and interacts directly with the myosin to diminish crossbridge attachment and cycling.

Testosterone and other trophic hormones play a permissive role in the erectile response. Testosterone is responsible for the development and the maintenance of male secondary sexual characteristics, including growth of penile tissue. Insufficient production of testosterone can lead to erectile dysfunction.

OUTCOME

Treatment of erectile dysfunction is based on augmenting the processes involved in the normal erectile response. One approach is to diminish vasoconstriction of the penile vasculature. This is accomplished through use of endothelin receptor blockers. Alternatively, sympathetic nervous system responses can be diminished by drugs that act in the central nervous system or drugs that act directly to block the α_1-adrenergic receptors in the corpus cavernosa.

A more common approach is to augment the vasodilation mediated by NO. Normally, NO has a very short half-life because cyclic GMP is rapidly degraded by phosphodiesterases. Sildenafil inhibits predominantly phosphodiesterase-5, the isoform found in the corpus cavernosa. Blockade of cyclic GMP degradation results in an enhanced vasodilation response to NO.

Sildenafil will potentiate the action of all NO effects and enhance the biologic half-life of NO. Consequently, using nitroglycerin may cause a marked peripheral vasodilation and drop in blood pressure. In addition, sildenafil has a small crossover to the type 6 phosphodiesterase found in rods and cones of the retina.

FURTHER READING

Text Sources
Carroll RG: Elsevier's Integrated Physiology. Philadelphia, Elsevier, 2007.

Copstead L, Banasik J: Pathophysiology, 3rd ed. Philadelphia, Saunders, 2005.

Guyton AC, Hall JE: Textbook of Medical Physiology, 11th ed. Philadelphia, Saunders, 2006.

McPhee SJ, Papadakis MA, Tierney LM Jr: Current Medical Diagnosis and Treatment, 46th ed. New York, McGraw-Hill, 2007.

Wein AJ, Kavoussi LR, Novick AC, et al: Campbell-Walsh Urology Review Manual, Philadelphia, Saunders Elsevier, 2007.

Practice Questions and Answers

Richard H. Ray*

PRACTICE QUESTIONS

These practice questions were designed to assess your understanding and ability to apply the medical physiology concepts illustrated by the cases in this book. The questions are framed in patient vignettes and use the disease process to illustrate the underlying mechanisms of symptom development and treatment options. Importantly, interpretation of diagnostic data is a hallmark of the question format, so the question stems are detailed and rich in information. There are two questions related to each case, and each question addresses a different aspect of the associated case. All questions are written in a "single best answer" format, with the number of options determined in part by the number of reasonable options for the question.

DIRECTIONS: Select the ONE letter answer that is the BEST response to each question.

Questions 1-2 are linked to Case 1:

A 42-year-old man comes to his primary care physician complaining of awkwardness when running or walking. The weakness began in his right leg 4 months ago, and now the left leg is beginning to show signs of weakness.

1. Neuromuscular examination reveals a positive Babinski sign on the right foot but not the left foot. The most likely explanation for the positive Babinski sign is:

    A. Death of the upper motor neurons of the motor cortex of the left hemisphere

    B. Death of the upper motor neurons of the motor cortex of the right hemisphere

    C. Impaired nerve transmission along the axons originating in the left motor cortex

    D. Impaired nerve transmission along the axons originating in the right motor cortex

    E. Death of the lower motor neurons of the spinal cord ventral horn

2. During testing of the right leg for the patellar tendon stretch reflex, what finding would be consistent with a diagnosis of an upper motor neuron defect?

    A. Spastic contraction

    B. Hyporeflexia

    C. Normal reflexes

    D. Diminished reflexes

    E. Flaccid paralysis

Questions 3-4 are linked to Case 2:

A 54-year-old woman returns to her oncologist for continuing treatment of recurrent ovarian cancer. It is now 2 days since treatment, and she is now complaining of paresthesia of the hands and feet and difficulty in fastening buttons due to muscle weakness in the hands. She began treatment for recurrent ovarian cancer 2 months ago, a treatment regimen of paclitaxel, 150 mg/m^2; gemcitabine, 800 mg/m^2; and cisplatin, 75 mg/m^2 three times weekly for six cycles.

3. Complete evaluation of the neuromuscular junction of this patient would reveal what electrical changes?

    A. Docking and fusion of the acetylcholine vesicles will be impaired.

    B. Amplitude of miniature end plate potentials would be diminished.

    C. The number of the acetylcholine receptors on the postsynaptic membrane would be increased.

    D. The number of acetylcholine receptors on the postsynaptic membrane would be decreased.

    E. The amplitude of the end plate potential would be diminished.

*Professor of Physiology, Brody School of Medicine, East Carolina University

4. Histologic study of the presynaptic nerve terminal would reveal what vesicular change?

A. The number of acetylcholine vesicles would be increased.

B. The number of acetylcholine vesicles would be decreased.

C. The amount of acetylcholine per vesicle would be increased.

D. The amount of acetylcholine per vesicle would be decreased.

E. Acetylcholine vesicles would be completely absent from most presynaptic nerve terminals.

Questions 5-6 are linked to Case 3:

A 35-year-old woman comes to her primary care physician complaining of difficulty in walking. On questioning, the patient indicates she had trouble walking for 5 days last month and also that she has experienced pain and prickly sensations that come and go, as well as occasional muscle weakness.

5. For each motor unit, how would the strength of the muscles innervated by the alpha-motor neuron be affected?

A. 10% of the muscle fibers in a motor unit would function normally and 90% abnormally.

B. 25% of the muscle fibers in the motor unit would function normally and 75% abnormally.

C. 50% of the muscle fibers in the motor unit would function normally and 50% abnormally.

D. 75% of muscle fibers in the motor unit would function normally and 25% abnormally.

E. 100% of the muscle fibers in a motor unit would function abnormally.

6. An MRI indicated Gd-enhancing brain lesions, as well as one infratentorium lesion and three periventricular lesions in the brain. Analysis of cerebrospinal fluid showed an oligoclonal IgG band. During the initial stages of this disease, how would the velocity of action potential transmission be altered within the central nervous system?

A. Myelinated axons would show a decreased conduction velocity, and unmyelinated axons would show a decreased conduction velocity.

B. Myelinated axons would show a decreased conduction velocity, and unmyelinated axons would show an increased conduction velocity.

C. Myelinated axons would show an increased conduction velocity, and unmyelinated axons would show a decreased conduction velocity.

D. Myelinated axons would show an increased conduction velocity, and unmyelinated axons would show an increased conduction velocity.

E. Myelinated axons would show a decreased conduction velocity, and unmyelinated axons would show no change in conduction velocity.

Questions 7-8 are linked to Case 4:

A 48-year-old man comes to the emergency department complaining of trouble seeing, and he has difficulty swallowing. Symptoms began 3 hours ago and are increasing in severity.

7. The patient is visiting friends who live on a commune and indicates that approximately 24 hours earlier he ate some green beans that were canned at the commune. Symptoms began 3 hours ago, and the decision to come to the emergency department was made because of his difficulty in swallowing. The patient is now anxious and easily excited. Physical examination reveals double vision and drooping of the eyelids. The patient is slurring his speech and has difficulty swallowing. Physical examination shows signs of muscle weakness. Study of the neuromuscular junction would show what abnormality?

A. Docking and fusion of the acetylcholine vesicles will be impaired.

B. Amplitude of miniature end plate potentials would be diminished.

C. The number of the acetylcholine receptors on the postsynaptic membrane would be increased.

D. The number of acetylcholine receptors on the postsynaptic membrane would be decreased.

E. The amplitude of the end plate potential would be diminished.

8. Stool sample tests positive for *Clostridium botulinum*. If the infection is left untreated, recovery of muscle function will likely occur within:

A. One hour

B. Four to 6 hours

C. 24 to 48 hours

D. Three to 5 days

E. Three to 5 weeks

Questions 9-10 are linked to Case 5:

A 65-year-old man comes to his primary care physician complaining of a decreasing ability to read that is more pronounced in the evening. Reading difficulty was due to a combination of diplopia and blurred vision.

9. The patient has a 15-year history of hypertension that is being managed with diuretics and a low-salt diet. He began using bifocals for reading about 10 years ago, and his current eyeglass prescription allows him to see comfortably. Edrophonium (Tensilon) test was positive. Plasma testing revealed the presence of antibodies directed against the acetylcholine receptor (normal < 0.03 mmol/L). After administering edrophonium, neuromuscular transmission recovers because of increased:

    A. Release of acetylcholine for the presynaptic terminal

    B. Concentration of acetylcholine in the synaptic cleft

    C. Binding affinity of the nicotinic receptor for acetylcholine

    D. Numbers of nicotinic receptors

    E. Calcium release following binding of acetylcholine to the nicotinic receptor

10. Plasma testing revealed the presence of antibodies directed against the acetylcholine receptor. In this patient, following a normal synaptic release of acetylcholine, the end plate potential on the postsynaptic membrane will be:

    A. Completely eliminated

    B. Diminished

    C. Normal

    D. Slightly enhanced

    E. Greatly enhanced

Questions 11-12 are linked to Case 6:

A 3-year-old boy is brought to the clinic for physical examination. His mother reports that the child has difficulty in walking and he appears clumsy compared with other boys of the same age.

11. The patient learned to stand and walk about 8 months after the three boys in his play group, who

are the same age. Both parents appear normal, and there is no known family history of musculoskeletal problems. The mother was adopted and does not know the medical history of her family of origin. Muscle biopsy confirmed the diagnosis of Duchenne muscular dystrophy, and the mother was a carrier of the gene. If the couple has another child, the chance of the child also developing Duchenne muscular dystrophy is:

    A. 50% for both boys and girls

    B. 50% for boys and 0% for girls

    C. 100% for boys and 0% for girls

    D. 100% for boys and 50% for girls

    E. 0% for boys and 0% for girls

12. Muscle coordination is low for this boy's age. Muscles are weak, and grip strength is weak. Plasma analysis showed elevated creatine kinase level, and muscle biopsy confirmed the diagnosis of Duchenne muscular dystrophy. The abnormal protein in this child normally serves what function?

    A. Connecting actin to myosin

    B. Connecting actin to titin

    C. Connecting myosin to titin

    D. Connecting titin to the cytoskeleton

    E. Connecting the cytoskeleton to the extracellular matrix

Questions 13-14 are linked to Case 7:

A 31-year-old man arrived by ambulance at the emergency department after an industrial accident that cut the femoral artery, causing the loss of 1.5 L of blood. Bleeding was controlled by direct pressure, and the patient received 2 L of 0.9% saline during transport. The patient is pale, diaphoretic, and anxious. Vital signs: BP 80/60 mm Hg, P 120/min and weak, R 22/min and shallow, T 35.5°C.

13. Which of the following changes in this patient is contributing to the narrowed arterial pulse pressure?

	Stroke Volume	Heart Rate	Total Peripheral Resistance
A.	Increased	Increased	Increased
B	Increased	Increased	Decreased
C	Increased	Decreased	Increased
D.	Increased	Decreased	Decreased
E.	Decreased	Increased	Increased

14. Fluid resuscitation will result in what changes in blood composition?

	Plasma Proteins	Plasma Cl⁻	Hematocrit
A.	Increased	Increased	Increased
B.	Decreased	Increased	Decreased
C.	Increased	Decreased	Increased
D.	Increased	Decreased	Decreased
E.	Decreased	Increased	Increased

Questions 15-16 are linked to Case 8:

A 68-year-old man comes to his primary care physician complaining of tiredness and difficulty in sleeping. Six months earlier, the patient experienced myocardial infarction of the anterior wall of the left ventricle. A stent was placed in the occluded coronary artery, reestablishing perfusion. The patient now complains of difficulty sleeping at night, awakening with shortness of breath.

15. Vital signs: T 37°C, P 80/min, R 18/min and shallow, BP 100/70 mm Hg, BMI 29. Physical examination: A third heart sound is evident. Auscultation reveals crackles at the base of the lung, and there is dullness to percussion at the base of the lung. The low arterial blood pressure is likely due to diminished:

    A. Preload
    B. Afterload
    C. Contractility
    D. Heart rate
    E. Total peripheral resistance

16. The patient reports that he is able to sleep better using pillows to elevate his chest and head. The shortness of breath is primarily due to diminished:

    A. Alveolar ventilation
    B. Blood oxygen transport capability
    C. Pulmonary blood flow
    D. Oxygen uptake across the alveolar-capillary barrier
    E. Tidal volume

Questions 17-18 are linked to Case 9:

A 45-year-old man comes to the emergency department complaining of sharp, stabbing chest pain beneath the sternum. Jugular veins are distended and enlarged during inspiration (Kussmaul sign). Imaging confirms the existence of a pericardial tamponade. Blood pressure is 105/55 mm Hg during expiration and 90/40 mm Hg during inspiration (pulsus paradoxus).

17. The patient is anxious, and cognitive abilities are slightly impaired. All heart sounds are muffled. A pericardial rub can be heard on the lower left sternal border. The drop in blood pressure during inspiration is caused by:

    A. Stretching of the pericardium by the negative intrathoracic pressure
    B. Increased venous return from the negative intrathoracic pressure
    C. Decreased ventricular filling from the negative intrathoracic pressure
    D. Increased pulmonary vascular resistance during inspiration
    E. Decreased pericardial fluid pressure during inspiration

18. Pulse is 85/min, and respiration rate is 22/min and shallow. Pericardiocentesis was performed under echocardiographic guidance. 300 mL of fluid was removed, relieving the symptoms. The patient was admitted to the hospital for treatment and observation. The major cardiovascular benefit of the pericardiocentesis was an increase in:

    A. Preload
    B. Afterload
    C. Contractility
    D. Heart rate
    E. Total peripheral resistance

Questions 19-20 are linked to Case 10:

A 58-year-old woman comes to her primary care physician complaining of shortness of breath and difficulty sleeping at night, especially while lying down. She complains of coughing at night that awakens her. The patient first reports having symptoms 3 days ago. The symptoms do not appear to be worsening. The patient has a systolic murmur that is heard best at the apex of the heart. The intensity of the murmur is constant throughout systole. The patient has rales during inspiration bilaterally in the base of the lung. There is no sign of peripheral edema.

19. Vital signs: T 37°C, P 80/min, R 15/min, BP 100/70 mm Hg, BMI 24. The valvular abnormality that most likely accounts for the murmur is:

    A. Tricuspid stenosis
    B. Tricuspid regurgitation
    C. Pulmonic stenosis

D. Pulmonic regurgitation

E. Mitral regurgitation

20. What cardiac or vascular region would be expected to have a change in dimension visible on imaging?

A. Vena cava enlargement

B. Right atrial enlargement

C. Right ventricular enlargement

D. Left atrial enlargement

E. Left ventricular enlargement

Questions 21-22 are linked to Case 11:

A 4-day-old female infant is seen by the cardiologist, having been referred because of suspicion of a patent ductus arteriosus. The infant was delivered by cesarean section at 32 weeks' gestational age because of preeclampsia in the mother. APGAR score was 7 at 1 minute and improved to 9 at 5 minutes. The pediatrician noted a machine-like murmur extending through both systole and diastole.

21. Vital signs: P 115/min, R 35/min, BP 65/35 mm Hg. Physical examination: The infant still exhibits the systolic and diastolic murmur but otherwise appears healthy. Cyanosis is not present. What region of the circulation would be expected to show an abnormal oxygen content?

A. Decreased oxygen content in the right atrium

B. Decreased oxygen content in the right ventricle

C. Increased oxygen content in the pulmonary artery

D. Increased oxygen content in the left ventricle

E. Decreased oxygen content in the aorta

22. The infant's Doppler echocardiogram reveals a continuous flow of blood from the aorta into the pulmonary artery through the ductus arteriosus. Treatment with indomethacin, a drug that blocks prostaglandin synthesis, will cause:

A. A reduction of the murmur and a reduction in the arterial P_{O_2}

B. A reduction of the murmur and no change in the arterial P_{O_2}

C. A reduction of the murmur and an increase in the arterial P_{O_2}

D. No change in the murmur and a reduction in the arterial P_{O_2}

E. No change in the murmur and no change in the arterial P_{O_2}

Questions 23-24 are linked to Case 12:

A 73-year-old man comes to the emergency department complaining of chest pain, shortness of breath on exertion, and syncope. The patient has poorly managed hypercholesterolemia and a 10-year history of hypertension. A systolic murmur is present, loudest over the aorta and peaking at mid systole. Palpitation of the carotid upstroke reveals a pulse that is both decreased and late relative to the apical impulse. Palpation of the chest reveals an apical impulse that is laterally displaced. Lungs are clear and there are no rales. The left atrium and left ventricle chambers are enlarged, and left ventricular hypertrophy is present.

23. Vital signs: T 37°C, P 85/min, R 18/min, BP 100/75 mm Hg. ECG: left axis deviation but no abnormalities in the ST segment. Chest radiograph: enlarged left ventricle and calcification of the aortic valve. Doppler ultrasonography: a greatly increased velocity of flow during the systolic portion of the cardiac cycle. Compared with an individual with a ventricular mean electrical axis of 90 degrees, this patient will have what change in the QRS complexes of the ECG?

A. QRS complexes will be smaller in lead aVF and larger in lead II.

B. QRS complexes will be smaller in lead aVL and larger in lead II.

C. QRS complexes will be smaller in lead aVR and larger in lead II.

D. QRS complexes will be larger in lead aVF and larger in lead I.

E. QRS complexes will be larger in lead aVL and larger in lead I.

24. Compared with normal, what valve will show an increase in the pressure gradient during the cardiac cycle?

A. Aortic valve during systole

B. Aortic valve during diastole

C. Mitral valve during systole

D. Mitral valve during diastole

E. Pulmonic valve during systole

Questions 25-26 are linked to Case 13:

A 22-year-old female college student comes to the university clinic complaining of palpitations. The patient has had occasional incidences of rapid heart rates but never lasting for more than 2 minutes. In this instance, the heart rate has been elevated for 15 minutes.

25. ECG shows ventricular tachycardia, characterized by narrow QRS complexes at a rate of 180/min. Atrial P waves are also present at a rate of 180/min, but the QRS complexes precede the P wave. What other abnormality of the P wave would be expected?

    A. P wave and QRS complex would have negative deflection in lead aVR.

    B. P wave and QRS complex would have negative deflection in lead II.

    C. P wave and QRS complex would have negative deflection in lead aVF.

    D. P wave would have a negative deflection and QRS complex a positive deflection in lead aVR.

    E. P wave would have a negative deflection and QRS complex a positive deflection in lead II.

26. The patient has only been sleeping 4 hours a night while studying for examinations and is consuming "more than the usual amount" of coffee to help her remain alert. ECG shows ventricular tachycardia, characterized by narrow QRS complexes at a rate of 180/min. Carotid sinus massage causes pulse rate to abruptly decrease to 80 beats/min. This effect is due to activation of:

    A. Parasympathetic nerves supplying the sinoatrial node

    B. Parasympathetic nerves supplying the atrioventricular node

    C. Sympathetic nerves supplying the sinoatrial node

    D. Sympathetic nerves supplying the atrioventricular node

    E. Sympathetic nerves supplying the ventricular muscle

Questions 27-28 are linked to Case 14:

A 45-year-old man presents at the clinic after having a reading of an elevated blood pressure at a health department screening. His blood pressure is 160/110 mm Hg and is equal in both arms and legs.

27. The patient's blood pressure has been consistently elevated (in the same range) for the last four times it was checked. If nitric oxide were used to acutely change blood pressure to 140/100 mm Hg, what would be the baroreceptor-mediated change in autonomic nervous system activity?

    A. Increased sympathetic nervous system activity and increased parasympathetic nervous system activity

    B. Increased sympathetic nervous system activity and no change in parasympathetic nervous system activity

    C. Increased sympathetic nervous system activity and decreased parasympathetic nervous system activity

    D. Decreased sympathetic nervous system activity and increased parasympathetic nervous system activity

    E. Decreased sympathetic nervous system activity and no change in parasympathetic nervous system activity

28. The patient indicates that he is too busy to exercise. There is a family history of heart disease but no family history of diabetes. Compared with the period before he developed hypertension, what change is there now in cardiac output and total peripheral resistance?

    A. Cardiac output is increased and total peripheral resistance is increased.

    B. Cardiac output is increased and total peripheral resistance is not changed.

    C. Cardiac output is increased and total peripheral resistance is decreased.

    D. Cardiac output is not changed and total peripheral resistance is increased.

    E. Cardiac output is not changed and total peripheral resistance is not changed.

Questions 29-30 are linked to Case 15:

A 66-year-old woman presents to the emergency department complaining of shortness of breath and chest pain that extends to her neck. The patient is pale and diaphoretic. She is immediately treated with morphine, nitroglycerin, and aspirin and placed on supplemental oxygen.

29. The patient's pulse oxymetry shows O_2 saturations of 98%. She had been taking captopril, an angiotensin I converting enzyme (ACE) inhibitor to control her blood pressure. She ran out of captopril 2 weeks ago and has not refilled the prescription. Vital signs: P 108/min, R 23/min, BP 135/105 mm Hg. Which of the vital signs indicates that the patient is at risk for myocardial ischemia?

    A. Elevated diastolic blood pressure

    B. Elevated heart rate

    C. Elevated systolic blood pressure

    D. Elevated respiratory rate

    E. Decreased pulse pressure

30. The patient's pulse oxymetry shows O_2 saturations of 98% and arterial P_{O_2} is 300 mm Hg. The expected P_{O_2} of a sample of blood from the coronary venous sinus would be:

A. 10

B. 40

C. 60

D. 100

E. 260

Questions 31-32 are linked to Case 16:

A 67-year-old man presents to his physician complaining of sharp cramps and pains in his legs while exercising. The cramping is occurring in the calf area and occurs at any exercise intensity greater than walking at a moderate pace. He states that the pain is relieved by rest but begins again when he begins to exercise again.

31. Segmental blood pressure readings show a marked decrease in blood pressure when measured at the calf. What combination of vascular flow and resistances characterizes the cramping period?

    A. Low blood flow, precapillary sphincters dilated

    B. Low blood flow, precapillary sphincters constricted

    C. Adequate blood flow, precapillary sphincters dilated

    D. Adequate blood flow, precapillary sphincters constricted

32. Contrast angiography revealed widespread arterial calcifications in the arteries below the knee. The vascular consequences of the calcifications are:

    A. Diminished vascular resistance in the region

    B. Increased sympathetic tone to the region

    C. Decreased velocity of flow through the stenosis

    D. Decreased volume of flow through the stenosis

    E. Decreased pressure gradient across the stenosis

Questions 33-34 are linked to Case 17:

A 60-year-old woman being treated for hypertension returns to her physician's office for treatment. Renal artery ultrasound now indicates that the size of the left kidney is decreased; there is an increase in blood flow velocity at the left proximal renal artery and a decreased blood flow through the left renal artery. Renal arteriography confirmed the presence of the stenosis on the left renal artery.

33. Past radiologic studies identified cholelithiasis, which was treated by laparoscopic surgery. Radiologic

findings at that time include an abnormal finding of an asymmetric left kidney. The progression of the hypertension would be the same if the stenosis was located on the:

A. Aorta above the origin of both renal arteries

B. Aorta between the origin of the left and right renal artery

C. Aorta beneath the origin of both renal arteries

D. Right renal vein

E. Left renal vein

34. During physical examination, the aorta is palpated superior to the navel. The patient has abnormalities of the optic fundi showing hypertensive retinopathy. The patient has been treated in the past for hypertension and is currently experiencing intolerance to her angiotensin I converting enzyme (ACE) inhibitor. Abdominal ultrasound ruled out an abdominal aortic aneurysm. Compared with the right kidney, the left kidney will have an increased:

A. Glomerular capillary pressure

B. Glomerular filtration rate

C. Rate of renin secretion

D. Rate of urine formation

E. Rate of sodium excretion

Questions 35-36 are linked to Case 18:

A 40-year-old man comes to his primary care physician complaining of blurred vision and a headache. The patient does not remember urinating during the past day and is unable to provide a urine sample for analysis.

35. The patient has a 6-year history of hypertension and hyperlipidemia. The hypertension has been poorly controlled because of noncompliance. Blood pressure is 210/150 mm Hg. A presystolic murmur (fourth heart sound) is evident. Funduscopic examination shows swelling of the optic nerve in both eyes (papilledema). The headache and blurred vision are likely due to:

A. Cerebral edema caused by the elevated blood pressure

B. Hyperlipidemia causing fatty plaques

C. Increased creatinine because of the low rate of urine production

D. Metabolic acidosis caused by the renal failure

E. Hyponatremia caused by the renal failure

36. The patient's blood pressure is 210/150 mm Hg and is the same in all four extremities. He is anxious and complains of an inability to concentrate because of the headaches. Laboratory test results are as follows:

SMA-12: BUN 160 mg/dL (normal: 7-20 mg/dL)

Creatinine 8.2 mg/dL (normal: 0.8 to 1.4 mg/dL)

Blood gas analysis: P_{O_2} 90 mm Hg, P_{CO_2} 33 mm Hg, HCO_3^- 12 mEq, pH 7.30

Plasma renin activity: 25 ng/mL/hr (normal: 1.9 to 3.7 ng/mL/hr)

ECG: normal sinus rhythm, left-axis deviation, no shift in ST segment

Cardiac enzymes (myosin, CK-MB): normal

The abnormal laboratory result that is only indirectly related to renal failure is:

A. Creatinine

B. Blood urea nitrogen

C. P_{CO_2}

D. HCO_3^-

E. Renin

Questions 37-38 are linked to Case 19:

A 45-year-old man comes to the emergency department complaining of severe pain on his right flank. The patient describes the colicky pain that has a sudden onset. There is no evidence of injury. The patient has been working in the yard all day and appears dehydrated. He is capable of providing a small volume of urine for analysis. Urine pH is 4.3, and osmolality is 1200 mOsm/L.

37. The high urine osmolarity as a consequence of:

A. Hypertension

B. Hypotension

C. Dehydration

D. Pain

E. Sodium depletion

38. Abnormal findings include microscopic hematuria (red blood cells) and small calcium oxalate crystals (kidney stones). The kidney stones appearing in the urine likely originated in the:

A. Collecting duct

B. Ureter

C. Bladder

D. Urethra

E. Renal calyx

Questions 39-40 are linked to Case 20:

A 5-year-old boy presents to the urgent care clinic because his mother noticed that the child is not going to the bathroom and the child's feet are swollen. Two weeks ago, the child was treated for strep throat with penicillin. The mother admits to ceasing administering the medication to the child after a couple of days because she thought the child was better. The patient is oliguric and has a slight fluid accumulation in the lower extremities and periorbital region. There is palpable peripheral edema in both feet.

Urinalysis: significant findings include very dark urine, presence of red blood cells, red blood cell casts, and protein (>3 g/day)

Serum complement C3, C4, CH50 levels: Low

ASO titer: 250 Todd units/mL (normal: <160 units/mL)

Anti-DNase-B level: >60 units

BUN: 32 mg/dL (normal: 7-18 mg/dL)

Creatinine: 2.0 mg/dL (normal: 0.6-1.2 mg/dL)

39. The appearance of protein in the urine is indicative of damage to the:

A. Tubular epithelium

B. Glomerular endothelium

C. Basement membrane of the glomerulus

D. Ureter

E. Bladder

40. Vital signs: T 37°C, P 78/min, R 15/min, BP 120/90 mm Hg. In this patient, the peripheral edema is due to:

A. Increased arterial blood pressure

B. Increased capillary blood pressure

C. Increased capillary permeability

D. Decreased capillary albumin concentration

E. Lymphatic obstruction

Questions 41-42 are linked to Case 21:

A 42-year-old woman experiencing peripheral edema is referred to the nephrologist for evaluation of renal function. The patient was diagnosed with type 1 diabetes mellitus at the age of 12 and has been managing her blood glucose with three daily injections of insulin. Over the past 5 years, the blood glucose level has not been as well managed, and 2 years ago urinalysis showed microalbuminuria.

Plasma analysis:
Fasting glucose 180 mg/dL (normal: 60-110 mg/dL)
BUN: 32 mg/dL (normal: 7-18 mg/dL)
Creatinine: 2.0 mg/dL (normal: 0.6-1.2 mg/dL)
Plasma albumin: 1.5 g/dL (normal: 3.5-5 g/dL)
Glycosylated hemoglobin A1c (HbA1c) levels: 7.8 (normal: <6)
Urinalysis:
Glucose: +3 (normal: 0)
Albuminuria: 200 mg/24 hr (normal: 0)

41. The major action of insulin on the renal handling of glucose is to:

    A. Increased apical membrane glucose transporters in the proximal tubule

    B. Increased basolateral membrane glucose transporters in the proximal tubule

    C. Decreased glomerular capillary permeability to glucose

    D. Decreased glomerular filtration rate

    E. Decreased glomerular filtered load of glucose

42. A reduction of plasma glucose to normal values for 24 hours will result in a correction in which of the above abnormal values?

    A. Creatinine

    B. Plasma albumin

    C. Urinary glucose

    D. Urinary albumin

    E. Glycosylated hemoglobin A1c

Questions 43-44 are linked to Case 22:

A 70-year-old woman, admitted 3 days earlier to the cardiac care unit after angioplasty, has gone into renal failure. Serial imaging with a contrast agent indicates that one of the three vessels is again stenosing. The patient was diagnosed 5 years ago with non–insulin-dependent diabetes mellitus (type 2), which has been managed with diet and exercise. Plasma analysis shows elevations in blood urea nitrogen and creatinine, increasing progressively with each daily measurement and reaching 50% above normal by day 3. Urinalysis shows muddy brown epithelial cell casts and debris. Urine production is 300 mL/day (oliguria). Fractional excretion of sodium is 3%, and urine osmolarity is 200 mOsm/kg.

43. Abnormal renal epithelial tubular cell function is indicated by:

    A. Elevated blood urea nitrogen

    B. Elevated plasma creatinine

    C. Oliguria

    D. Fractional excretion of sodium of 3%

    E. Urine osmolarity of 200 mOsm/L

44. The tubular concentration of the contrast media could be reduced by:

    A. Enhancing proximal tubule reabsorption of a contrast agent

    B. Decreasing glomerular filtration rate

    C. Infusion of isotonic saline

    D. Decreasing renal perfusion pressure

    E. Decreasing plasma sodium concentration

Questions 45-46 are linked to Case 23:

A 38-year-old man presents to his primary care physician complaining of difficulty in voiding for the past 6 months. The patient was diagnosed with insulin-dependent diabetes mellitus at age 15. He has managed his diabetes with daily injections of insulin and has been able to achieve good plasma glucose control. Cystoscopy shows no obstruction, but cystometry showed a weak contraction of the detrusor muscle.

45. Impaired detrusor muscle contraction will impede micturition by:

    A. Increasing parasympathetic nerve activity

    B. Inhibiting the alpha-motor neuron to the external bladder sphincter

    C. Occluding the ureter

    D. Occluding the urethra

    E. Diminishing the tension on the bladder wall

46. Which of the following changes in bladder volume will most likely occur in this patient?

    A. Decreased postvoid residual volume

    B. Increased rate of filling from the ureters

    C. Increased pre-void volume

    D. Increased rate of emptying through the urethra

Questions 47-48 are linked to Case 24:

A 48-year-old woman in an inpatient psychiatric hospital complains of polyuria and polydipsia. The patient was admitted to the hospital 1 year ago and was diagnosed with bipolar affective disorder. Lithium has been used successfully for the past year to control the psychiatric problems.

Plasma analysis:
Sodium: 150 mEq/L (normal: 135 to 145 mEq/L)
Potassium: 4.8 mEq/L (normal: 3.5 to 5 mEq/L)
Chloride: 115 mEq/L (normal: 101 to 112 mEq/L)
pH: 7.48 (normal venous: 7.31 to 7.41)
Osmolality: 320 mOsm/kg (normal: 275 to 293 mOsm/kg)
Urinalysis:
Urine osmolality 200 mOsm/kg (normal: 100 to 900 mOsm/kg)
24-Hour sample: 4.8 L (normal: < 2 L/24 hr)

47. An individual with the plasma osmolarity of 320 mOsm/kg would be expected to have a urine osmolarity of:

    A. 50 mOsm/kg

    B. 150 mOsm/kg

    C. 320 mOsm/kg

    D. 900 mOsm/kg

    E. 1800 mOsm/kg

48. The patient appears dehydrated, and the plasma osmolality is 320 mOsm/kg (normal: 275 to 293 mOsm/kg). During a water deprivation test there was little increase in urine osmolarity after 6 hours. Desmopressin injection had little effect. Plasma and kidney tissue analysis would be expected to show:

    A. Increased levels of ADH and increased V2 receptor activity

    B. Increased levels of ADH and normal V2 receptor activity

    C. Increased levels of ADH and decreased V2 receptor activity

    D. Decreased levels of ADH and increased V2 receptor activity

    E. Decreased levels of ADH and normal V2 receptor activity

Questions 49-50 are linked to Case 25:

A 58-year-old man comes to the emergency department complaining of bleeding in his mouth. The patient has multiple small bleeding sites on the mucous membranes of the mouth and nose. The bleeding began 24 hours ago and has been continuous in spite of compression. The patient suffered a myocardial infarction 18 months earlier and since that time has stopped smoking, begun a moderate exercise program, and is on a low dose of warfarin (Coumadin) as a "blood thinner." One month ago he began taking herbal supplements containing garlic and ginkgo biloba extract. Hematocrit is 35% (normal males: 42%), and a stool sample tested positive for blood. Prothrombin time (PT) is 35 seconds (normal: 11-15 seconds) and partial thromboplastin time (PTT) is 48 seconds (normal: 26-35 seconds).

49. Plasma analysis should show a decrease in:

    A. Erythropoietin

    B. Thrombopoietin

    C. Plasminogen

    D. Thrombin

    E. Antithrombin 3

50. What aspect of hemostasis is still functioning normally?

    A. Intrinsic clotting pathway

    B. Extrinsic clotting pathway

    C. Platelet plug formation

    D. Thrombin formation

    E. Fibrin formation

Questions 51-52 are linked to Case 26:

A 3-year-old boy is brought to the pediatrician by his parents who have noted excessive bleeding around the knees and elbows. The parents have noted that the toddler bleeds very easily when the skin is scratched. Family history is significant for the presence of hemophilia in the mother's family. Physical examination reveals erythematic lesions, particularly around the knees and elbows and purpura on the elbows.

CBC:

Hemoglobin	10.9 g/dL (13.4-17.4 g/dL)
Hematocrit	32% (40%-54%)
Platelets	200,000/mm^3 (150,000-400,000/mm^3)

Coagulation studies:

Platelets	412 (150-440)
Prothrombin time	12.5 sec (11-15 sec)
APTT	42 sec (26.4-35 sec)

Bleeding time	6 minutes (2-8 minutes)
Factor VIII:C level	5% (25-100%)
vWF antigen	145% (71-210%)

51. The coagulation studies are consistent with a defect in:

    A. The intrinsic clotting pathway

    B. The extrinsic clotting pathway

    C. Platelet plug formation

    D. Plasminogen formation

    E. Heparin formation

52. The inheritance pattern for this disease is characterized as:

    A. Autosomal dominant

    B. Autosomal recessive

    C. X-linked dominant

    D. X-linked recessive

    E. Multifactorial

Questions 53-54 are linked to Case 27:

A 25-year-old woman comes to her primary care physician complaining of oral bleeding. The patient has been on low molecular weight heparin for the past 2 years after the diagnosis of pulmonary embolism. Physical examination shows purpura, petechiae, and hemorrhagic bullae in the mouth. A blood sample is positive for heparin-induced thrombocytopenia (HIT) antibody.

53. The patient should have a high level of:

    A. Erythropoietin

    B. Thrombopoietin

    C. Vasopressin

    D. Oxytocin

    E. Growth hormone

54. The antibody diminishes platelet plug formation by binding to antigens on the surface of the:

    A. Megakaryocytes

    B. Platelets

    C. Red blood cells

    D. Fibrin mesh

    E. Capillary endothelium

Questions 55-56 are linked to Case 28:

A 50-year-old man comes to his family physician complaining of fatigue. The patient indicates that climbing the stairs leaves him short of breath, and this has been progressively worse over the past month. He smokes, drinks 6 cups of coffee a day, and has two or three alcoholic drinks after work. The patient has been taking aspirin for the past 6 months for frequent stomach pain. He has cut down on his caloric intake for the past 3 months in an effort to lose weight, with moderate success. Upper and lower endoscopy reveals a bleeding gastric ulcer.

55. Vital signs: T 36°C, P 105/min, R 24/min, BP 90/75 mm Hg, BMI 33, hematocrit 28. A blood smear would show what kind of red blood cells?

    A. Normal

    B. Hypochromic and microcytic

    C. Macrocytic

    D. Sickled

    E. Hypochromic

56. Vital signs: T 36°C, P 105/min, R 24/min, BP 90/75 mm Hg, BMI 33. Hematocrit: 30%. Red blood cell smear shows microcytic hypochromic cells. Serum iron values: 27 µg/dL. Transferrin saturation: 13%. Serum ferritin: 20 µg/L. Stool is positive for occult blood. If the iron deficiency is corrected, what percentage of the red blood cells will be synthesized each day?

    A. 0.5%

    B. 1%

    C. 3%

    D. 5%

    E. 10%

Questions 57-58 are linked to Case 29:

A 58-year-old man is transported to the emergency department after being awakened by a crushing pain in his chest that radiated down to the left arm. The patient is immediately treated with morphine, nitroglycerin, and aspirin and placed on supplemental oxygen. Pulse oximetry shows O_2 saturations of 98%. The patient is pale and diaphoretic, is anxious, and continues to complain of pain that was only partially relieved by the morphine.

57. The patient has a past history of hypertension that has been controlled with diuretics. A thrombus formed in the left anterior descending coronary artery can embolize and become trapped in:

    A. The main coronary artery

    B. The coronary vein

C. A distal section of the left anterior descending coronary artery

D. The proximal section of the left anterior descending coronary artery

E. The pulmonary circulation

58. Vital signs: T 36°C, P 118/min, R 28/min, BP 85/70 mm Hg, BMI 33.

ECG: Wide Q wave in leads I and aVL, ST segment elevation in leads I, aVL and V_{2-5}.

Blood test (CBC, chem panel, cardiac markers): elevated troponin I, elevated troponin T and normal CK-MB

Lipid panel: Total cholesterol high, HDL low, LDL high

What agent will allow rapid restoration of blood flow to the ischemic area?

A. Nitroglycerin

B. Tissue plasminogen activator

C. Heparin

D. Protamine

E. Dicumarol

Questions 59-60 are linked to Case 30:

A 55-year-old man comes to the clinic complaining of fatigue and persistent shortness of breath, which becomes worse during exercise. He has a history of respiratory infections and has a chronic cough that is worse in the morning. The patient has smoked cigarettes since he was a teenager; currently he estimates smoking one pack of cigarettes a day. He is in mild respiratory distress, with an elevated respiratory rate and shallow breaths. An end-expiratory wheeze is heard on auscultation.

59. Pulmonary function test: FEV_1 was 70% of predicted and peak expiratory flow was 60% of predicted. Forced vital capacity was 90% of predicted. The breathing pattern and the pulmonary function tests are consistent with:

A. An obstructive disease process only

B. A restrictive disease process only

C. A combined obstructive and restrictive disease

D. Emphysema

E. Chronic bronchitis

60. This patient's chest radiograph is normal and arterial blood gases are Po_2 75 mm Hg, Pco_2 42 mm Hg, and pH 7.32. In this patient, ventilation is being stimulated by afferent inputs from what structures?

A. Aortic arch chemoreceptors only

B. Carotid body chemoreceptors only

C. Central chemoreceptors only

D. Aortic arch and carotid body chemoreceptors but not central chemoreceptors

E. Aortic arch and central chemoreceptors but not carotid body chemoreceptors

Questions 61-62 are linked to Case 31:

A 29-year-old man is transported by the rescue squad to the emergency department in acute respiratory distress after being stabbed in the left lateral chest. Air can be heard entering the thorax through the stab wound during inspiration, and bubbles form at the stab wound during exhalation.

61. The patient has a 3-cm puncture wound on the left lateral chest between the third and fourth rib. He is conscious, is able to speak, and complains of chest pains associated with each breath and has difficulty breathing. At the end of inspiration, what is the pressure in the left intrapleural space?

A. −8 mm Hg

B. −6 mm Hg

C. 0 mm Hg

D. 6 mm Hg

E. 8 mm Hg

62. Air movement was minimized by placing a compression bandage at the site of injury before transport. Pulse oximetry shows 85% oxygen saturation. The hemodynamic event contributing to the low oxygen saturation is the:

A. Low perfusion of the left lung

B. Low perfusion of the right lung

C. Enhanced perfusion of the left lung

D. Enhanced perfusion of the right lung

E. Low cardiac output

Questions 63-64 are linked to Case 32:

A 10-year-old boy is brought to the emergency department because of difficulty breathing that developed during soccer practice. The boy has a history of allergies, including pollen, but never previously showed this level of respiratory difficulty. He now complains of tightness in the chest. Vital signs: T 37°C, P 120/min, R 30/min and shallow, BP 110/95 mm Hg. The patient is wheezing, anxious, and short of breath. The wheezing is more prominent on exhalation, and there is an extended forced expiratory phase.

63. Forced spirometry taken at this time would show:

    A. Increased vital capacity

    B. Increased peak expiratory flow

    C. Decreased FEV_1/FVC ratio

    D. Decreased tidal volume

    E. Decreased total lung capacity

64. During testing 1 week later, spirometry showed normal values. When challenged with methacholine, spirometry now showed decreased FEV_1, decreased FVC, and increased residual volume. Forced spirometry flow-volume loop showed scooping and diminished peak flow. The action of methacholine was to:

    A. Constrict the large airways

    B. Dilate the large airways

    C. Constrict the mid-sized airways

    D. Dilate the mid-sized airways

    E. Constrict the terminal bronchioles

Questions 65-66 are linked to Case 33:

A 38-year-old man is transported to the emergency department after being found unconscious and in respiratory depression in an apartment.

65. The patient was intubated and manually ventilated and transported to the emergency department. On arrival, an arterial blood sample is obtained for blood gas analysis and for drug screen. Findings showed Po_2 60 mm Hg, Pco_2 80 mm Hg, HCO_3^- 26 mEq/L, and pH 7.22. The acid-base disturbance is:

    A. Compensated metabolic acidosis

    B. Acute metabolic acidosis

    C. Compensated respiratory acidosis

    D. Acute respiratory acidosis

    E. Compensated metabolic alkalosis

66. On arriving at the emergency department, the patient is placed on a ventilator with supplemental oxygen. The patient is in a coma and does not respond to painful stimuli. Pupils are small and reactive. Muscle tone is flaccid, and the deep tendon reflexes are depressed. There is a positive Babinski sign. Drug screen is positive for short-acting barbiturate. The respiratory depression in this patient is due to diminished activity in the:

    A. Cerebral motor cortex

    B. Limbic system

    C. Autonomic nervous system

    D. Brain stem

    E. Reticular activating system

Questions 67-68 are linked to Case 34:

A 62-year-old man comes to the clinic at a ski resort on a mountain peak (14,000 ft, barometric pressure 420 mm Hg) complaining of dyspnea, headache, dizziness, and inability to sleep. He was short of breath while climbing the stairs at the lodge and noticed that he was breathing rapidly even when sitting down.

67. The patient arrived at the resort yesterday from a sea-level town and reports no current health issues or medications. End-tidal gas analysis will show:

    A. Increased CO_2 and increased O_2

    B. Increased CO_2 and decreased O_2

    C. Decreased CO_2 and increased O_2

    D. Decreased CO_2 and decreased O_2

68. The arterial blood gas abnormality contributing to the headache is:

    A. Increased O_2

    B. Decreased O_2

    C. Increased CO_2

    D. Decreased CO_2

    E. Increased HCO_3^-

Questions 69-70 are linked to Case 35:

A 68-year-old man comes to the clinic complaining of difficulty breathing. The patient suffered a myocardial infarction involving the anterior wall of the left ventricle 6 months earlier. The patient indicates that he has difficulty sleeping when lying down, which has been getting worse over the past month.

69. Inspiratory crackles are present, particularly at the base of the lungs. Chest radiograph: blurry fluid buildup in the lung space appearing in a typical "butterfly" shape. The primary cause for the difficulty breathing is:

    A. Increased pulmonary artery pressure

    B. Decreased pulmonary artery pressure

    C. Increased pulmonary capillary pressure

    D. Decreased pulmonary capillary pressure

    E. Increased alveolar pressure

70. Vital signs: T 37°C, P 80/min, R 26/min and shallow, BP 100/65 mm Hg. Inspiratory crackles are present, particularly at the base of the lungs. Chest radiograph shows a blurry fluid buildup in the lung space appearing in a typical "butterfly" shape. The primary gas exchange defect is:

    A. Impaired oxygen exchange because of the low oxygen gradient between the alveoli and the pulmonary capillaries

    B. Impaired oxygen exchange because of the low solubility of oxygen in interstitial fluid

    C. Impaired oxygen exchange because of the decreased distance between the alveolar air and the capillary

    D. Impaired carbon dioxide exchange because of the decrease in surface area

    E. Impaired carbon dioxide exchange because of the low CO_2 gradient between the alveoli and the pulmonary capillaries

Questions 71-72 are linked to Case 36:

A 28-year-old man is brought to the emergency department complaining of headache, vertigo, dizziness, and confusion. It is a cold winter evening. The patient lives alone in a rural area and was using a kerosene heater to heat his house. He was found by a neighbor walking outside the house without a jacket. There was an odor of kerosene and some smoke in the house.

71. Vital signs: T 35°C, P 90/min, R 22/min, BP 120/90 mm Hg. The patient remains confused and complains of chest pain and weakness. Carboxyhemoglobin level is 40%. Increasing alveolar minute ventilation will have the greatest effect on:

    A. Arterial P_{O_2}

    B. Mixed venous P_{O_2}

    C. Arterial P_{CO_2}

    D. Mixed venous P_{CO_2}

    E. Arterial blood O_2 content

72. Vital signs: T 35°C, P 90/min, R 22/min, BP 120/90 mm Hg. The patient remains confused and complains of chest pain and weakness.
    Arterial blood gases: Po2 of 95 mm Hg, Pco2 of 40 mm Hg, pH 7.4
    Mixed venous blood gases: P_{O_2} 22 mm Hg, P_{CO_2} of 43 mm Hg, and pH of 7.37
    Carboxyhemoglobin level: 40%
    Hematocrit: 42%

The decrease in mixed venous blood oxygen values is due to:

    A. Enhanced tissue uptake of oxygen

    B. Decreased arterial P_{O_2} levels

    C. Diminished cardiac output

    D. Decreased hematocrit

    E. Decreased arterial blood oxygen content

Questions 73-74 are linked to Case 37:

A 57-year-old man comes to the cardiovascular rehab clinic to begin an exercise program after a myocardial infarction.

73. The patient is able to walk at a brisk pace for 20 minutes. In contrast, jogging or climbing stairs causes him to become short of breath. Vital signs: T 37°C, P 80/min, R 17/min, BP 130/90 mm Hg, BMI 33. There are some crackles heard at the base of both lungs on inspiration. The increase in ventilation that occurs while walking at a brisk pace is due to stimulation of the brain stem ventilatory centers by:

    A. Decreased arterial P_{O_2}

    B. Increased arterial P_{CO_2}

    C. Decreased arterial pH

    D. Descending stimulation from higher brain centers

    E. Decreased central nervous system P_{O_2}

74. The patient begins a cardiovascular stress test on a treadmill during which the speed and inclination of the treadmill are increased every 10 minutes. Heart rate is monitored through an electrocardiogram, arterial oxygen saturation is monitored through a pulse oximeter, and blood pressure is taken at regular intervals. At low exercise intensity, arterial pressure increases to 140/85 mm Hg, heart rate increases to 120/min, and respiratory rate increased to 30/min. Pulse oximetry decreased to 95%. After 10 minutes, an increase in exercise intensity causes little change in arterial pressure but pulse oximetry fell to 91%. The decrease in pulse oximetry is due to:

    A. Low arterial blood pressure

    B. Low cardiac output

    C. Inadequate alveolar ventilation

    D. Impaired oxygen diffusion

    E. Diminished blood oxygen-carrying capacity

Questions 75-76 are linked to Case 38:

A 17-year-old boy is brought to the emergency department by his coworkers because of "abnormal behavior." The patient is working for the summer in a plastics factory. He has been working there for 1 month, but today he appeared confused, sleepy, and complained of dizziness and headaches. Vital signs: T 37°C, P 120/min, R 30/min and shallow, BP 100/90 mm Hg. The skin appears unusually pink. Retinal arteries and veins both appear pink. Patient's mental status is confused and lethargic. Patient appears weak from a loss of muscle strength. A bitter almond smell is detected on the patient's breath.

75. The pigmentation changes are primarily due to:

    A. Increased arterial P_{O_2}

    B. Increased arterial P_{CO_2}

    C. Increased venous P_{O_2}

    D. Increased venous P_{CO_2}

    E. Increased arterial lactate concentration

76. Arterial blood gases: P_{O_2} 105 mm Hg, P_{CO_2} 18 mm Hg, pH 7.32, wide anion gap

    Pulse oxymetry: 98%

    Mixed venous blood gases: P_{O_2} 60 mm Hg, P_{CO_2} 20 mm Hg, pH 7.30

    Plasma lactate concentration: 18 mmol/L (elevated)

    Plasma analysis shows cyanide.

    The impaired ability of the carotid body to utilize oxygen is indicated by what vital sign?

    A. Increased respiratory rate

    B. Increased heart rate

    C. Decreased systolic arterial pressure

    D. Decreased diastolic arterial pressure

    E. Decreased temperature

Questions 77-78 are linked to Case 39:

A 66-year-old woman is brought into the clinic by her husband when she began to complain of severe chest pain, which was exacerbated with inspiration.

77. The patient states that she began feeling pain in her chest and thought she was having a heart attack. She states that the pain was increased when she inhaled. The patient feels like she can't breathe and complains that her heart won't stop racing. Prior medical history reveals that she had been treated for clots in her legs 6 months ago. The patient states that she got better and stopped taking the warfarin she was prescribed because she didn't like the way it made her feel. She admits to having bouts of calf pain over the last few weeks but thought it was a result of her recent attempts to improve her health by taking evening walks. Spiral CT is positive for medium-sized pulmonary embolism. The chest pain is likely due to a clot that initially formed in a/the:

    A. Peripheral vein

    B. Vena cava

    C. Pulmonary artery

    D. Pulmonary vein

    E. Coronary artery

78. The patient shows dyspnea with intermittent bouts of coughing. Grimacing is evident on inspiration with a guarding action of holding her chest. Auscultation of the lungs reveals significant rales. There is localized wheezing and a pleural friction rub. Spiral CT is positive for medium-sized pulmonary embolism. The ventilation/perfusion mismatch is characterized as:

    A. Anatomic dead space

    B. Physiologic dead space

    C. Intrapulmonary shunt

    D. Extrapulmonary shunt

    E. Hypoxic pulmonary vasoconstriction

Questions 79-80 are linked to Case 40:

A 24-year-old man presents to his primary care physician complaining of fever and chills that have persisted for 1 week. During this time, he has had an unproductive cough and shortness of breath when he exerts himself. His chest now hurts when he coughs, and the sputum has a greenish yellow tint. There are altered breath sounds and rales in the upper right lobe, noted during chest auscultation. The upper right lobe is also dull to percussion. An increase in fremitus is evident.

79. In contrast to the lower lobes, the upper lobes of the lung are often the site of infection because of high:

    A. Ventilation

    B. Perfusion

    C. Alveolar P_{O_2}

    D. Alveolar P_{CO_2}

    E. Diffusion capability

80. The patient has a general feeling of malaise and has noticed a decrease in appetite. He has been using an over-the-counter cold medicine for symptom relief, but symptoms return when the medication wears off. Vital signs: T 40°C, P 90/min, R 25/min, BP 112/70 mm Hg. Physical appearance includes a pale sunken face. Breathing pattern is rapid and shallow, with some dyspnea during deep breaths. The breathing pattern is characteristic of:

    A. Obstructive lung disease

    B. Restrictive lung disease

    C. Mixed venous hypoxia

    D. Mixed venous hypercapnia

    E. Diffusion limitation

Questions 81-82 are linked to Case 41:

A 19-year-old male college student is transported to the emergency department by ambulance after hitting his head in a fall from a balcony. Witnesses indicate that he landed on his head and shoulder and immediately lost consciousness. The paramedics found the student not breathing and unresponsive to verbal commands.

81. The abnormal respiration is indicative of damage to what region of the brain?

    A. Thalamus

    B. Hypothalamus

    C. Cortex

    D. Pons

    E. Medulla oblongata

82. The patient was intubated and ventilated. His head and neck were immobilized and he was transported to the emergency department. Vital signs: T 34°C, P 15/min, R 10/min, BP 60/30 mm Hg. The patient is unresponsive and in decerebrate posture, with adduction and flexion of the arms, wrists pronated and fingers flexed, and legs and feet extended. Pupils are fixed and dilated bilaterally. Glasgow Coma Scale score: 3 (severe) (normal: 15). Radiograph of head and cervical spine shows a compression fracture of the skull overlying the temporal lobe. The altered pupil reflex is consistent with damage to what region of the brain?

    A. Thalamus

    B. Hypothalamus

    C. Motor cortex

    D. Sensory cortex

    E. Medulla oblongata

Questions 83-84 are linked to Case 42:

A 27-year-old man is brought to the emergency department after having been involved in a motor vehicle collision. The patient does not wear prescriptive lenses nor does he have a history of visual problems.

83. A tumor located in the lateral geniculate body of the left thalamus would produce a visual field defect:

    A. Limited to the left eye

    B. Limited to the left visual field of both eyes

    C. Impacting peripheral vision bilaterally

    D. Impacting central vision bilaterally

    E. Limited to the right visual field of both eyes

84. The patient is currently taking topiramate (Topamax) for migraines and eszopiclone (Lunesta) for insomnia brought on because of stress. Vital signs: T 37°C, P 90/min, R 28/min, BP 135/85 mm Hg. Physical examination indicates no apparent head trauma from the collision. Reflexes were normal. Goldmann field examination shows that central vision is intact but peripheral vision is missing bilaterally. CT reveals an intracranial tumor located near the optic chiasm. A tumor located more rostrally along the left eye optic nerve would have a visual field defect:

    A. Limited to the left eye

    B. Limited to the left visual field

    C. Impacting peripheral vision bilaterally

    D. Impacting central vision bilaterally

    E. Limited to the right eye

Questions 85-86 are linked to Case 43:

An 8-year-old boy is brought by his parents to the pediatrician because of an increasing pattern of clumsiness and headaches. The parents have noted that the child is having difficulty in grabbing or picking up objects, such as crayons, with his right hand. His ability to draw lines is greatly diminished. The child's teacher first brought this to the parents' attention 3 weeks ago, and it has been getting progressively worse. An intention tremor is present when moving the right hand to pick up an object. There is no tremor at rest, and moving the left hand to pick up an object does not generate an intention tremor.

85. Diagnostic testing should focus on what regions of the cerebellum?

    A. Flocculonodular lobe

    B. Vestibulocerebellum

C. Midline portions of the right vermis

D. Midline portions of the left vermis

E. Intermediate zone of right hemisphere

86. During the past 4 days, the child has been complaining of headaches. The child has been properly immunized and has reached all developmental milestones. Vital signs: T 37°C, P 85/min, R 20/min, BP 95/80 mm Hg. Some swelling of the optic nerve is observed by funduscope, with no visual disturbances. Muscle strength is not diminished. Romberg test is negative. MRI shows a laterally located cyst at the junction of the vermis and hemisphere of the posterior lobe of the right cerebellum. As the cyst expands and impacts the flocculonodular lobe, additional symptoms will appear related to:

A. Balance

B. Fine motor skills

C. Gross motor skills

D. Planning motor activities

E. Evaluating proprioceptive input

Questions 87-88 are linked to Case 44:

A 68-year-old man comes to the physician's office complaining of trembling in his hands and difficulty walking. Neurologic examination shows the patient has a resting tremor of the left hand that diminishes when performing a task. During passive movement of the left arm, the muscles are rigid, causing "cogwheel" motion during stretching. The patient's facial expressions are reduced. When walking, the patient has difficulty taking the first step but then is able to walk smoothly with a shuffling gait.

87. These symptoms are consistent with damage to the:

A. Striatum

B. Substantia nigra

C. Thalamus

D. Globus pallidus

E. Subthalamic nucleus

88. MRI is normal. Symptomatic relief may be obtained by drugs that help restore levels of what neurotransmitter?

A. GABA

B. Acetylcholine

C. Norepinephrine

D. Glutamate

E. Dopamine

Questions 89-90 are linked to Case 45:

A 19-year-old college student comes to student health services complaining of a sporadic loss of memory. The periods of amnesia occur while he is awake and occasionally in class. During those times, his classmates report that he begins smacking his lips and fumbling around, disrupting the class. When confronted by his teacher, he has no recollection of those events and is confused and disoriented. He rests for about 30 minutes and then feels fine. The student did suffer a head injury while playing sports 6 months earlier but does not indicate any cognitive defects. Vital signs: T 37°C, P 76/min, R 18/min, BP 118/76 mm Hg.

89. An electroencephalogram (EEG) would be useful to detect:

A. Areas of ischemia

B. Areas of depressed brain function

C. Synchronized firing of groups of neurons

D. Epilepsy during the time in between seizures

E. Action potentials in individual neurons

90. The patient is evaluated for epilepsy. The EEG tracing indicates waves of moderate amplitude and frequency of 8 to 13 waves per second. This tracing is indicative of:

A. Slow wave sleep

B. Rapid eye movement sleep

C. Emotional stress

D. Calm consciousness

E. Alert consciousness

Questions 91-92 are linked to Case 46:

A 74-year-old woman is brought to her physician's office by her daughter, who complains that her mother is behaving oddly. The woman lives in a house in a small town and has lived alone for the 5 years since her husband died. She admits to forgetting about food while its cooking on the stove but says it is because she is so busy. She can remember events 20 years ago but has difficulty recalling recent events. She has begun to call her grandchildren by her children's names.

91. These memories are typically transferred to long-term storage in neurons of the:

A. Cerebellum

B. Basal ganglia

C. Amygdala

D. Medial temporal lobe

E. Prefrontal lobe

92. The patient is healthy and is not on any current medications. Vital signs: T 37°C, P 72/min, R 15/min, BP 118/65 mm Hg, BMI 22. Physical examination shows no significant findings. CT reveals significant atrophy of the parietal, temporal, and frontal lobes of the cerebral cortex and degeneration of the cingulate gyrus. Histologic examination of the brain would likely show:

A. Focal necrosis

B. Lewy bodies

C. Amyloid-beta plaques

D. Mitochondrial swelling

E. Demyelination

Questions 93-94 are linked to Case 47:

A 53-year-old man is brought to the emergency department by ambulance because of difficulty speaking. The patient tried to explain to his wife that something was wrong but was unable to speak clearly. He is, however, able to communicate in writing on a limited basis.

93. A CT scan will likely show damage to what region of the brain?

A. Broca's area of the left hemisphere

B. Broca's area of the right hemisphere

C. Wernicke's area of the left hemisphere

D. Wernicke's area the right hemisphere

E. Purkinje area of the left hemisphere

94. The patient has been on β blockers to control hypertension and has type 2 diabetes that is being managed with diet and exercise. Vital signs: T 36.5°C, P 85/min, R 18/min, BP 134/88 mm Hg, BMI 31. The patient is anxious but able to respond to spoken commands. CT shows an occlusion in the left hemisphere of a branch of the anterior main division of the middle cerebral artery supplying the frontal cortex. The area of damage can be minimized by prompt treatment with:

A. Heparin

B. Warfarin (Coumadin)

C. Tissue plasminogen activator

D. Anti-thrombin III

E. Protamine

Questions 95-96 are linked to Case 48:

A 50-year-old man comes to the physician's office complaining of a persistent and disabling sense that he is spinning even while he is sitting still. The sensation has become progressively worse since it was first noted about 5 months ago. He has stopped social drinking, but with no sign of improvement. He also indicates his left ear is problematic, with mild ear pain, a gradual decrease in hearing, and often a constant ringing (tinnitus).

95. These symptoms are associated with modalities transmitted along which cranial nerve?

A. VI

B. VII

C. VIII

D. IX

E. X

96. Vital signs: T 37°C, P 72/min, R 15/min, BP 126/80 mm Hg. The patient appears confused and has a mild slurred speech. During the examination, the patient exhibits a positive Romberg test and ataxia, along with vertical nystagmus. The nystagmus is indicative of damage to:

A. Cranial nerve I

B. Cranial nerve II

C. Cranial nerve III

D. Cranial nerve IV

E. The vestibular apparatus

Questions 97-98 are linked to Case 49:

A 37-year-old man comes to the physician's office complaining of chronic pain in the upper and middle back, headaches, muscle weakness in the hands, and loss of sensitivity to hot and cold temperature.

97. A defect limited to one side of the spinal cord anterior lateral pathways would cause:

A. Ipsilateral loss of temperature sensation below the site of the lesion

B. Contralateral loss of temperature sensation below the side of the lesion

C. Bilateral loss of temperature sensation above the side of the lesion

D. Ipsilateral loss of temperature sensation above the side of the lesion

E. Contralateral loss of temperature sensation above the side of the lesion

98. Radiography of the skull and cervical spine shows thoracic scoliosis and osteoporosis. MRI reveals focal cord enlargement due to an intramedullary neoplasm. Obstruction of the spinal cord canal can cause what combination of CSF pressure changes?

Above the Tumor	Below the Tumor
A. Increase	Increase
B. Increase	Decrease
C. Decrease	Increase
D. Decrease	Decrease

Questions 99-100 are linked to Case 50:

A 45-year-old man comes to his physician complaining of a drooping eyelid and facial twitching on the left side of his face. He first noticed the symptoms about 6 hours ago, but they have continued to worsen. He is now having trouble tasting and is drooling from the left corner of his mouth. The patient has extreme left-sided facial weakness and paralysis. He is unable to blink his left eye.

99. The altered sensory and motor modalities are transmitted along:

    A. Cranial nerve I

    B. Cranial nerve II

    C. Cranial nerve V

    D. Cranial nerve IV

    E. Cranial nerve VII

100. The patient has not had any neurologic problems in the past, although he did have the flu 3 weeks ago. Vital signs: T 38.2°C, P 80/min, R 18/min, BP 120/76 mm Hg. Output from what region of the motor cortex is no longer reaching the facial muscles?

    A. Medial portions of the left hemisphere motor cortex

    B. Lateral portions of the left hemisphere motor cortex

    C. Medial portions of the right hemisphere motor cortex

    D. Lateral portions of the right hemisphere motor cortex

Questions 101-102 are linked to Case 51:

A 22-year-old woman presents to the university health clinic complaining of weakness, tingling, and intense pain in her right hand. The tingling and numbness is particularly intense on the palmar thumb side, upper right hand, and wrist. The pain is increasing in intensity and is now waking her at night. She describes the pain as a burning sensation, which can be diminished by moderate movement and stretching of the wrist.

101. This pain modality is transmitted along:

    A. Large myelinated axons

    B. Small myelinated axons

    C. Unmyelinated axons

102. The patient appears healthy and is not in acute distress. Vital signs: T 37°C, P 66/min, R 15/min, BP 118/76 mm Hg. There is pain when assessing range of motion of the right wrist.

    Bilateral hand x-rays: Negative for fracture or arthritis

    Phalen's maneuver: Positive (symptoms reappear)

    Tinel's test: Positive (symptoms radiate along the medial nerve)

    The patient's symptoms are caused by:

    A. Degeneration of the median nerve

    B. Compression of the median nerve

    C. Hypersensitivity within the spinal cord

    D. Hypersensitivity within the thalamus

    E. Hypersensitivity of the pain receptors

Questions 103-104 are linked to Case 52:

An 80-year-old woman is brought to her primary care physician by her adult daughter because she is losing weight and unable to keep food down. During the past several months, the patient has lost weight and has had difficulty in swallowing both solid and liquid food. She frequently regurgitates undigested food both during the day and at night while sleeping.

103. Esophageal manometry is ordered to assess the pressure changes that occur during peristalsis. In a normal individual, how will balloon dilation of the esophagus change the tone of the smooth muscle on the oral (toward the mouth) and aboral (toward the stomach) portions of the esophagus?

    A. Contraction of the smooth muscle oral to the balloon and contraction of the smooth muscle aboral to the dilation

    B. Contraction of the smooth muscle oral to the balloon and relaxation of the smooth muscle aboral to the dilation

C. Relaxation of the smooth muscle oral to the balloon and contraction of the smooth muscle aboral to the dilation

D. Relaxation of the smooth muscle oral to the balloon and relaxation of the smooth muscle aboral to the dilation

104. Chest radiograph shows an air-fluid interface in an enlarged, fluid-filled esophagus. Endoscopy results were normal with no sign of distal stricture or carcinoma. Esophageal manometry confirms complete absence of peristalsis in the lower third of the esophagus and elevated lower esophageal sphincter pressure with incomplete relaxation during swallowing. Application of a calcium channel blocker to the smooth muscle of the lower esophageal sphincter will cause:

A. Contraction and lower esophageal sphincter

B. No change in lower esophageal sphincter tone

C. Relaxation of the lower esophageal sphincter

D. Recovery of the peristaltic reflex

E. Inhibition of the peristaltic reflex

Questions 105-106 are linked to Case 53:

A 55-year-old man comes to the primary care physician complaining of burning abdominal pain that begins shortly after eating. The patient has experienced pain associated with eating for the past few months. In the past, the pain had been relieved by antacids but not by NSAIDs. The patient has smoked one pack of cigarettes a day for 40 years and drinks 4 cups of coffee daily.

105. The periods of pain are associated with an increased secretion from:

A. Gastric enterochromaffin-like cells

B. Gastric chief cells

C. Mucus neck cells

D. Pancreatic alpha cells

E. Pancreatic delta cells

106. The patient reports an 8-pound weight loss over the past 3 months without intentional diet or exercise. During the physical examination, the patient reports epigastric tenderness to deep palpation. Fecal analysis: positive for occult blood and positive fecal antigen assay for *Helicobacter pylori*. The most likely source of the occult blood is the:

A. Esophagus

B. Stomach

C. Ileum

D. Colon

E. Rectum

Questions 107-108 are linked to Case 54:

A 54-year-old man comes to the emergency department at 2 o'clock in the morning after being awakened by an intense left-sided chest pain radiating to his back. The patient spent the evening at a college reunion where he sampled several spicy dishes and consumed a moderate quantity of beer. His past medical history includes an appendectomy at age 18 and a cholecystectomy at age 34. Vital signs: T 36.4°C, P 80/min, R 18/min, BP 130/90 mm Hg. The abdomen is not tender, and he denies nausea or vomiting. The patient is anxious but is not pale or diaphoretic.

107. The severity of the symptoms related to the sphincter tone in this patient would be:

A. Increased after nitric oxide administration

B. Decreased after nitric oxide administration

C. Increased after acetylcholine administration

D. Decreased after acetylcholine administration

E. Increased after norepinephrine administration

108. Plasma analysis results were within normal limits. ECG showed a normal sinus rhythm. Cardiac enzymes, troponin, and CK-MB levels were normal. Endoscopy was normal. The pain is most directly associated with what change in luminal pH?

A. Increased pH of the esophagus

B. Increased pH of the stomach

C. Increased pH of the duodenum

D. Decreased pH of the esophagus

E. Decreased pH of the stomach

Questions 109-110 are linked to Case 55:

A 65-year-old woman comes to the clinic complaining of weakness and lethargy. The patient indicates that for the past 6 years she has had rheumatoid arthritis and the pain is managed by daily ingestion of an NSAID. During the past 6 months, she noted a decrease in stamina. Vital signs: T 36°C, P 80/min, R 18/min, BP 90/70 mm Hg, BMI 22. The patient is pale and thin. Physical examination is otherwise unremarkable.

   Blood analysis: Hematocrit 25%

Blood smear: Megaloblastic cells (MCV 120 fL) and hypersegmented neutrophils.

109. The deficient vitamin in this individual is normally absorbed in what section of the gastrointestinal tract?

    A. Stomach

    B. Duodenum

    C. Jejunum

    D. Ileum

    E. Colon

110. Serum Vitamin B_{12}: 90 pg/mL. Schilling test: Lack of absorption of vitamin B_{12}. This patient's symptoms are due to an impaired secretion of cells in the:

    A. Esophagus

    B. Stomach

    C. Ileum

    D. Colon

    E. Pancreas

Questions 111-112 are linked to Case 56:

111. A 38-year-old male patient comes to the emergency department complaining of an abrupt, severe epigastric pain and is evaluated for acute pancreatitis. Pancreatic proteases are secreted as inactive zymogens with the initial activation in the duodenum mediated by the enzyme:

    A. Trypsin

    B. Enterokinase

    C. Carboxypeptidase

    D. Amylase

    E. Lipase

112. A 38-year-old male patient comes to the emergency department complaining of an abrupt, severe epigastric pain after an afternoon drinking binge. He describes his pain as radiating to his back, and he feels nauseated. The patient recently vomited and is sweating profusely. Vital signs: T 39°C, P 98/min, R 17/min, BP 95/70 mm Hg. The patient's pain worsens with walking and lying supine. His pain lessens if he sits up or leans forward. On palpation, his upper abdomen is tender, without guarding, rigidity, or rebound. His abdomen is distended. He exhibits overall weakness, pallor, and cool, clammy skin. The patient has mild jaundice as well. An elevation in serum lipase would confirm damage to what cell population?

    A. Salivary ducts

    B. Pancreatic acinar cells

    C. Gastric chief cells

    D. Hepatocytes

    E. Pancreatic islet beta cells

Questions 113-114 are linked to Case 57:

A 26-year-old woman presents with fatigue and loose "sawdust-like" bowel movements as often as three times per day. She also notes an occasional rash over her joints that is extremely itchy.

113. If the patient tests positive for a wheat allergy, the diarrhea would be classified as:

    A. Secretory

    B. Osmotic

    C. Hypermotility

    D. Reabsorptive

114. The patient delivered a full-term infant 9 months ago. Her symptoms began approximately 1 month post partum. The patient also has a family history of autoimmune disease. Vital signs: T 37°C, P 80/min, R 16/min, BP 90/60 mm Hg, BMI 17.

    Serologic antibody test is negative for anti-gliadin antibody and positive for anti-endomysial antibody. Upper endoscopy biopsy reveals shortening of the villi and crypt hyperplasia. Loss of the villi will result in:

    A. Impaired nutrient absorption

    B. Increased bile secretion

    C. Decreased sodium secretion

    D. Decreased water secretion

    E. Increased chyme osmolarity

Questions 115-116 are linked to Case 58:

A 38-year-old man comes to the clinic complaining of abdominal cramping and diarrhea. The patient has a 20-year history of alcohol abuse. He is complaining over the past 6 months of passing pale and malodorous stools that are difficult to flush. Vital signs: T 37°C, P 72/min, R 15/min, BP 120/80 mm Hg. The patient is malnourished, and his liver appears cirrhotic. There is jaundice of the sclera. Plasma analysis shows:

    Plasma K: 3.3 mEq/L (normal: 3.5-5.0 mEq/L)
    Serum calcium: 1.9 mEq/L (normal: 2.1-2.8 mEq/L)
    pH: 7.30 (normal: 7.35-7.45)

HCO_3^-: 18 mEq/L (normal: 22-28 mEq/L)
Serum triglyceride: 30 mg/dL (normal: 35-160 mg/dL)
Cholesterol: 130 mg/dL (normal: < 200 mg/dL).
Fecal analysis: Positive for fat

115. The patient's acid-base disturbance is characterized as:

    A. Respiratory acidosis

    B. Respiratory alkalosis

    C. Metabolic acidosis

    D. Metabolic alkalosis

116. Compared with a normal individual, during the postprandial period, this patient will show the most significant decrease in the amount of chylomicrons in the:

    A. Hepatic portal vein

    B. Intestinal lymphatics

    C. Hepatic vein

    D. Arteries

    E. Colonic lumen

Questions 117-118 are linked to Case 59:

A 46-year-old man comes to the clinic complaining of abdominal cramping and severe diarrhea that has persisted for 36 hours. The patient just returned from a camping trip in the mountains. Both of his companions are also experiencing severe diarrhea. The diarrhea initially had loose feces but now is composed mostly of watery stools. The patient indicates he has not eaten in the past 24 hours, but he has consumed 2 L of a sports drink (Gatorade). The patient does not report nausea or a history of fever.

117. Compared to the amount of fluid normally secreted into the intestinal lumen, the amount of the sports drink ingested is:

    A. Much less

    B. Approximately equal

    C. Much greater

118. Physical examination had no significant findings.

    Vital signs: T 37°C, P 105/min, R 15/min, BP 90/70 mm Hg, BMI 29

    Sodium: 141 mEq/L (normal: 136-145 mEq/L)

    Potassium: 3.4 mEq/L (normal: 3.5-5.0 mEq/L)

    Chloride: 105 mEq/L (normal: 95-105 mEq/L)

Fecal analysis is negative for the presence of leukocytes or blood but positive for the presence of enterotoxigenic *E. coli*. The decrease in plasma potassium is likely due to:

    A. Increased aldosterone release

    B. Cellular uptake of potassium

    C. Renal potassium excretion

    D. Intestinal loss of potassium

    E. Diminished potassium intake

Questions 119-120 are linked to Case 60:

A 56-year-old man comes to his family physician complaining of fecal incontinence. The patient had surgery 6 months previously to treat rectal hemorrhoids. The surgery was successful, but over the past 2 months the patient indicates difficulty in determining when he needs to have a bowel movement.

119. Normal defecation involves:

    A. Voluntary relaxation of the external anal sphincter

    B. Voluntary contraction of the external anal sphincter

    C. Voluntary relaxation of the internal anal sphincter

    D. Voluntary contraction of the internal anal sphincter

    E. Reverse peristalsis

120. Physical examination shows no apparent abnormalities. Digital examination of the rectum does not show any signs of rectal prolapse. Vital signs: T 37°C, P 76/min, R 15/min, BP 130/90 mm Hg, BMI 27. Anal manometry shows a decreased tone in the internal anal sphincter but normal tone in the external anal sphincter. Proctosigmoidoscopy shows muscle damage to the internal anal sphincter. Anal electromyography will likely show damage to what nerve population?

    A. Sensory afferents

    B. Sympathetic efferents

    C. Parasympathetic afferents

    D. Sympathetic afferents

Questions 121-122 are linked to Case 61:

A 6-year-old boy is brought to the pediatrician by his mother, who indicates the child is not well. The patient is a generally healthy child who is up-to-date on all of his immunizations. Over the past few weeks his mother has noticed that her son has been losing weight even though there is an increase in his thirst and appetite. The patient says that he doesn't feel well, is tired, and can't keep up with the other kids and that he has "to pee a lot." Physical examination shows slightly decreased skin turgor. Patient had until recently been at the 50th percentile for weight and height.

Vital signs: T 36.8 C, P 80/min, R 22/min, BP 104/76 mm Hg, weight 46 lb (21 kg, 30th percentile), height 48 in (122 cm, 50th percentile)

Urinalysis:
Color: light yellow (normal: colorless to dark yellow)
Specific gravity: 1.050 (normal:1.006 to 1.030)
pH: 4.5 (normal: 4.6-8.0, average 6.0)
Glucose: Positive (+1) (normal: negative)
RBCs: Negative (normal: negative)
Protein: Negative (normal: negative)
Ketones: Positive (normal: negative)
Leukocytes: Negative (normal: negative)

121. A blood test would likely show what change in insulin, glucose, and C peptide?

	Insulin	Glucose	C Peptide
A.	Increase	Increase	Increase
B.	Increase	Increase	Decrease
C.	Increase	Decrease	Increase
D.	Increase	Decrease	Decrease
E.	Decrease	Increase	Decrease

122. Blood tests (fasting):

Glucose: 250 mg/dL (normal: 64-128 mg/dL)

C peptide: 0.1 ng/mL (normal: 0.4-2.2 ng/mL)

The tissue that would show the greatest defect in glucose uptake is:

A. Small intestine

B. Liver

C. Brain

D. Skeletal muscle

E. Kidney

Questions 123-124 are linked to Case 62:

A 54-year-old unresponsive man is brought to the emergency department.

123. The patient is a known type 1 diabetic, and Accu-Chek indicates a glucose level of 36 mg/dL (normal: 64-128 mg/dL). In this patient, the hepatocyte handling of glucose is characterized by:

A. Increased hexokinase activity

B. Glycogenolysis

C. Gluconeogenesis

D. Lipolysis

E. Suppressed glucose uptake

124. The patient is a business executive and was late for an important meeting. He was found unconscious on his office floor by his assistant, who confirmed that the patient was breathing and then dialed 911. The ambulance crew arrived and provided supportive care, including initiating an intravenous line of lactated Ringers during transport to the local emergency department. Vital signs: T 36.9°C, P 110/min, R 28/min, BP 90/70 mm Hg, BMI 31. Physical examination shows no apparent trauma. The patient is responsive to deep painful stimuli only. Glucose (Accu-Chek): 36 mg/dL (normal: 64-128 mg/dL)

A blood test would likely show what concentration of insulin, glucose, and C peptide?

	Insulin	Glucose	C Peptide
A.	Increase	Increase	Increase
B.	Increase	Increase	Decrease
C.	Increase	Decrease	Increase
D.	Increase	Decrease	Decrease
E.	Decrease	Increase	Increase

Questions 125-126 are linked to Case 63:

A 30-year-old woman visits her primary care physician with concerns about a growth on her neck. She also complained about anxiety and irritability. She noticed a 6-pound loss of weight over the past 2 months despite an increase in her appetite. Patient also complains of feeling uncomfortable when in a warm room. Vital signs: T 38°C, P 110/min, R 18/min, BP 140/90 mm Hg, BMI 26.

125. The cellular mechanisms of action for the hormone that is elevated in this patient involves binding to a:

A. Cell membrane receptor and activating adenylate cyclase

B. Cell membrane receptor and activating guanylyl cyclase

C. Cell membrane receptor and activating a tyrosine kinase

D. Perinuclear receptor and altering DNA transcription

E. Cell membrane receptor and increasing sodium permeability

126. The patient's thyroid gland is enlarged symmetrically. The skin is warm and moist to the touch. Exophthalmos is evident by the patient's protruding eyes. Onycholysis is present in her nails. Blood analysis (thyroid panel) shows the following:

Serum TSH: 0.1 mIU/mL (normal: 0.4-6.0 mIU/mL)

Thyroxine: 40 µg/dL (normal: 4.5-11.2 µg/dL)

Triiodothyronine: 280 ng/dL (normal: 95-190 ng/dL)

TSH receptor antibody: positive (normal: negative)

In this patient, thyroid hormone secretion can be suppressed by:

A. Inhibiting hypothalamic TRH release

B. Inhibiting TSH release from the anterior pituitary

C. Inhibiting TSH release from the posterior pituitary

D. Inhibiting both TSH and ACTH release from the anterior pituitary

E. Immunosuppression

Questions 127-128 are linked to Case 64:

A 48-year-old woman patient visits her family practitioner complaining of fatigue, weakness, and weight gain. She also states that she experiences frequent muscle cramping and always feels cold. When questioned, she indicates that she has experienced an increase in constipation and headaches during the past 2 months. Vital signs: T 36°C, P 50/min, R 16/min, BP 100/64 mm Hg, BMI 32. The patient is an overweight postmenopausal female. Her skin is pale, dry, and thin, and her hair is brittle.

127. A dietary deficiency of what compound would produce symptoms similar to those described above?

A. Iron

B. Intrinsic factor

C. Iodide

D. Calcium

E. Magnesium

128. This patient's laboratory studies showed the following:

RBC count: 3.9 million cells/µL (normal: 4.2 to 5.4 million cells/µL)

Blood analysis (thyroid panel):

Serum TSH: 6.4 mIU/mL (normal: 0.4-6.0 mIU/mL)

Thyroxine: 3.9 µg/dL (normal: 4.5-11.2 µg/dL)

Triiodothyronine: 80 ng/dL (normal: 95-190 ng/dL)

TSH receptor antibody: Negative (normal: negative)

Thyroid antibodies: Positive (normal: negative)

Her symptoms could be reversed by treatment with:

A. Hypothalamic thyroid hormone–releasing hormone

B. Thyroid-stimulating hormone (TSH)

C. Iodide

D. Thyroid hormone

E. TSH receptor antibodies

Questions 129-130 are linked to Case 65:

A 58-year-old woman is referred to an internist because of high calcium levels found during treatment for a fracture of her femur, which was fractured at the midshaft by a compression. The injury should not have been severe enough to break the bone. During treatment, the patient was noted to have high calcium levels and was referred for further study.

129. If there is no disease present, this patient would be expected to have:

A. Inadequate dietary calcium

B. Increased renal excretion of calcium

C. Decreased parathyroid hormone levels

D. Decreased vitamin D levels

E. Decreased osteoclast activity

130. The patient appears healthy and exercised regularly before the injury. The left femur is immobilized, and the injury appears to be healing well. Vital signs: T 37°C, P 80/min, R 15/min, BP 116/76 mm Hg, BMI 26. Plasma analysis showed the following:

Serum calcium: 14.2 mg/dL (normal: 8.4-10.2 mg/dL)

Serum phosphorus (inorganic): 2.1 mg/dL (normal: 3.0-4.5 mg/dL)

PTH levels: 2200 pg/mL (normal: 230-630 pg/mL)

These data indicate that the bone weakness was caused by:

A. Osteoporosis

B. Dietary calcium deficiency

C. Excessive renal calcium excretion

D. Excessive osteoclast activity

E. Excessive osteoblast activity

Questions 131-132 are linked to Case 66:

A 16-year-old girl is brought to a physician by her parents because of the girl's dramatic weight loss. The patient dances 4 days a week at a private studio. During the past 2 months, she has not been interested in eating and now is weak and unable to complete the dance regimens. Her last menstrual period was 4 months ago. Vital signs: T 35.5°C, P 55/min, R 15/min, BP 90/66 mm Hg, BMI 15. The patient is thin with minimal subcutaneous fat stores. Leg muscles are well toned, but arm and upper body muscles are weak. Complexion is pale and capillary refill after compression of a finger nailbed is slow.

131. In this patient, which of the metabolic hormones is likely elevated?

    A. Insulin

    B. Glucagon

    C. Epinephrine

    D. Growth hormone

    E. Cortisol

132. The patient denies that there is any problem. Pregnancy test is negative, and hematocrit is 33% (low). In this patient, mitochondrial metabolism is been supported by:

    A. Glucose from glycogen stores

    B. Glucose from gluconeogenesis

    C. Free fatty acids from adipose stores

    D. Free fatty acids from lipogenesis

Questions 133-134 are linked to Case 67:

A 23-year-old woman comes to her family physician complaining about weight gain. The patient has gained 20 pounds since graduating from college 2 years ago and is now finding routine activities, such as climbing stairs, difficult.

133. The increase in weight may be explained by an increase in the activity of neurons that use the neurotransmitter:

    A. α-Melanocyte-stimulating hormone

    B. Cocaine- and amphetamine-related transcript (CART)

    C. Neuropeptide Y

    D. Leptin

    E. Insulin

134. The patient was active in intramural sports while in college but has not found an organized physical activity since graduating. She works for a publishing firm and spends most of her time sitting at a desk. Her job requires a lot of overtime hours, and she admits to having a poor diet while working. Vital signs: T 37.2°C, P 82/min, R 15/min, BP 130/85 mm Hg, BMI 31. Which of the following intermediary metabolism processes are active in this individual?

    A. Glycogenolysis

    B. Glycolysis

    C. Adipolysis

    D. Gluconeogenesis

    E. Ketolysis

Questions 135-136 are linked to Case 68:

An 18-year-old girl comes to the university clinic complaining of fever, chills, headache, and aching joints. Prior to today, the patient has been generally healthy and is up to date on all immunizations. Vital signs: T 39°C, P 96/min, R 26/min, BP 105/85 mm Hg. The patient has a sore throat and a nonproductive cough. Her skin is dry, and she appears mildly dehydrated. Influenza antigen test from throat swab showed positive for influenza type A.

135. Related to temperature balance, the early signs of an infection include:

    A. Shivering

    B. A decrease in core temperature

    C. Sweating

    D. Cutaneous vasodilation

    E. A decrease in heart rate

136. In this patient, a temporary drop in body core temperature would occur following:

    A. Shivering

    B. Cutaneous vasoconstriction

    C. Prostaglandin synthesis inhibition

    D. Interleukin-1 production

    E. Interferon production

Questions 137-138 are linked to Case 69:

A 20-year-old man is brought to the emergency department after camping with some friends. He became cold and wet during a rainstorm during the night, and in the morning his friends had difficulty waking him. Vital signs: T 32°C (rectal), P 50/min, R 8/min, BP 90/70 mm Hg, BMI 26.

137. Which mechanism of heat transfer accounts for the hypothermia?

    A. Conduction

    B. Convection

    C. Radiation

    D. Evaporation

    E. Metabolism

138. The patient is conscious but confused. His skin is pale, and his lips, fingers, and toes are cyanotic and cold. Corneal reflexes are diminished. The patient is shivering uncontrollably and has difficulty speaking. ECG shows sinus bradycardia. The cyanosis in the fingers is due to:

    A. Low alveolar P_{O_2}

    B. Low blood flow

    C. Diminished blood buffering capacity

    D. High tissue P_{CO_2}

    E. Increased hemoglobin affinity for oxygen

Questions 139-140 are linked to Case 70:

A 38-year-old man is transported to the emergency department after having fainted at home.

139. During evaluation for Addison's disease, a plasma cortisol sample taken at 4 PM showed a cortisol concentration of 55 nmol/L, when the normal range is 82 to 413 nmol/L. A plasma sample taken at 8 AM the next morning showed a plasma level of 85 nmol/L, indicating that:

    A. The patient is recovering.

    B. The patient is getting worse.

    C. The patient is still hypocortisolemic, because cortisol is normally higher in the morning.

    D. The patient is hypercortisolemic, because cortisol is normally lower in the morning.

    E. Plasma levels of cortisol-binding protein are diminished in the morning.

140. The patient had tuberculosis 2 years earlier, which was managed medically. He has had vomiting and diarrhea for the past 24 hours, and his family reports a weight loss of about 15 pounds during the past 3 months. Vital signs: T 39.5°C, P 120/min, R 28/min, BP 80/65 mm Hg. The patient is disoriented and is having difficulty remaining conscious. He is sweating and appears malnourished. Excessive pigmentation is present on the lips and gums

and in the palmar creases of the hands. Infusion of an ACTH analogue, tetracosactide, resulted in a plasma cortisol increase to 100 nmol/L (normal response is an increase > 330 nmol/L). A blood sample taken before the tetracosactide test would have shown what combination of ACTH, CRH, and cortisol?

	ACTH	CRH	Cortisol
A.	Increased	Increased	Increase
B.	Increased	Increased	Decrease
C.	Increased	Decreased	Increase
D.	Increased	Decreased	Decrease
E.	Decreased	Increased	Increase

Questions 141-142 are linked to Case 71:

A 35-year-old female patient comes in with a complaint of recent rapid weight gain and excessive sweating. Her face looks swollen compared to the rest of her body.

141. The patient complains of recent weakness, backaches, and headaches, and her periods have been irregular lately. Over the past month, she has noticed frequent bruising with slow healing. She is not on any birth control or using any medication except for acetaminophen for the headaches. Vital signs: T 37°C, P 68/min, R 14/min, BP 130/86 mm Hg, BMI 33. Her face is round and her trunk is swollen, but the arms and legs are thin. She has supraclavicular fat pads.

Glucose tolerance: Abnormal consistent with insulin resistance.

Plasma cortisol levels at 4 PM: 25 µg/dL (normal: 3-15 µg/dL)

An increase in what metabolic pathway accounts for the muscle weakness?

    A. Glycogenolysis

    B. Gluconeogenesis

    C. Lipolysis

    D. Adipose synthesis

    E. Glycolysis

142. A 35-year-old woman with suspected Cushing's syndrome comes to the office for testing. The following results were obtained:

Pregnancy test (hCG): Negative

Glucose tolerance: Abnormal consistent with insulin resistance

Plasma cortisol levels at 4 PM: 25 µg/dL (normal: 3-15 µg/dL)

Dexamethasone is given orally at 11 PM. At around 8 AM the next morning, cortisol levels are 35 μg/dL (normal: <5 μg/dL).

A 24-hour urine collection for free cortisol is abnormally high.

Plasma ACTH: 7 pg/mL (normal: >20 pg/mL)

These results are consistent with an overproduction of:

A. CRH from the hypothalamus

B. ACTH from an anterior pituitary tumor

C. ACTH from a posterior pituitary tumor

D. Cortisol from the adrenal cortex

E. Cortisol from an adrenal tumor

Questions 143-144 are linked to case 72:

A 45-year-old woman comes in for her regular checkup and complains about having a constant thirst and getting up frequently in the night to urinate. The patient has a history of high blood pressure. Her blood pressure has remained high regardless of medications prescribed or dosage. Vital signs: T 37°C, P 85/min, R 17/min, BP 145/110 mm Hg, BMI 32.

Basic metabolic panel:
Glucose: 95 mg/dL (normal: 70-110 mg/dL)
Calcium: 9.2 mg/dL (normal: 8.4 to 10.2 mg/dL)
Sodium: 146 mEq/L (normal: 136 to 145 mEq/L)
Chloride: 100 mEq/L (normal: 95-105 mEq/L)
Potassium: 3.2 mEq/L (normal: 3.5 to 5.0 mEq/L)
Plasma aldosterone (recumbent): 25 ng/dL (normal: 2-16 ng/dL)
Plasma renin activity: 0.8 ng/mL/hr (normal: 1.9 to 3.7 ng/mL/hr)

143. The decreased plasma renin activity is due to:

A. Increased sympathetic activity

B. Hypertension

C. Obesity

D. Hyperaldosteronism

E. Hypovolemia

144. It is possible that the patient may be noncompliant with her medications because her blood pressure has remained high regardless of the medications she was prescribed or the dosage. The most important plasma component in indicating hyperaldosteronism is the:

A. Glucose

B. Calcium

C. Sodium

D. Potassium

E. Chloride

Questions 145-146 are linked to Case 73:

A 56-year-old woman presents to the emergency department with chest pain, sweating, extreme anxiety, abdominal pain, pale skin, and racing heart. The patient has experienced these symptoms intermittently over the past month, and they usually subside after 15 to 20 minutes. She states that her hobby is gardening, and she noticed that these episodes occur when she is lifting a heavy bag of soil or when she runs to answer the phone. These episodes happen several times a week. Vital signs: T 98.7°F, P 128/min, R 17/min, BP 146/95 mm Hg, BMI 25.

145. The majority of the cardiac symptoms may be prevented by treatment with a drug that blocks:

A. α_1-Adrenergic receptors

B. α_2-Adrenergic receptors

C. β_1-Adrenergic receptors

D. β_2-Adrenergic receptors

E. β_3-Adrenergic receptors

146. This time the symptoms are more severe.

Blood studies:

Epinephrine: 80 mg/dL (normal: 20 mg/dL)

Norepinephrine: 400 mg/dL (normal: 60 ng/dL)

24-hour urine specimen:

Metanephrine: 1235 ug/24 hours (normal: 24-96 μg/24 hr)

Total urine catecholamines: 1420 μg/24 hr (normal: 14-110 μg/24 hr)

A problem exclusive of adrenal medullary chromaffin cell origin is indicated by which of the above results?

A. Hypertension

B. Tachycardia

C. Elevated plasma epinephrine

D. Elevated plasma norepinephrine

E. Elevated total urinary catecholamines

Questions 147-148 are linked to Case 74:

A 33-year-old woman visits her primary care physician complaining of amenorrhea, headaches, profuse sweating, and joint pains associated with changes in the size of her hands and feet. The patient reports significant increase in the size of her hands and feet, as well as protrusion of her lower jaw. She first noticed these changes about 6 months ago when she was home for the holidays and saw some high school and early college pictures of herself. After that, she says she became more aware of her bodily changes. Her husband and she are also trying to conceive and have been unsuccessful due to amenorrhea for the past 8 months.

147. The usual mechanism of hypothalamic control of the abnormal hormone in this patient is by:

    A. A releasing hypothalamic hormone

    B. An inhibitory hypothalamic hormone

    C. Both releasing and inhibitory hypothalamic hormones

    D. Release of a pro-hormone

    E. Release of a pre-prohormone

148. A 33-year-old woman visits her primary care physician to be evaluated for acromegaly. The major biologic action of the hormone that is abnormal in this patient is:

    A. Stimulated lipolysis

    B. Increased insulin-dependent uptake of glucose in skeletal muscle

    C. Stimulated gluconeogenesis

    D. Inhibited free fatty acid metabolism

    E. Inhibited glycogenolysis

Questions 149-150 are linked to Case 75:

The 42-year-old man comes to his physician because of a decrease in sexual desire and erectile dysfunction. The patient has noticed visual problems and headaches during the past month. The decrease in sexual desire began about 2 months ago and was accompanied by erectile dysfunction. Vital signs: T 37°C, P 76/min, R 15/min, BP 128/86 mm Hg, BMI 28. There is a small amount of growth of the breasts (gynecomastia). Stimulation of the nipples produces a small amount of milk (galactorrhea). Testicular size is small (hypogonadism).

149. The hypogonadism is a result of:

    A. Prolactin suppression of gonadotropin-releasing hormone

    B. Excessive estrogen production

    C. Excessive progesterone production

    D. Growth hormone suppression

    E. High levels of somatostatin

150. Laboratory studies showed the following:

Testosterone: 300 ng/dL (normal: 500-900 ng/dL)

Thyroxine: 8 µg/dL (normal: 5-12 µg/dL)

Prolactin: 300 ng/mL (normal: < 20 ng/mL)

Pituitary MRI: macroprolactinoma 8 cm in diameter

As the tumor grows in size there will be a decrease in the release of the other pituitary hormones because of:

    A. Negative feedback inhibition

    B. Positive feedback inhibition

    C. Destruction of the hypothalamohypophyseal portal system

    D. Destruction of the anterior pituitary gland

    E. Destruction of the posterior pituitary gland

Questions 151-152 are linked to Case 76:

A 28-year-old female visits the obstetrician complaining of amenorrhea and milk discharge from her nipples. The patient was involved in a motorcycle accident 3 months ago, and the impact was sufficient to break her helmet. She indicated she just has not felt right since the accident. The patient is constantly tired, has gained 5 pounds, and drinks fluids and urinates more than before the accident. Vital signs: T 36.5°C, P 84/min, R 15/min, BP 95/60 mm Hg, BMI 29. A small amount of white fluid can be expressed from the nipples. The patient appears otherwise healthy. Gynecologic examination does not reveal any evidence of pregnancy.

151. Plasma analysis will likely show an increase in:

    A. Estrogen

    B. Progesterone

    C. Human chorionic gonadotropin

    D. Prolactin

    E. Follicle-stimulating hormone (FSH)

152. Her pregnancy test was negative. Additional laboratory findings included:

FSH levels: 2 mIU/mL (normal: 4-30 mIU/mL)

LH levels: 2 mIU/mL (normal: 5-30 mIU/mL)

Cortisol level: 2 µg/dL (normal: 3-15 µg/dL)

Thyroxine (T$_4$): 3 µg/dL (normal: 5-12 µg/dL)

Triiodothyronine (T$_3$): 60 ng/dL (normal: 115-190 ng/dL)

Prolactin levels: 70 ng/mL (normal: < 20 ng/mL)

The low FSH levels are likely due to:

A. Negative feedback inhibition from plasma estrogen levels

B. Negative feedback inhibition from plasma progesterone levels

C. GnRH secretion because of the elevated prolactin

D. Inadequate GnRH delivery to the anterior pituitary

E. Damage to the FSH secreting cells of the anterior pituitary

Questions 153-154 are linked to Case 77:

A 50-year-old female presents to the office for her annual physical examination. The patient complains of night sweats, hot flashes, and vaginal dryness. She also reports irregular menstruation. She lives with her husband and is concerned about menopause. Vital signs: T 98°F, P 70/min, R 16/min, BP 130/90 mm Hg, BMI 33, weight 125. The pelvic examination is unremarkable.

153. Plasma analysis will likely show what combination of reproductive hormones?

	Estrogen	FSH	LH
A.	Increased	Increased	Increased
B.	Increased	Increased	Decreased
C.	Increased	Decreased	Increased
D.	Increased	Decreased	Decreased
E.	Decreased	Increased	Increased

154. The patient has a history of mild hypothyroidism, obesity, and eczema. She is currently taking levothyroxine and topical corticosteroids.

CBC: Within normal limits

CHEM-7: Within normal limits

FSH: 80 U/L (normal premenopausal: 4-30 U/L)

LH: 170 U/L: (normal premenopausal: 5-150 U/L)

The increased pulsatile secretion of GnRH is due to:

A. Impaired negative feedback inhibition by FSH

B. Impaired negative feedback inhibition by LH

C. Impaired negative feedback inhibition by estrogen

D. Inhibitory descending signals from the thalamus

E. Inhibitory descending signals from the reticular activating system

Questions 155-156 are linked to Case 78:

A 17-year-old girl comes to the pediatrician because of an 8-month absence of a menses. The patient joined a cross country team at high school 3 years ago and is training for the upcoming state championships. She had ranged between the 25th and 55th percentile for both height and weight since her second birthday, but she has progressively lost weight during the past 2 years. All other developmental milestones were met at an appropriate age. Both parents are of normal height and stature. Vital signs: T 37°C, P 90/min, R 22/min, BP 100/80 mm Hg, BMI 17.

155. Analysis of hypothalamic hormone secretion should show a depressed secretion of:

A. Growth hormone–releasing hormone

B. Gonadotropin-releasing hormone

C. Pituitary hormone inhibiting hormone

D. Somatostatin

E. Prolactin inhibiting hormone

156. Physical examination reveals a well-toned female athlete with minimal subcutaneous body fat.

Pregnancy test (hCG): negative

Radiographic imaging: Normal hypothalamus and pituitary

LH: 0.4 IU/mL (normal: 0.9 to 10.6 IU/mL)

Prolactin: 12 ng/mL (normal: < 20 ng/mL)

Injection of GnRH stimulates the release of both FSH and LH.

The primary hormone secretion deficiency in this patient is in the:

A. Hypothalamus

B. Anterior pituitary

C. Posterior pituitary

D. Ovary

E. Adrenal cortex

Questions 157-158 are linked to Case 79:

A 24-year-old woman presents to her gynecologist with concern regarding her menstrual cycle. She complains of very irregular menstrual periods (< 8 a year), which are very heavy. The patient also noticed dark, coarse hair growing on her face, upper arms, chest, and abdomen, which she stated is extremely embarrassing.

She also complains of persistent acne on her face. She is married without children. She and her husband have been trying for a pregnancy for about 3 months but have been unsuccessful. Vital signs: T 98.8°F, P 82/min, R 14/min, BP 125/80 mm Hg, height 5 ft 3 in, weight 145 lb, BMI of 26, with the majority of the excess fat centralized around her abdominal area.

157. The endocrine abnormality accounting for this patient's symptoms is excessive:

    A. Estrogen production

    B. Progesterone production

    C. Androgen production

    D. Cortisol production

    E. Aldosterone production

158. A 24-year-old woman is referred to her gynecologist because of a tentative diagnosis of polycystic ovarian disease. Transvaginal ultrasound showed a 2- to 5-fold ovarian enlargement with thickened tunica albuginea with approximately 20 follicles that are 1 to 5 mm in diameter without a dominant follicle and a thin endometrium.

    Blood test: Elevated LH/FSH ratio > 2.5

    Prolactin level: Elevated

    Testosterone and DHEA levels: Increased

    Glucose tolerance test: Abnormal

    Thyroid hormone level: Normal

    In a normal ovarian cycle, multiple follicular maturations are prevented by:

    A. GnRH secretion

    B. A surge in FSH

    C. A surge in LH

    D. Estrogen secretion from the dominant follicle

    E. Inhibition of LH and FSH secretion

Questions 159-160 are linked to Case 80:

A 28-year-old nulliparous woman visits her gynecologist complaining of pelvic pain accompanying her menses. The patient states that the pain begins around 1 week before her menses and becomes increasingly severe until flow slackens, at which time the pubic pain subsides. The intervals of pain have been getting progressively worse over the past few months. She states that her menses are no longer regular or consistent, and that they "feel heavier than they used to be."

159. The hormone responsible for the pain is secreted by the:

    A. Dominant follicle

    B. Anterior pituitary

    C. Posterior pituitary

    D. Hypothalamus

    E. Corpus luteum

160. The patient also complains of some discomfort during intercourse. She states that all of these symptoms have started within the past 6 months and that previously she only had mild cramping with menstruation. Vital signs: T 98.6°F, P 70/min, R 16/min, BP 120/70 mm Hg, weight 125 lb. Pelvic examination is unremarkable.

    MRI: Lesions along the uterus

    Laparoscopy and tissue biopsy: Endometrial tissue on the ovaries and uterine tubes

    What form of contraceptive control will be most useful to diminish the symptoms?

    A. Condoms

    B. Diaphragm

    C. Spermicidal gel

    D. Intrauterine device

    E. Oral estrogen

Questions 161-162 are linked to Case 81:

A 24-year-old woman comes to the emergency department complaining of severe left lower quadrant pelvic pain and abnormal vaginal bleeding. She states that the pain began abruptly 1 hour ago. The patient describes pain as 10 on a scale of 0 to 10 and states it radiates to her lower back. She denies nausea or vomiting. She has a history of abnormal periods and pelvic inflammatory disease, with the last period ending 8 weeks ago. Vital signs: T 99°F, P 92/min, R 22/min, BP 142/76 mm Hg. There is tenderness in the left inguinal region on palpation.

161. A normal pregnancy would be confirmed by the presence of a blastocyst in the:

    A. Ovary

    B. Fallopian tube

    C. Uterus

    D. Vagina

    E. Peritoneum

162. Additional laboratory studies showed the following:

CBC: Hematocrit 37% (normal: 38% to 42%), leukocytosis

β-hCG: Positive (2000 mIU/mL)

Progesterone level: 12 ng/mL

Transvaginal and transabdominal ultrasound: No intra-uterine pregnancy. Normal intrauterine sac; swollen left fallopian tube with an apparent mass

At this time, progesterone is being secreted by the:

A. Corpus luteum under control of LH

B. Corpus luteum under control of β-hCG

C. Corpus luteum under control of chorionic somato-mammotropin

D. Placenta under control of LH

E. Placenta under control of β-hCG

Questions 163-164 are linked to Case 82:

A 40-year-old pregnant woman visits her obstetrician after noting vaginal bleeding. The bleeding is a small volume and had begun during the previous night. Fetal age is estimated at 32 weeks' gestation. Chorionic villi sampling did not reveal any genetic abnormalities. There have been two prior pregnancies, one ending in a 10-week miscarriage and the other a normal labor and vaginal delivery 3 years earlier. The mother had developed gestational diabetes at week 34, four weeks before delivery. Vital signs: T 99°F, P 84/min, R 24/min, BP 130/90 mm Hg, weight 145 lb. Patient looks normal for 32 weeks' gestation. There is localized uterine pain.

163. Fetal distress can be indicated by which of the changes in fetal heart rate?

A. Bradycardia and tachycardia

B. Increased heart rate during uterine contractions

C. Variability in heart rate

D. Decreased heart rate during fetal movement

164. The following studies were done:

Fetal:

Ultrasound: Fetus is normal for gestational age.

Fetal heart rate: Normal

Maternal:

Glucose tolerance test: Borderline elevated

Estriol levels: Normal for gestational age

Estriol provides an assessment of the viability of the:

A. Placenta and fetal adrenal

B. Placenta and maternal adrenal

C. Maternal and fetal adrenal

D. Placenta only

E. Fetal adrenal only

Questions 165-166 are linked to Case 83:

A pregnant 34-year-old woman arrives in the emergency department by ambulance after suffering a seizure. The patient is at 29 weeks' gestation, and this is her third pregnancy. She has a history of hypertension and diabetes but managed these conditions well during her previous pregnancies. However, with this pregnancy, the patient experienced excessive swelling, in comparison to the past two pregnancies and reports a decrease in urine production. She had an acute decrease in visual acuity 2 days ago and had a seizure while in the waiting room at the optometrist's office and arrived at the emergency department 45 minutes later.

165. The decrease in urine production is indicative of:

A. Hypotension

B. Increased ADH secretion

C. Declining renal function

D. Increased cardiac output

E. Edema

166. The patient is anxious and recovering from the unexpected seizure. Vital signs: T 98°F, P 100/min, R 20/min, BP 160/110 mm Hg. Ophthalmoscope shows retinal hemorrhage. The patient has edema of the hands and feet. The remainder of the physical examination is appropriate for 29 weeks' gestation.

Ultrasound: Fetal growth restriction.

Blood tests:

Platelets: 80,000/mL (normal: 150,000-350,000/mL)

Aspartate aminotransferase: 80 IU/L (normal: 7-27 IU/L)

Lactate dehydrogenase: 650 IU/L (normal: 50-150 IU/L)

Alanine aminotransferase: 40 IU/L (normal: 1-21 IU/L)

Uric acid: 12 mg/dL (normal: 2-7 mg/dL)

Fasting blood glucose level: 105 mg/dL (normal: 70-110 mg/dL)

24-hour urine collection:

300 mL (normal: > 500 mL/24 hr)

8g protein (normal: < 1 g/24 hr)

Fetal growth restriction is due to:

A. Inadequate placental function

B. Impaired maternal hepatic function

C. Impaired maternal renal function

D. Maternal edema

E. Maternal hypertension

Questions 167-168 are linked to Case 84:

A 32-year-old woman visits her gynecologist for a normal prenatal checkup. She is pregnant with gestational age estimated at 32 weeks. This is her first pregnancy. Her mother is overweight and has recently been diagnosed with type 2 diabetes. Vital signs: T 38.5°C, P 85/min, R 22/min, BP 130/90 mm Hg, BMI 33. The patient presents as a typical 32-week pregnant female. Glucose tolerance test is abnormal, indicating insulin resistance.

167. The increase in plasma glucose is due to:

A. Impaired glucose uptake by skeletal muscle

B. Impaired glucose uptake by the liver

C. Impaired glucose uptake by the brain

D. Impaired reabsorption of glucose by the kidney

E. Excessive glucose uptake by the intestine

168. Compared with normal, the expected growth consequence will be:

A. Increased placental growth

B. Decreased placental growth

C. Increased fetal growth

D. Decreased fetal growth

E. Increased maternal growth

Questions 169-170 are linked to Case 85:

A 17-year-old boy comes to the pediatrician with an absence of signs of puberty. Physical examination reveals a normal prepubertal male in spite of his age, with no signs of secondary sexual characteristic development. The patient appears underdeveloped with little muscle mass, and his voice is high-pitched. Pubic and axillary hair is sparse, the testes are underdeveloped (volume < 4 mL), and the phallus is small. Evaluation of cranial nerve I shows normal smelling ability.

169. Injection of what hormone will result in the appearance of those characteristics associated with puberty?

A. Gonadotropin releasing hormone (GnRH)

B. Follicle-stimulating hormone (FSH)

C. Prolactin

D. Luteinizing hormone (LH)

E. Testosterone

170. Additional studies were done:

LH: 0.6 IU/mL (normal: 0.9 to 10.6 IU/mL)

Testosterone: 80 ng/dL (normal: 300-1000 ng/dL)

Injection of 100 µg GnRH stimulates a lower than normal release of both FSH and LH. Which of the characteristics of pubertal development will not be corrected by treatment with exogenous testosterone?

A. Growth of the external genitalia

B. Growth spurt followed by closure of the epiphyseal plates

C. Growth of facial hair

D. Growth of axillary hair

E. Development of the mature sperm

Questions 171-172 are linked to Case 86:

A 1-year-old boy is referred to the surgeon because of bilateral absence of testes within the scrotum. The absence of the testes was noted at birth and has persisted through the first year of life.

171. In utero, the regression of the primordial fallopian tube is mediated by the hormone:

A. Testosterone

B. Relaxin

C. Inhibin

D. Anti-müllerian hormone

E. Anti-wolffian hormone

172. All other developmental aspects are normal. Vital signs: T 37°C, P 90/min, R 22/min, BP 88/40 mm Hg. Physical examination reveals that the scrotal sac is empty to palpation. Ultrasound indicates that the testes are located within the inguinal canal. Failure of the testes to descend impairs what aspect of reproductive function?

A. Testosterone production

B. Inhibin production

C. Maturation of spermatogonia

D. Growth of the penis

E. Impairment of erectile response

Questions 173-174 are linked to Case 87:

A 65-year-old man comes to the clinic complaining of difficulty urinating. He states that over the past month he has had to get out of bed three to five times a night to urinate and his bladder does not completely empty during voiding. The patient states that he finds himself "stopping and starting again several times while urinating."

173. If these symptoms are caused by benign prostatic hyperplasia, the patient will also exhibit:

A. Increased tone in the internal urethral sphincter

B. Increased tone in the external urethral sphincter

C. Increased pressure within the bladder during micturition

D. Decreased pressure within the ureter

E. Decreased pressure within the renal calyx

174. The patient also describes his urinary stream as "weak." He states that he had two urinary tract infections within the last 3 months. Vital signs: T 37°C, P 72/min, R 18/min, BP 128/80 mm Hg, BMI 28. Examination of lower abdomen shows a distended bladder but no pain on palpation. Digital rectal examination reveals a smooth, firm, and elastic enlargement of the prostate, with no induration.

Urinalysis: Negative hematuria and negative urinary tract infection

Plasma: Prostate specific antigen (PSA) levels normal.

The obstruction of the urethra as it passes through the prostate is due to:

A. Growth of a testosterone-sensitive cancer within the prostate

B. Growth of an estrogen-sensitive cancer within the prostate

C. Prostate hypertrophy stimulated directly by dihydrotestosterone

D. Prostate hypertrophy stimulated directly by testosterone

E. α_1-Adrenergic-stimulated hypertrophy of urethral smooth muscle

Questions 175-176 are linked to Case 88:

A 60-year-old man comes to his primary care physician concerned about erectile dysfunction.

175. Which of the following observations would suggest a psychological rather than a vascular cause of erectile dysfunction?

A. Lack of a vasodilator response to nitric oxide

B. Lack of a vasodilator response to the nonadrenergic, noncholinergic parasympathetic nerves

C. The presence of nocturnal erections

D. Diminished vasoconstriction response to α_1-adrenergic agonists

E. Diminished vasodilator response to α_1-adrenergic antagonists

176. A 60-year-old man visits his primary care physician concerned about the inability to have sex with his wife. He reports an inability to achieve erections in at least 75% of intercourse attempts over the past 6 months and a complete absence of nocturnal erections. The patient has a 3-year history of hypertension, which has been controlled by a calcium channel blocker. In addition, he has mild hyperlipidemia that is controlled with dietary modification. The patient has a 1-year history of chest pain with moderate physical exertion and is being treated with aspirin and nitroglycerin. He is a social drinker and smokes one pack of cigarettes per day. The biologic action of nitroglycerin will be potentiated by drugs used to treat erectile dysfunction that increase the half-life of what cellular second messenger?

A. cAMP

B. ATP

C. Phosphokinase A

D. cGMP

E. GTP

ANSWERS TO PRACTICE QUESTIONS

Question Number	Answer Choice	Page Number*	Question Number	Answer Choice	Page Number
1	C	35	40	D	62
2	A	5	41	E	65
3	E	7	42	C	65
4	B	7	43	D	67
5	E	10	44	C	67
6	E	10	45	E	70
7	A	12	46	C	70
8	E	14	47	D	73
9	B	15	48	C	73
10	B	15	49	D	78
11	B	16	50	C	78
12	E	16	51	A	80
13	E	22	52	D	80
14	B	22	53	B	82
15	C	27	54	B	82
16	D	27	55	B	84
17	C	30	56	B	84
18	A	30	57	C	86
19	E	33	58	B	86
20	D	33	59	C	93
21	C	35	60	D	93
22	B	35	61	C	95
23	E	38	62	A	95
24	A	38	63	C	97
25	E	40	64	C	97
26	B	40	65	D	99
27	C	42	66	D	99
28	D	42	67	D	101
29	B	45	68	D	101
30	A	45	69	C	103
31	A	48	70	B	103
32	D	48	71	C	105
33	B	54	72	E	105
34	C	54	73	D	107
35	A	56	74	D	107
36	C	56	75	C	109
37	C	59	76	A	109
38	E	59	77	A	111
39	C	62	78	B	111

*Explanations in support of the answer choice can be found in these pages.

Question Number	Answer Choice	Page Number	Question Number	Answer Choice	Page Number
79	C	113	121	E	165
80	B	113	122	D	165
81	E	117	123	A	168
82	E	117	124	D	168
83	E	119	125	D	170
84	A	119	126	E	170
85	E	121	127	C	172
86	A	121	128	D	172
87	B	123	129	B	174
88	E	123	130	D	174
89	C	126	131	E	176
90	D	126	132	B	176
91	D	128	133	C	178
92	C	128	134	B	178
93	A	131	135	A	181
94	C	131	136	C	181
95	C	133	137	A	183
96	E	133	138	B	183
97	B	135	139	C	189
98	B	135	140	B	189
99	E	137	141	B	191
100	D	137	142	E	191
101	C	139	143	B	193
102	B	139	144	D	193
103	B	144	145	C	195
104	C	144	146	C	195
105	A	146	147	C	198
106	B	146	148	A	198
107	A	150	149	A	201
108	D	150	150	C	201
109	D	152	151	D	203
110	B	152	152	D	203
111	B	153	153	E	208
112	B	153	154	C	208
113	B	155	155	B	210
114	A	155	156	A	210
115	C	157	157	C	212
116	B	157	158	D	212
117	A	159	159	E	214
118	D	159	160	E	214
119	A	161	161	C	216
120	A	161	162	B	216

Question Number	Answer Choice	Page Number	Question Number	Answer Choice	Page Number
163	A	218	170	E	224
164	A	218	171	D	226
165	C	220	172	C	226
166	A	220	173	C	229
167	A	222	174	C	229
168	C	222	175	C	231
169	E	224	176	D	231

Credits (Figures and Tables)

After the title of the credited text, the number of the figure or table used in Problem-Based Physiology is listed along with the page number from the credited text.

Berne RM, Levy MN, Koeppen BM, et al: Physiology, 5th ed. St. Louis, Mosby, 2003.
43-1, p. 180.

Boron W, Boulpaep E: Medical Physiology. Philadelphia, Saunders, 2005.
2-1, p. 220; 4-3, p. 223.

Carroll RG: Elsevier's Integrated Physiology. Philadelphia, Elsevier, 2007.
I-1, p. 44; II-1, p. 84; II-2, p. 92; 11-1, p. 200; III-1, p. 121; 19-1, p. 24; 20-1, p. 124; 20-2, p. 125; 22-4, p. 130; 23-2, p. 136; 25-1, p. 58; 25-2, p. 62; V-1, pp. 100 & 101; VII-1, p. 142; 53-4, p. 150; 58-1, p. 154; 61-1, p. 170; 62-1, p. 172; 63-1, p. 164; 64-1, p. 163; 65-1, p. 164; 66-2, p. 173; 68-1, p. 9; IX-1, p. 160; IX-2, pp. 166 & 167; 70-2, p. 168; 71-1, p. 169, 71-2, p. 172; 74-1, p. 162; 74-2, p. 173; 76-1, p. 161; X-1, p. 190; 78-1, p. 185; 78-2, p. 178; 80-1, p. 184; 81-1, p. 198; 84-1, p. 172; 86-1, p. 191; 86-2, p. 193; 87-1, p. 194; 88-1, p. 41. Table 69-1, p. 8; Table IX-1, p. 162.

Copstead L, Banasik J: Pathophysiology, 3rd ed. Philadelphia, Saunders, 2005.
10-1, p. 481; 12-1, p. 483; VI-1, p. 1061; 41-1, p. 1106; 42-1, p. 1159; 46-1, p. 1129; 46-3, p. 1129; 49-1, p. 1084; 73-1, p. 1066.

Guyton AC, Hall JE: Textbook of Medical Physiology, 11th ed. Philadelphia, Saunders, 2006.
I-2, p. 81; I-3, p. 78; 1-1, p. 677; 1-2, p. 680; 1-3, p. 690; 3-1, p. 69; 4-1, p. 86; 4-2, p. 88; 6-1, p. 91, 6-2, p. 75; 7-1, p. 209; 7-2, p. 375; 7-3, p. 112; 7-4, p. 185; 7-5, p. 375; 7-6, p. 280; 7-7, p. 282; 8-1, p. 234; 8-2, p. 265; 8-3, p. 497; 8-4, p. 499; 9-1, p. 107; 11-2, p. 274; 11-3, p. 271; 13-1, p. 124; 13-2, p. 153; 14-1, p. 210; 14-2, p. 138; 14-3, p. 375; 14-4, p. 225; 15-1, p. 250; 15-2, p. 142; 15-3, p. 143; 16-1, p. 196; 16-2, p. 198; III-2, p. 349; 17-1, p. 218; 17-2, p. 226; 18-1, p. 400; 18-2, p. 324; 19-2, p. 356; 21-1, p. 331; 22-1, p. 333; 22-2, p. 335; 22-3, p. 338; 23-1, p. 313; 26-1, p. 462; 27-1, p. 458; 31-1, p. 472; 32-1, p. 526; 33-1, p. 506; 34-1, p. 496; 35-1, p. 488; 37-1, p. 520; 42-2, p. 641; 45-1, p. 742; 45-2, p. 744; 47-1, p. 717; 48-1, p. 693; 48-2, p. 652; 48-3, p. 657; 49-2, p. 764; 50-1, p. 686; 50-2, p. 686; 51-1, p. 600; 52-1, p. 782; 53-1, p. 796; 53-2, p. 800; 53-3, p. 820; 54-1, p. 798; 57-1, p. 772; 57-2, p. 772; 59-1, p. 788; 60-1, p. 790; 66-1, p. 874; 67-1, p. 869; 69-1, p. 891; 70-1, p. 956; 75-1, p. 1040; 77-1, p. 1022; 77-2, p. 1022; 82-1, p. 1030; 83-1, p. 316; 85-1, p. 1007; 85-2, p. 1005. Table 7-1, p. 754; Table 34-1, p. 538; Table 67-1, p. 869.

Koeppen B, Stanton B: Berne & Levy Physiology, 6th ed. Philadelphia, Mosby, 2008.
44-1, p. 189; 44-2, p. 190.

Nolte J: Elsevier's Integrated Neuroscience. Philadelphia, Mosby, 2007.
46-2, p. 219.

INDEX

Note: Page numbers followed by f indicate figures; those followed by t indicate tables.

A

ACE inhibitor. *See* Angiotensin I converting enzyme inhibitor
Acetazolamide, 102
Acetylcholine
  botulism toxicity and exocytosis of, 12–14
  myasthenia gravis attacking, 15
  myasthenia gravis, edrophonium impacting, 15
  myasthenia gravis, pyridostigmine treating, 16
  Taxol-induced peripheral neuropathy, release of, 7–8
Achalasia
  case of, 144
  esophagus failure causing, 144, 145
  laboratory studies for, 144
  physical examination for, 144
  practice questions for, 251–252
  treating, 145
Acid secretion. *See also* Gastric acid
  mechanisms stimulating, 150f, 151
  peptic ulcer from imbalance of, 146–147, 147f
  in stomach, 146, 146f
Acoustic neuroma. *See also* Vertigo, 134
  treating, 134
Acromegaly
  case of, 198
  GH overproduction in, 198–199
  laboratory studies for, 198
  physical examination for, 198
  practice questions for, 259–260
  treating, 199
ACTH. *See* Adrenocorticotropic hormone
Activity, Pulse, Grimace, Appearance, and Respiration (APGAR), 36
Acute adrenal insufficiency
  ACTH overproduction in, 189
  ACTH used in testing for, 190
  case of, 189
  damage from, 190
  laboratory studies for, 189
  physical examination for, 189
  practice questions for, 258
  symptoms of, 189
Acute mountain sickness
  acetazolamide treating, 102

Acute mountain sickness *(Continued)*
  arterial hypoxia initiating, 101–102, 101t
  case of, 101
  HAPE, HACE developed by, 101
  headache in, 102
  laboratory studies for, 101
  physical examination for, 101
  practice questions for, 245
  sleep impacted by, 102
Acute tubular necrosis
  case of, 67
  creatinine and BUN elevated in, 68
  death from, 68
  hyperkalemia, hyperphosphatemia encountered in, 68, 69f
  laboratory studies for, 67
  physical examination for, 67
  practice questions for, 241
  treating, 68–69
  tubular system, fluid modified by, 67, 68f
Addisonian crisis. *See* Acute adrenal insufficiency
Adenosine diphosphate (ADP), 78
Adenosine triphosphate (ATP), 78
  cyanide poisoning impacting production of, 109
  exercise increasing, 48, 48f
ADH. *See* Antidiuretic hormone
Adipose, 192
ADP. *See* Adenosine diphosphate
Adrenal gland, 186–188
Adrenal insufficiency. *See* Acute adrenal insufficiency
Adrenocorticotropic hormone (ACTH)
  acute adrenal insufficiency, overproduction of, 189
  acute adrenal insufficiency testing using, 190
  aldosterone secretion increased by, 190f, 193
  cortisol, interaction with, 190
Advanced trauma life support (ATLS), 99–100
Alcohol, 153
Aldosterone
  ACTH increasing secretion of, 190f, 193
  Conn's syndrome impacting, 193
  function of, 190, 190f
ALS. *See* Amyotrophic lateral sclerosis
Alveoli
  COPD impairing ventilation in, 93
  exercise increasing ventilation of, 107, 107f

Alveoli *(Continued)*
  gas pressure functions in, 90, 90f, 91
  pneumonia, bacteria transported into, 113
Alzheimer's disease
  case of, 128
  cognitive decline in, 128
  laboratory studies for, 128
  memory impacted by, 128
  physical examination for, 128
  practice questions for, 249–250
  treating, 128
Amiloride, 74
Amyotrophic lateral sclerosis (ALS)
  Babinski's Sign's, presence in, 4–5
  case of, 4
  death from, 5
  diagnosing, 4
  Hyperreflexia in, 4, 5f
  laboratory studies for, 4
  physical examination for, 4
  practice questions for, 233
  progression of, 5
  riluzole treating, 5
Anemia. *See* Iron deficiency anemia
Angiotensin I converting enzyme inhibitor (ACE inhibitor)
  essential hypertension treated with, 44
  malignant hypertension, problems of treatment with, 56, 57f
Angiotensin II, 43, 44, 44f
Anorexia nervosa. *See* Starvation
Antidiuretic hormone (ADH)
  distal tubule, water reabsorption stimulated by, 73
  lithium impacting water reabsorption and, 74
  nephrogenic diabetes insipidus impairing, 74
  synthesis of, 73
Aortic valve stenosis
  case of, 38
  cause of, 31f, 38
  chest pain from, 38–39
  laboratory studies for, 38
  murmurs of, 38
  physical examination for, 38
  practice questions for, 237
  shortness of breath, syncope from, 39
  treating, 39
  ventricle pressure increased in, 38, 39f

W